Right Ventricular Function and Failure

Editors

JERRY D. ESTEP
MIRIAM S. JACOB

CARDIOLOGY CLINICS

www.cardiology.theclinics.com

May 2020 • Volume 38 • Number 2

ELSEVIER

1600 John F. Kennedy Boulevard • Suite 1800 • Philadelphia, Pennsylvania, 19103-2899

http://www.theclinics.com

CARDIOLOGY CLINICS Volume 38, Number 2
May 2020 ISSN 0733-8651, ISBN-13: 978-0-323-76000-3

Editor: Stacy Eastman
Developmental Editor: Donald Mumford

Cardiology Clinics (ISSN 0733-8651) is published quarterly by Elsevier Inc., 360 Park Avenue South, New York, NY 10010-1710. Months of issue are February, May, August, and November. Business and Editorial Offices: 1600 John F. Kennedy Blvd., Ste. 1800, Philadelphia, PA 19103-2899. Customer Service Office: 3251 Riverport Lane, Maryland Heights, MO 63043. Periodicals post-age paid at New York, NY and additional mailing offices. Subscription prices are $352.00 per year for US individuals, $706.00 per year for US institutions, $100.00 per year for US students and residents, $432.00 per year for Canadian individuals, $885.00 per year for Canadian institutions, $466.00 per year for international individuals, $885.00 per year for international institutions, $100.00 per year for Canadian students/residents and $220.00 per year for international students/residents. To receive student/resident rate, orders must be accompanied by name of affiliated institution, data of term, and the *signature* of program/residency coordinator on institution letterhead. Orders will be billed at individual rate until proof of status is received. Foreign air speed delivery is included in all *Clinics* subscription prices. All prices are subject to change without notice. **POSTMASTER:** Send address changes to *Cardiology Clinics*, Elsevier Health Sciences Division, Subscription Customer Service, 3251 Riverport Lane, Maryland Heights, MO 63043. **Customer Service: 1-800-654-2452 (U.S. and Canada); 314-447-8871 (outside U.S. and Canada). Fax: 314-447-8029. E-mail: journalscus-tomerservice-usa@elsevier.com (for print support); journalsonlinesupport-usa@elsevier.com (for online support).**

Reprints. For copies of 100 or more, of articles in this publication, please contact the Commercial Reprints Department, Elsevier Inc., 360 Park Avenue South, New York, NY 10010-1710. Tel.: 212-633-3874; Fax: 212-633-3820; E-mail: reprints@elsevier.com.

Cardiology Clinics is also published in Spanish by McGraw-Hill Interamericana Editores S. A., P.O. Box 5-237, 06500, Mexico D. F., Mexico; in Portuguese by Reichmann and Alfonso Editores Rio de Janeiro, Brazil; and in Greek by Dimitrios P. Lagos, 8 Pondon Street, GR115-28 Ilissia, Greece.

Cardiology Clinics is covered in *MEDLINE/PubMed (Index Medicus), Excerpta Medica, The Cumulative Index to Nursing and Allied Health Literature* (CINAHL).

Printed in the United States of America.

Contributors

EDITORIAL BOARD

JAMIL A. ABOULHOSN, MD, FACC, FSCAI
Director, Ahmanson/UCLA Adult Congenital
Heart Center, Streisand/American Heart
Association Endowed Chair, Divisions of
Cardiology and Pediatric Cardiology, David
Geffen School of Medicine at UCLA, Los
Angeles, California

DAVID M. SHAVELLE, MD, FACC, FSCAI
Associate Professor, Keck School of Medicine
of USC, Director, General Cardiovascular
Fellowship Program, Director, Cardiac
Catheterization Laboratory, LAC + USC
Medical Center, Division of Cardiovascular

Medicine, University of Southern California,
Los Angeles, California

TERRENCE D. WELCH, MD, FACC
Assistant Professor, Department of Medicine,
Section of Cardiology, Dartmouth-Hitchcock
Medical Center, Lebanon, New Hampshire;
Department of Internal Medicine, Geisel School
of Medicine at Dartmouth, New Hampshire

AUDREY H. WU, MD
Assistant Professor, Internal Medicine,
University of Michigan, Ann Arbor, Michigan

EDITORS

JERRY D. ESTEP, MD
Department of Cardiovascular Medicine,
Cleveland Clinic Sydell and Arnold Miller Family
Heart, Vascular and Thoracic Institute, Kaufman
Center for Heart Failure Treatment and
Recovery, Cleveland Clinic, Cleveland, Ohio

MIRIAM S. JACOB, MD
Department of Cardiovascular Medicine,
Cleveland Clinic Sydell and Arnold Miller Family
Heart, Vascular and Thoracic Institute, Kaufman
Center for Heart Failure Treatment and
Recovery, Cleveland Clinic, Cleveland, Ohio

AUTHORS

HASAN ASHRAF, MD
Cardiovascular Diseases Fellow, Department
of Cardiovascular Diseases, Mayo Clinic,
Scottsdale, Arizona

WILLIAM R. AUGER, MD, FCPP
Director, Pulmonary Hypertension and CTEPH
Research Program, Temple Heart and Vascular
Institute, Temple University, Adjunct Professor
of Medicine, Lewis Katz School of Medicine,
Philadelphia, Pennsylvania

EVAN L. BRITTAIN, MD, MSc
Assistant Professor of Medicine, Division of
Cardiovascular Medicine, Department of
Medicine, Vanderbilt University Medical
Center, Nashville, Tennessee

STEVEN J. CASSADY, MD
Division of Pulmonary and Critical Care Medicine,
Department of Medicine, University of Maryland
School of Medicine, Baltimore, Maryland

KALYAN R. CHITTURI, DO
Houston Methodist DeBakey Heart & Vascular
Center, Houston, Texas

REBECCA COGSWELL, MD
Assistant Professor, Department of Medicine,
Division of Cardiology, University of Minnesota,
Minneapolis, Minnesota

MILAD C. EL HAJJ, MD
Department of Medicine, Internal Medicine,
Medical University of South Carolina,
Charleston, South Carolina

ASHRITH GUHA, MD, MPH, FACC
Houston Methodist DeBakey Heart & Vascular
Center, Houston, Texas

JESSICA H. HUSTON, MD
Advanced Heart Failure Fellow, Division of
Cardiovascular Medicine, Department of
Medicine, Vanderbilt University Medical
Center, Nashville, Tennessee

CHRISTINE JELLIS, MD, PhD
Department of Cardiovascular Medicine, Heart
and Vascular Institute, Cleveland Clinic,
Cleveland, Ohio

RANJIT JOHN, MD
Professor, Department of Surgery, Division of
Cardiothoracic Surgery, University of
Minnesota, Minneapolis, Minnesota

PAYTON KENDSERSKY, MD
Duke University Medical Center, Durham,
North Carolina

FRANCIS D. PAGANI, MD, PhD
Department of Cardiac Surgery, Otto Gago MD
Endowed Professor of Cardiac Surgery,
Director, Center for Circulatory Support,
Frankel Cardiovascular Center, University of
Michigan, Ann Arbor, Michigan

GAUTAM V. RAMANI, MD
Division of Cardiovascular Medicine,
Department of Medicine, University of
Maryland School of Medicine, Baltimore,
Maryland

IVAN M. ROBBINS, MD
Professor of Medicine, Division of Allergy,
Pulmonary, and Critical Care Medicine,
Vanderbilt University Medical Center,
Nashville, Tennessee

JULIE L. ROSENTHAL, MD
Assistant Professor of Medicine, Department
of Cardiovascular Diseases, Mayo Clinic,
Scottsdale, Arizona

ANDREW SHAFFER, MD
Assistant Professor, Department of Surgery,
Division of Cardiothoracic Surgery, University
of Minnesota, Minneapolis,
Minnesota

THIDA TABUCANON, MD, MSc
Kaufman Center for Heart Failure Treatment
and Recovery, Heart, Vascular, and Thoracic
Institute, Cleveland Clinic, Cleveland,
Ohio

WAI HONG WILSON TANG, MD
Kaufman Center for Heart Failure Treatment
and Recovery, Heart, Vascular, and Thoracic
Institute, Department of Cardiovascular
Medicine, Cleveland Clinic, Cleveland,
Ohio

RYAN J. TEDFORD, MD
Department of Medicine, Division of
Cardiology, Medical University of South
Carolina, Charleston, South Carolina

RAJARAJAN A. THANDAVARAYAN, PhD
Houston Methodist DeBakey Heart & Vascular
Center, Houston, Texas

MICHAEL C. VIRAY, MD
Department of Medicine, Division of
Cardiology, Medical University of South
Carolina, Charleston, South
Carolina

TOM KAI MING WANG, MBCHB, MD(res)
Department of Cardiovascular Medicine, Heart
and Vascular Institute, Cleveland Clinic,
Cleveland, Ohio

CARY WARD, MD
Division of Cardiovascular Medicine, Duke
University Medical Center, Durham, North
Carolina

Contents

Right-sided heart failure (RHF) occurs from impaired contractility of the right ventricle caused by pressure, volume overload, or intrinsic myocardial contractile dysfunction. The development of subclinical right ventricle (RV) dysfunction or overt RHF is a negative prognostic indicator. Recent attention has focused on RV-specific inflammatory growth factors and mediators of myocardial fibrosis to elucidate the mechanisms leading to RHF and potentially guide the development of novel therapeutics. This article focuses on the distinct changes in RV structure, mechanics, and function, as well as molecular and inflammatory mediators involved in the pathophysiology of acute and chronic RHF.

For many years, the importance of the right heart was neglected, and the right ventricle was viewed as merely a conduit for transmitting blood to the lungs. However, the realization that right ventricular function is a key determinant of prognosis in left heart failure, pulmonary hypertension, and after implantation of left ventricular assist devices renewed interest in accurate quantification of right ventricular function. This article reviews traditional and gold-standard hemodynamic assessments of the right ventricle in health and disease.

Right heart failure is a complex and diverse syndrome with unique causes and pathophysiology. The right heart is being recognized as a structurally discrete and functionally independent predictor of mortality. Renewed interest in the right heart has led to efforts to consolidate definitions of right heart failure in an effort to standardize nomenclature and unify epidemiologic studies. Improvements in imaging in particular have contributed to epidemiologic studies, as well as understanding of right heart physiology, which has subsequently led to improved diagnostics and management. This article describes the various causes of right heart disease and its epidemiology.

Cardiorenal syndrome is a complex interplay of dysregulated heart and kidney interaction that leads to multiorgan system dysfunction, which is not an uncommon occurrence in the setting of right heart failure. The traditional concept of impaired perfusion and forward flow recently has been modified to include the recognition of systemic venous congestion as a contributor, with direct and indirect mechanisms, including elevated renal venous pressure, reduced renal perfusion pressure, increased renal interstitial pressure, tubular dysfunction, splanchnic congestion, and neurohormonal and inflammatory activation. Treatment options beyond diuretics and vasoactive drugs remain limited and lack supportive evidence.

Right ventricular dysfunction is increasingly being recognized as a marker of poor prognosis in a variety of cardiovascular diseases. Hence, identification and accurate quantification of the degree of impairment is crucial. Although echocardiography remains the mainstay for right ventricular evaluation, multimodality noninvasive cardiac imaging provides additional useful corroborative assessment. Cardiac MRI is particularly useful for accurate quantification of right ventricular volumes and function, as well as myocardial tissue characterization. This article outlines the clinically useful applications of multimodality imaging for comprehensive assessment of the right heart and associated structures in the setting of right ventricular failure.

Right ventricular failure after left ventricular assist device (LVAD) implantation remains common in the contemporary, continuous-flow era. Clinically meaningful, reproducible, and consensus definitions of both early and late right ventricular failure after LVAD are needed for progress in advanced heart failure. Right ventricular failure after LVAD implantation and post-LVAD vasoplegia share similar risk factors and physiology. The relative right ventricular failure that accompanies right ventricular vasoplegia can be treated with temporary right ventricular assist device support.

Durable left ventricular assist device therapy is an increasingly accepted surgical therapy for advanced heart failure refractory to guideline-directed medical therapy. Right heart failure is a known and frequent complication after durable left ventricular assist device implantation and remains an important clinical challenge. Medical management of right heart failure after left ventricular assist device therapy focuses on improving right ventricular contractility and optimizing right ventricular preload and afterload. Mechanical circulatory support options include surgical and percutaneous devices options as well as the total artificial heart or heart transplantation. Early institution of therapy is necessary to reduce the morbidity and mortality.

Survivorship into adulthood of patients with congenital heart disease is due to improvements in prenatal detection, novel surgeries, and specialized adult congenital heart disease care. As patients survive further into adulthood, long-term complications of congenital and repaired physiology have been more clearly elucidated. The overall mortality of patients with adult congenital heart disease with heart failure is around 4%. Congenital malformations, palliations, residual defects, and resultant physiology impact the right ventricle. This relationship influences morbidity and mortality. For this discussion, focus on atrial septal defects, Ebstein anomaly, Tetralogy of Fallot, transposition of the great vessels, and single right ventricle physiology.

Right Heart Failure in Pulmonary Hypertension

Steven Cassady and Gautam V. Ramani

Right heart failure is a major cause of morbidity and mortality in pulmonary hypertension. Its pathophysiology is complex and involves both adaptive and maladaptive patterns of right ventricular change. In addition to the gold standard of right heart catheterization, noninvasive imaging such as echocardiography is useful in diagnosis and risk assessment. Management focuses on optimizing preload, reducing afterload, and supporting the function of the right ventricle with vasopressors and inotropes, if necessary. If required, mechanical support is increasingly used to facilitate recovery or as a bridge to transplant.

Surgical and Percutaneous Interventions for Chronic Thromboembolic Pulmonary Hypertension

William R. Auger

The treatment of chronic thromboembolic pulmonary hypertension has expanded considerably. The ability to endarterectomize chronic thromboembolic material, the availability of pulmonary hypertension medical therapy to treat inoperable chronic thromboembolic pulmonary hypertension and/or residual pulmonary hypertension, and the rebirth of pulmonary balloon angioplasty have changed the management landscape. Patient selection requires a multidisciplinary evaluation at an experienced center. What is inoperable chronic thromboembolic pulmonary hypertension to one group may be operable chronic thromboembolic pulmonary hypertension to another. The ultimate challenge then becomes which intervention provides the optimal long-term outcome for any individual patient.

Pulmonary Hypertension and Right Ventricular Failure: Lung Transplant Versus Heart-Lung Transplant

Jessica H. Huston, Evan L. Brittain, and Ivan M. Robbins

Pulmonary arterial hypertension is a highly morbid disease with limited treatment options that improve survival and currently the only curative treatment is transplantation. There is a small body of literature comparing the efficacy of lung and heart-lung transplantation in this population. The bulk of evidence suggests that most patients with severe right ventricular failure undergoing transplant will have recovery of right ventricular function after lung transplantation. Existing data suggest that, in the absence of complex congenital heart disease or significant left ventricular dysfunction, double-lung transplant is the surgical procedure of choice.

CARDIOLOGY CLINICS

SERIES OF RELATED INTEREST

Cardiac Electrophysiology Clinics
Heart Failure Clinics
Interventional Cardiology Clinics

THE CLINICS ARE AVAILABLE ONLINE!
Access your subscription at:
www.theclinics.com

Preface

Right Heart Failure: Underlying Pathophysiology, Causes, Diagnostic, and Treatment Considerations

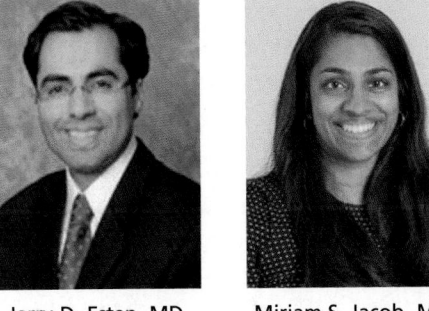

Jerry D. Estep, MD   Miriam S. Jacob, MD

Editors

Right heart failure accounts for significant morbidity and mortality in the world. The list of conditions that cause right ventricular (RV) dysfunction that can progress to significant right heart failure are many, and these causes are often different from the conditions that cause classic, predominantly left-sided heart failure. Solid-organ replacement by heart or heart-lung transplantation and assistance with mechanical devices for those with significant right heart failure are, for many patients, the only options to treat this devastating syndrome. This issue of *Cardiology Clinics* harnesses expertise across multiple disciplines to present a broad spectrum of topics, including underlying pathophysiology and hemodynamics that define right heart failure to guide the available medical and surgical treatment options. The goal of this issue is to provide health care providers with the diagnostic and treatment platform they need to care for these complex patients, many of whom suffer from multiorgan failure, including liver and/or renal disease.

We open with an excellent review that focuses on the distinct changes in RV structure and function, as well as molecular and inflammatory mediators involved in the pathophysiology of right heart failure. Subsequent reviews address the gold-standard hemodynamic assessments of the RV and the role of multimodality imaging to evaluate and manage these patients. In addition, a contemporary review is provided to highlight the epidemiology and, importantly, the causes of right heart failure. Independent of the underlying cause, cardiorenal syndrome, a complex interplay of dysregulated heart and kidney interaction that can lead to progressive multiorgan system dysfunction, is addressed.

In this issue, we also focus on right heart failure after congenital heart disease and after left ventricular assist device placement. We also highlight an underrecognized disease, chronic thromboembolic pulmonary hypertension (CTEPH) to heighten awareness of this potentially curable cause of right heart failure. Treatment options for CTEPH include pulmonary thromboendarterectomy, a unique cardiothoracic surgical procedure that can result in marked improvements in pulmonary hemodynamics and functional status in select patients with this condition. Novel percutaneous treatment options for CTEPH are also addressed.

Finally, the safety and efficacy of lung and heart-lung transplantation is reviewed. This review helps to better understand the implications of RV ventricular dysfunction prior to lung transplantation and the potential benefits of double-lung transplantation in comparison to the more complicated strategy of heart-lung transplantation. It is our hope that readers enjoy and learn from this issue that appropriately places the often underappreciated right ventricle front and center given the

Cardiol Clin 38 (2020) ix–x
https://doi.org/10.1016/j.ccl.2020.03.001
0733-8651/20/© 2020 Published by Elsevier Inc.

significant clinical implications associated with right heart failure.

Jerry D. Estep, MD
Department of Cardiovascular Medicine
Cleveland Clinic Sydell and Arnold Miller
Family Heart
Vascular and Thoracic Institute
Kaufman Center for Heart Failure
Treatment and Recovery
Cleveland Clinic
9500 Euclid Avenue Desk J3-4
Cleveland, OH 44122, USA

Miriam S. Jacob, MD
Department of Cardiovascular Medicine
Cleveland Clinic Sydell and Arnold Miller
Family Heart
Vascular and Thoracic Institute
Kaufman Center for Heart Failure
Treatment and Recovery
Cleveland Clinic
9500 Euclid Avenue Desk J3-4
Cleveland, OH 44122, USA

E-mail addresses:
estepj@ccf.org (J.D. Estep)
jacobm@ccf.org (M.S. Jacob)

Pathophysiology of Acute and Chronic Right Heart Failure

Rajarajan A. Thandavarayan, PhD, Kalyan R. Chitturi, DO,
Ashrith Guha, MD, MPH*

KEYWORDS

- Right heart failure • Pulmonary hypertension • Hypertrophy • Metabolism • Angiogenesis
- Inflammation • Mechanical circulatory support

KEY POINTS

- Right-sided heart failure occurs from impaired contractility of the right ventricle leading to the resultant clinical syndrome.
- The right heart is a thin-walled chamber that is poorly adapted to increases in afterload.
- Cardiomyocytes in the right ventricle are 15% smaller than in the left ventricle and contain more than 30% collagen, although they have similar protein composition and overlap in gene expression.

INTRODUCTION

Right-sided heart failure (RHF) occurs from impaired contractility of the right ventricle (RV) caused by pressure, volume overload, or intrinsic myocardial contractile dysfunction leading to the resultant clinical syndrome. Irrespective of underlying cause, the development of subclinical RV dysfunction or overt RHF is a negative prognostic indicator associated with increased morbidity and mortality. The distinct embryologic origins of the RV and pulmonary circulation predispose to RV dysfunction, although the mechanisms driving the pathophysiology of RHF remain incompletely understood. Recent attention has focused on RV-specific inflammatory growth factors and mediators of myocardial fibrosis to elucidate the mechanisms leading to RHF and potentially guide the development of novel therapeutics. This article is an overview of the distinct changes in RV structure, mechanics, and function, as well as molecular and inflammatory mediators involved in the pathophysiology of acute and chronic RHF. Although RV failure is a result of conditions that cause an increase in afterload (often experimentally induced by an increase in pressure), preload (often experimentally induced by valvular regurgitation), or a combination thereof, this article evaluates the animal models and relates them to patient conditions based on chronicity of pressure and volume overload states.

THE RIGHT HEART MILIEU

The origins and microenvironment of the RV and pulmonary circulation form the foundational basis of the structural and functional differences in the RV compared with the left ventricle (LV) and predispose to RV dysfunction and failure. This unique milieu also explains why the application of concepts involved in the pathogenesis of left-sided heart failure are not often reproduced in models of RHF.

For example, the right and left heart differ in embryologic origins and molecular composition. Derived from the anterior heart field, RV progenitors differ from their LV counterparts arising from the posterior mesoderm. Most of the cells comprising the future RV and atria depend on the expression of transcription factor LIM homeodomain islet-1

Houston Methodist DeBakey Heart & Vascular Center, 6550 Fannin Street, Houston, TX 77030, USA
* Corresponding author. Methodist DeBakey Cardiology Associates, 6550 Fannin MSB 1801, Houston, TX 77030.
E-mail address: gashrith@houstonmethodist.org

Cardiol Clin 38 (2020) 149–160
https://doi.org/10.1016/j.ccl.2020.01.009

(Isl-I), whereas cells giving rise to the future LV do not express this transcription factor.[1] In utero, the RV is the dominant chamber and the wall thickness between the 2 ventricles is equal, although pulmonary vascular resistance (PVR) deceases rapidly at birth and RV wall thickness regresses with increased compliance. Cardiomyocytes in the RV are 15% smaller than LV cardiomyocytes and contain more than 30% collagen, although they have similar protein composition and overlap in gene expression.[2] Given a thinner wall, the RV depends more on coronary perfusion pressure and is vulnerable to increases in RV pressure and systemic hypoperfusion. Probably an adaptation to ischemia and other myocardial stressors, the RV may have a higher activity of aerobic glycolytic metabolism than the LV because a rodent model showed higher expression of HK1 and HK2 messenger RNA (mRNA) and protein.[3]

Despite embryologic, genetic, and structural differences, the RV mostly shares similarities in function with the LV except for a few notable features. For example, RV contractility differs compared with the LV in that longitudinal shortening of subendocardial myocytes accounts for approximately 75% of RV contraction.[4] The adequacy of RV contractility to pressure-overload states also partly depends on optimal ventriculoarterial coupling, often approximated with either the ratio of RV elastance to pulmonary artery (PA) elastance (Ees/Ea) or the ratio between tricuspid annular plane excursion (TAPSE) and PA systolic pressure. Both measures compare surrogates for RV contractility and afterload.[5,6] However, overall the RV and LV share similarities in responses to acute increases in either preload or afterload with immediate increases in ventricular dilatation to preserve stroke volume.

ACUTE RIGHT HEART FAILURE

The development of acute RHF (ARHF) portends a worse prognosis, with an estimated mortality ranging from 6% to 14%.[7,8] Coupled to the high-compliance, low-resistance pulmonary circuit, the RV is much thinner in diameter and less muscular than the LV and has greater capacity to adapt to changes in volume rather than pressure.[9] Thus, ARHF most often occurs because of sudden increases in RV afterload or intrinsic myocardial dysfunction rather than volume overload. Abrupt increases in RV afterload, such as an acute massive pulmonary embolism (PE), may rapidly decrease RV stroke volume with minimal compensatory increase in RV systolic pressure, resulting in hemodynamic collapse. Impaired RV contractility caused by an acute RV myocardial infarction (RVMI) can lead to ARHF, with subsequent tricuspid regurgitation (TR), acute RV dilatation, and decreased LV filling from impaired ventricular interdependence possibly leading to cardiogenic shock.

Pressure Overload: Acute Pulmonary Embolism

The development of ARHF from a PE depends largely on a multitude of factors, including the size of the embolism and anatomic location (ie, within the larger segments of the pulmonary arteries), the release of humoral growth factors, and preexisting cardiopulmonary comorbidities. Initially, the occlusion of a major pulmonary arterial segment leads to an immediate increase in PVR, partly from physical obstruction but also from hypoxic vasoconstriction related to ventilation-perfusion mismatch and the local release of thromboxane A2 and serotonin from local platelets.[10,11] If more than 30% to 50% of the total cross-sectional area of the pulmonary arterial vasculature is decreased (either from blockage or resultant vasoconstriction), pulmonary arterial pressure (PAP) increases.[12] The resultant increase in PVR leads to RV strain from ventricular dilatation and hypokinesis, TR with tricuspid annular dilatation, and impaired RV contractility with reduced RV stroke volume. After a short period of adaptation, patients with an acute massive PE experience eventual circulatory collapse, because RV pressure overload leads to a leftward shift of the interventricular septum, impaired LV diastolic filling during diastole, and diminished cardiac output. The presence of shock portends a poor prognosis unless immediate reperfusion treatment along with circulatory and respiratory support is initiated.[13]

Contractile Dysfunction: Acute Right Ventricle Infarct

An acute RVMI significant enough to cause ARHF usually occurs in the setting of an inferior myocardial infarction (MI), because coronary blood flow needs to be disrupted to both the RV free wall and the interventricular septum, which accounts for a significant amount of contractility as well as in the LV. Often a dominant right coronary artery is occluded proximal to the major branches, leading to reduced RV systolic function and acute RV dilatation, although variations are possible depending on the coronary anatomy.[14] RV ischemia from decreased coronary perfusion leads to inadequate oxygen delivery to the RV myocardium and worsened contractility, RV dilatation, and dyskinesis.[15] Decreased RV compliance results in diminished RV stroke volume and increased diastolic pressures, worsening ventricular interdependence, which may eventually lead to hemodynamic collapse from biventricular diastolic dysfunction.[16,17] RV involvement portends worsened prognosis in inferior MI, because the multicenter randomized SHOCK (Should We Emergently Revascularize Occluded Coronaries for Cardiogenic Shock) and CORE (Collaborative Organization for RheothRx Evaluation) trials found patients with inferior MI and RV myocardial involvement remain at high risk of death, shock, and arrhythmia despite revascularization.[18]

Acute Volume Overload: Insights from Animal Models

In addition, ARHF related to acute volume overload occurs in a variety of clinical conditions, with tricuspid or pulmonary regurgitation and aggressive fluid resuscitation in the postsurgical or critical care setting being common scenarios. Several animal models have elucidated the mechanical processes involved in the pathophysiology of volume overload–related ARHF in various clinical settings. The details of the models and the changes are summarized in **Fig. 1**.

For example, an isolated ejecting canine heart model showed that increasing RV volume had a small but significant ventricular-interdependence effect on LV diastolic pressures, although it did not contribute to large acute pressure-volume shifts even with RV volumes at the physiologic limit.[19] A murine model of RV volume overload

with aortocaval shunting showed severe RV dilatation, increased RV stroke volume, and reduced RV EF.[20] In addition, a feline model of biventricular volume overload did not find impaired contractility inherent in either RV or LV cardiomyocyte hypertrophy secondary to substantial volume overloading when afterload is normal.[21] A novel ovine model of ARHF with functional TR showed that a combination of volume infusion, pulmonary hypertension (PH), or ischemia mediated significant RV and tricuspid annular enlargement, with neither process significant on its own.[22] The general conclusion that can be gained from these models is that volume overload is tolerated better than pressure overload in the RV and that preexisting conditions lower the threshold for developing volume overload–related ARHF.

Role of Cytokines and Impaired Metabolism in Acute Right Ventricular Overload

Preclinical models have shown that cytokine activation and impaired cellular metabolism are associated with the pathophysiology of ARHF from pressure overload. A rodent model of pressure-overload ARHF from acute PE showed a shift in cardiac physiology favoring the fetal gene expression pattern with upregulation of multiple CC and CXC chemokine genes, downregulation of fatty acid transporters and oxidative enzymes, and upregulation of stretch-sensing and hypoxia-inducible transcription factors.[23] A murine model of pressure-overload ARHF induced by pulmonary

↑ Preload (Volume Overload)
Sepsis, Aggressive Resuscitation, Tricuspid Regurgitation
↓ ERK1/2
↑ Chemokines (TNF-α, TGF-β)
↑ Glycolysis
↓ Fatty acid oxidation

↑ Afterload
Acute PE,
Acidosis,
Hypoxia,
ARDS,
Positive Pressure
Ventilation
↑ Chemokines
(CCL, CXCL, CCR₁,
CXCR₄, IL-1β, IL-6,
TNF-α)
↑ Neutrophils and
macrophages
↑ Hypoxia-inducible
factor
↓ Fatty acid
oxidation
↓ Ventriculoarterial
coupling

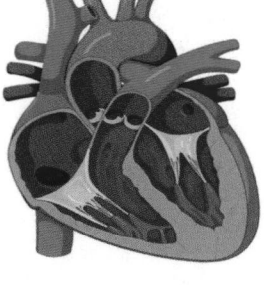

↓ Contractility
RVMI,
Myocarditis,
Postcardiotomy
Syndrome,
Post-LVAD,
Primary Graft
Dysfunction
↑ Chemokines
(TNF-α, IL-6)
↑ PDK
↑ Glycolysis
↓ Glucose oxidation
↓ (miR)-126
↓ (miR)-208
↓ Angiogenesis,
↓ Fatty acid
oxidation
↑ ROS

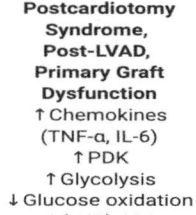

Fig. 1. ARHF: pathophysiology, causes, metabolic, and inflammatory pathways. Integral transcriptional, signal transduction, immunobiologic, and metabolic pathways involved in the pathophysiology of acute right heart failure. ARDS, acute respiratory distress syndrome; CCL, CC chemokine ligand; CCR₁, CC chemokine receptor type 1; CXCL, CXC chemokine ligand involved in neutrophil activation; CXCR₄, CXC chemokine receptor type 4 involved in lymphocyte chemotaxis; ERK1/2, phosphorylated extracellular regulated kinase; IL-1β, interleukin-1β; IL-6, interleukin-6; LVAD, left ventricular assist device; (miR)-126, microRNA expressed on endothelial cells involved in angiogenesis transcriptional processes; (miR)-208, microRNA involved in regulation of beta-myosin heavy chain production in development, stress-dependent growth factor; PDK, pyruvate dehydrogenase kinase; ROS, reactive oxygen species; RVMI, right ventricular MI; TGF-β, transforming growth factor-β; TNF-α, tumor necrosis factor-a.

arterial banding showed a downregulation of mitochondrial enzymes involved in cellular metabolism, including acetyl-coenzyme A acyltransferase 2, NADH dehydrogenase, NADH-ubiquinone oxidoreductase, succinate dehydrogenase complex, and ATP synthase.[24] Another rodent model of pressure-overload ARHF from acute PE showed that moderately severe PH was associated with increased expression of monocyte chemoattractant protein 1 (MCP-1); myeloperoxidase activity; mRNA cytokine-induced neutrophil chemoattractant 1 (CINC-1), cytokine-induced neutrophil chemoattractant 2 (CINC-2), macrophage inflammatory protein 2 (MIP-2), and macrophage inflammatory protein 1 alpha (MIP-1α) in the RV; and cardiomyocyte necrosis and phagocytosis via infiltration of neutrophils and monocytes.[25] A pressure-overload feline model of ARHF showed that activation of the calpain, a protease linked to the cleavage of cytoskeletal proteins, induced programmed cardiomyocyte cell death in the RV myocardium.[26]

Impaired metabolism and molecular markers have been discovered in models of volume-overload ARHF, although no actionable therapeutic targets have been identified. A porcine model of ARHF involving aggressive volume loading and induced iterative PE in animals with baseline chronic thromboembolic PH detected RV subendocardial and subepicardial focal ischemic lesions that express autophagy-related protein light chain 3-phosphatidyletanolamineconjugate (LC3-II) and increased circulating high-sensitivity troponin I on hemodynamic restoration.[27] A murine model of RV dysfunction from volume overload showed a decreased amount of phosphorylated extracellular regulated kinase (ERK1/2) in the RV and LV in response to increased preload.[20] In a study by Shah and colleagues[28] using an acute TR canine model, early RV volume overload was associated with RV dilatation and decreased RV contractility. This finding was coupled with an increase in sympathetic activation with no change in beta receptor density.

Another murine model of RV dysfunction from induced pulmonary insufficiency showed downregulation of genetic pathways involving tumor necrosis factor-α (TNF-α), transforming growth factor β1 (TGF-β1), p53, and extracellular matrix remodeling at 1 month before transition to upregulation at 3 months, highlighting that dynamic gene expression changes are involved in worsening RV dysfunction and possibly progression to ARHF.[29]

CHRONIC RIGHT HEART FAILURE

Chronic RHF (CRHF) is most commonly a consequence of continuing increase in RV pressure overload caused primarily by pulmonary arterial hypertension (PAH) and secondary PH (PH) as seen in pulmonary disease or left heart disease, although chronic volume overload from valvular lesions such as TR and pulmonic regurgitation, albeit less common, also lead to development of RV failure.[15,30–32] Because chronic RHF is predominantly caused by an increase in RV afterload (pressure-overload state), animal models have typically stimulated different pressure-overload states (either through drugs or surgery) to assess pathogenesis.

The right heart is a thin-walled chamber that is poorly adapted to increases in afterload.[30–36] Increases in afterload imposed on the RV initially stimulate compensatory myocyte hypertrophy to maintain sufficient cardiac output, which indicates an adaptation in the RV. The adaptive phenotype matches the clinical compensated stage, wherein the hypertrophied RV starts to progress through isovolumic phases of contraction and relaxation with increased RV systolic pressure and higher end-diastolic volume. However, if the pressure overload continues, then the RV transitions from an adapted to maladaptive molecular phenotype characterized by oxidative stress, inflammation, impaired angiogenesis, myocyte loss, and replacement/fibrosis.[15,31,36–38] In the decompensated phase, which matches the maladaptive molecular changes, there is a concurrent increase in PVR and right atrial pressure. Although PVR remains determinedly increased, cardiac output consequently decreases, followed by a decrease in pulmonary artery pressure PAP.[39,40]

CHRONIC RIGHT VENTRICLE VOLUME OVERLOAD

Patients with congenital heart disease (CHD), develop sequelae of chronic right ventricular volume overload from chronic pulmonic incompetence or TR. These patients have RV volume overload in addition to pressure overload, which significantly contributes to CRHF.[2] In many patients with right-sided obstructive lesions such as tetralogy of Fallot, pulmonary atresia and systemic RVs such as L-transposition of the great arteries, hypoplastic left heart syndrome, and corrected transposition, and single RV physiology, the RV is uniquely at risk.[24] During the past few decades, improvement in surgical approach has shifted CHD survivorship from early to middle adulthood. These patients thus have lived for a long time with abnormal cardiac loading conditions that predispose them to RHF.[41]

MOLECULAR CHANGES AFTER CHRONIC RIGHT VENTRICLE VOLUME OVERLOAD

Knowledge of the molecular changes in the RV in response to chronic volume overload is very limited, despite an increasing number of adult patients with CHD with common late sequelae of RV volume overload after RV outflow tract reconstruction, single RVs with an aortopulmonary shunt, and L-transposition of great arteries with atrioventricular regurgitation.

The animal models have typically been created to have volume overload by surgically creating pulmonic regurgitation, TR, or atrial septal defect to study the changes in RV over time. The details of the models and the changes are summarized in **Table 1**.[29,42–45]

Table 1
Molecular changes in RV in response to chronic volume overload in different animal models

Molecular Changes	RV Induction	Study Objective	Findings
Metabolic changes	Animals: 12-wk-old male, FVB mice Experimental model: pulmonary insufficiency was created by entrapping the pulmonary valve leaflets with sutures	Physiologic and molecular characteristics of the RV volume overload	• Genes related to mitochondrial pathways and G protein–coupled receptor signaling was downregulated • TNF-α, TGF-β1, p53-signaling, and ECM remodeling upregulated[42]
Angiogenesis	Animals: 4-mo-old sheep. Experimental model: TAP implantation and pulmonary valve distortion in the RVOT	Feasibility and efficacy of autologous UCMNC transplant on RV function	• Treatment with UCMNCs significantly improved RV diastolic function • Significant enhancement of angiogenesis after UCMNC transplant[43]
Hypertrophy	Animals: young adult cats Experimental model: interatrial septal defect	Quantitative structural study of myocardium hypertrophying after pressure and volume overload	• Volume density of cardiomyocytes, connective tissue, and collagen fibrils are not affected by volume overload • In the hypertrophied myocardium, diameter of the mean capillary was increased • No difference between hemodynamic overload, resultant hypertrophy in both pressure and volume overload models[44]
Oxidative stress	Animals: 8-wk-old, male, Wistar rats. Experimental model: aortocaval shunt	Acute effect of intravenous S-NO-HSA infusion on hemodynamic and oxidative stress alteration in chronic RV overload model	• Increased GSH/GSSG ratio in shunt group was significantly decreased in S-NO-has–treated group • S-NO-HSA treatment decreased PH and improved RV systolic/diastolic function and RV-arterial coupling by increasing energy reserve and reducing oxidative stress[45]

(continued on next page)

Table 1
(continued)

Molecular Changes	RV Induction	Study Objective	Findings
Neurohormonal response	Patients: 42 patients, aged 17–57 y (mean, 30 y). Clinical model: surgically corrected CHD	Examined the pressure and/or volume overload on RV function and correlated with the BNP levels in patients with surgically corrected CHD	• The RV volume over-loaded patients presented lower RV and LV ejection fraction compared with pressure-overloaded patients • The RV volume over-loaded patients presented increased BNP levels • Levels of BNP independently associated with degree of RV volume overload and function[46]

Abbreviations: BNP, B-type natriuretic peptide; ECM, extracellular matrix; FVB, Friend leukemia virus B; GSH/GSSG, glutathione reduced/oxidized; RVOT, RV outflow tract; S-NO-HSA, S-nitroso human serum albumin; TAP, transannular patch; UCMNC, umbilical cord blood mononuclear cell.

Overall it seems that chronic RV volume overload is characterized by mitochondrial dysfunction, increased oxidative stress, increased growth factors, natriuretic peptides, and extracellular matrix remodeling, which are phenotypically related to RV hypertrophy and fibrosis, which eventually lead to RV failure.

CHRONIC RIGHT VENTRICLE PRESSURE OVERLOAD

Chronic pressure overload is seen in PH and the resulting RHF is the leading cause of lung transplant and death in those patients.[38] Changes in chronic RV pressure overload have been best studied aspect of the pathophysiology of RHF because of the availability of several animal models.[46–49]

Adaptive Changes

Chronically increased pulmonary pressures do not immediately result in RV failure. During the initial period of exposure, the RV adapts to the increased afterload by altering its metabolism and morphology so as to meet the increased work requirement. Several interconnected adaptive mechanisms have been proposed, including myocyte hypertrophy, a switch in the primary fuel used for ATP generation, increased angiogenesis, and decreased production of mitochondrial reactive oxygen species.[46–49] Although the RV adaptation mechanism is initially successful in many cases, it is temporary, and the progressive increases in pressure overload lead to RHF.

Progression from Adaptive to Maladaptive Changes

The transition from adaptive to maladaptive changes in the RV is difficult to predict clinically, and patients with different causes of cardiac pulmonary disease progress to overt RHF over different periods of time. Because RHF is the primary determinant of outcomes in patients with PAH, understanding the major mediators of RV compensation, failure, and recovery is essential to improving patient survival. Initially the RV adapts by increasing its contractility through the synthesis of additional sarcomeres and extracellular matrix, and via cardiac hypertrophy (see **Fig. 1**).[38,50] However, at some point, adaptation is inadequate for the pressure overload, causing RV dilatation, RV systolic and diastolic dysfunction, and frank RHF.[50–53] This sequence of events is not well understood in the RV and the factors that initiate the switch from adaptive to maladaptive states are unknown. Several cellular and molecular changes (**Fig. 2**) involved in the RV maladaptive remodeling that could play a role have been proposed, including cardiac hypertrophy, fibrosis, oxidative stress, inflammation, angiogenesis, metabolism, neurohormonal modulation, and different signaling pathways.[31,39,54]

Right Ventricle Hypertrophy

RV hypertrophy is one of the central features to of compensation to chronic pressure overload.[55–57]

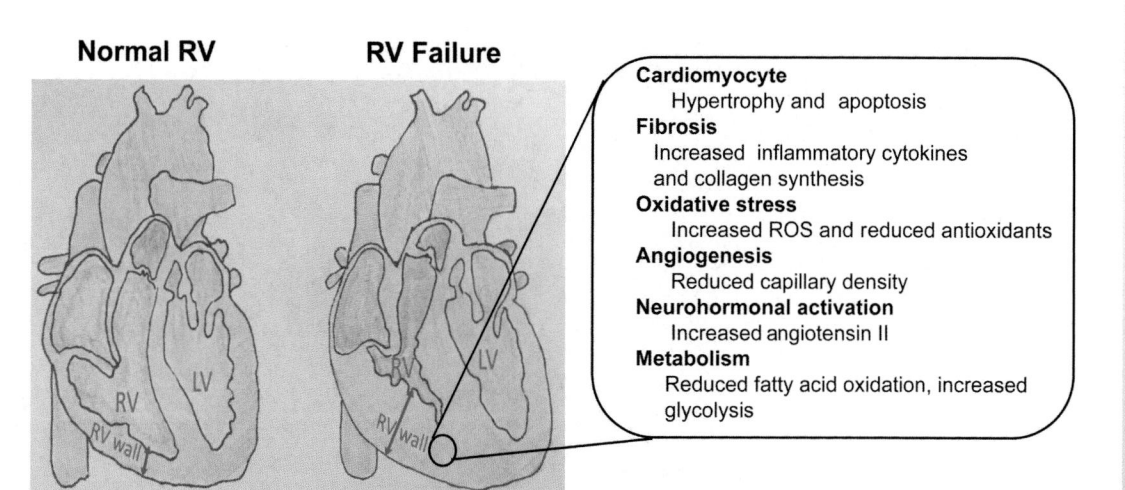

Normal RV   **RV Failure**

Cardiomyocyte
    Hypertrophy and apoptosis
Fibrosis
    Increased inflammatory cytokines
    and collagen synthesis
Oxidative stress
    Increased ROS and reduced antioxidants
Angiogenesis
    Reduced capillary density
Neurohormonal activation
    Increased angiotensin II
Metabolism
    Reduced fatty acid oxidation, increased
    glycolysis

Fig. 2. Chronic pressure-overload induced RHF: molecular and cellular mechanisms.

Chronic pressure overload provokes different responses in the LV and the RV because of their divergent embryonic origins. Both chambers characteristically start evolving at a 3.5-mm thickness prenatally but develop at diverse rates after birth. The LV grows in size to about 11 mm in thickness, whereas the RV is about 4 mm.[57,58] Thus, in order to acclimatize for the higher chronic PAP that are associated with the diverse types of PH, these 2 relative thicknesses change. In general, cardiomyocyte size increases through the synthesis of additional sarcomeres and, in addition, extracellular matrix increases as well, with secondary augmented cardiac fibrosis.[59,60] At some point, compensation is inadequate for the pressure overload, resulting in dilatation, decreased systolic and diastolic function, and frank RHF.[60]

A couple of therapeutic approaches have been used to target hypertrophy in the prevention and treatment of RHF in chronic pressure overload. In a recent RV chronic-pressure-overload model, spherical aggregation helped the ability of cardiac progenitor cells (CPCs), improved RV contractile function, and reduced RV hypertrophy and fibrosis.[61] Although a phase I study of CPC therapy in children with hypoplastic left heart syndrome is underway, there is a potential for rapid translation of this therapy to the clinic, especially in patients that do not respond to traditional cell therapy. Another study shows that upregulation of ADAMTS8 in pulmonary artery smooth muscle cells (PASMCs) contributes to the pathogenesis of PAH, which involves proliferation and migration of PASMCs, enhanced matrix metalloproteinase activity, and mitochondrial dysfunction.[62] ADAMTS8 inhibition in PASMCs is a novel strategy to prevent the

development of PH by ameliorating RV hypertrophy and failure in response to increased PA pressure, and mebendazole treatment reduced ADAMTS8 expression and RV hypertrophy and ameliorated RHF in rodents.[62]

Right Ventricle Angiogenesis

Angiogenesis is one of the main drivers of RV adaptation in the setting of chronic pressure overload.[63] In the early stage of PAH, RV hypertrophy is accompanied by increased angiogenesis as an adaptive response. However, as RV hypertrophy continues to progress without additional angiogenesis, it leads to to cardiomyocyte apoptosis and RHF.[63,64] This impaired angiogenic reaction leads to an inadequate supply of oxygen and nutrients, thus resulting in cardiomyocyte contractile dysfunction. In a preclinical pulmonary artery banding, RV pressure–overload model, child CPC spherical aggregation significantly improved the ability of CPCs to improve RV contractile function, increase RV angiogenesis, and reduce RV hypertrophy and RV fibrosis.[61,65] This improvement is mainly attributed to increased Notch1 signaling, by enhancing CPC differentiation.[61,65] Patients who have PH associated with systemic sclerosis are predisposed to RV failure because of endothelial injury and impaired angiogenesis, which leads to RV ischemia.[63,66] Accordingly, the angiogenesis-deficient RV cannot maintain its normal function during chronic pressure overload. Collectively, impaired angiogenesis may be one of the key processes leading to RV decompensation, and regulating angiogenic signaling pathways might be a novel approach to maintain, extend, or even reestablish adaptive RV remodeling.

Right Ventricle Fibrosis and Inflammation

RV fibrosis increases myocardial stiffness, which contributes to functional impairment.[67] However, a certain level of fibrosis may be helpful because it offers mechanical support to cardiomyocytes nearby and averts excessive RV dilatation and distortion caused by pressure overload.[68] In patients with chronic RV pressure overload, less than 10% of ventricular volume is fibrosed and fibrosis is often limited to the RV septal insertion points.[39] Although the RV is facing the pressure overload, it uses NO to lessen the afterload by stimulating pulmonary vasodilation. In a recent preclinical study, 3 weeks after PA banding, NO synthase 2 (NOS2) expression was increased 2-fold in the hypertrophied RV with increased NO production. In addition, NOS2 is localized in interstitial and perivascular cardiac fibroblasts after PA banding. In the hypertrophied RV, NOS2 induction was accompanied by an increased formation of reactive oxidants blocked by ex vivo NO synthase inhibition. On a cellular level, this study indicates that NOS2 induction promotes collagen deposition from the cardiac fibroblast, causative of the pathogenesis of RV fibrosis and its impaired function.[69] In a chronic-pressure-overload Rat model of PH, ASK1 inhibition reduced RV fibrosis and inflammatory gene expression, and improved RV function.[47] However, in another preclinical study, treatment with the antifibrotic compound pirfenidone did not diminish the progress of fibrosis or RV hypertrophy, or improve RV function. In addition, pirfenidone showed no adverse effects on the RV, likely suggesting that it may be safe in patients with RHF.[70] Fibrosis may thus have ventricular-specific features that require further investigation of its pathophysiologic consequence and therapeutic responsiveness in RV failure.

Right Ventricle Metabolism

Imbalances of RV metabolism related to RHF caused by pressure overload has been observed in various experimental studies[58,71,72] and is confirmed in many studies in patients with PAH.[58,73,74] Under conditions of increased pressure overload, there is an initial increased oxidative metabolism associated with increased glucose use. Accompanying this process, a metabolic switch is also observed that leads to inhibition of the fatty acid pathway and activation of the glycolytic pathway. Different groups have observed upregulated glycolysis with suppression of fatty acid oxidation and associated modulation of different transcriptional profiles advancing glucose oxidation and downregulation of PPARα target genes.[75] Pyruvate dehydrogenase kinase (PDK), an inhibitor of pyruvate dehydrogenase, has been linked to the metabolic switch and is upregulated in RV hypertrophy. This PDK-mediated metabolic switch is associated with decreased RV myocyte contractility and cardiac output.[76] To compensate for increased glycolysis, glucose uptake is accelerated, and can be assessed by PET, both in experimental PH and RHF,[77] and in patients with PAH.[78] Another study showed that mutant bone morphogenetic receptor type 2 (BMPR2) expression in the RV may impair hypertrophic responses in part because of fatty acid oxidation defects in multiple experimental models.[73] This study extended these findings to human heritable PAH RVs, in which alteration in expression of genes associated with fatty acid oxidation and lipid deposition in mice showed that RV lipid deposition is reversible using metformin.[73] This finding might suggest that an impaired metabolic compensatory mechanism plays a role in the maladaptive hypertrophic response in BMPR2. These findings suggest that early interventions to prevent RHF may be directed toward preservation of intracardiac lipid composition.

Lipotoxicity has been recognized in the pressure-loaded RV in a model of BMPR2 mutation.[72] However, myocardial shortage of lipids has also been suggested to have negative effects on cardiac remodeling and function.[72] Interestingly, RHF caused by chronic pressure overload is associated with decreased intracardiac unsaturated lipid levels, especially in the most abundant form of cardiolipin. These changes were accompanied by preserved mitochondrial capacity for fatty acid oxidation, with an increased mitochondrial capacity for glucose oxidation, and early expression of oxidative stress markers.[72] Together these observations emphasize the relevance of a deeper understanding of RV dysfunction induced by different types of disease and the therapeutic potential of lipid modulation therapies.

Right Ventricle Neurohormonal Modulation

In response to chronic pressure overload, RV neurohormonal systems are activated and involved in RV structural and functional changes,[79–81] although it is necessary for maintaining the cardiac output for the enhancement of cardiac contractility and hypertrophy in the earlier stage of pressure overload. However, the progressive overstimulation of the adrenergic system and the renin-angiotensin-aldosterone system

(RAAS) might be associated with the transition of RV adaptation to RV maladaptation and subsequent RHF.[79–81] Angiotensin-converting enzyme (ACE) converts angiotensin I to angiotensin II, which in turn activates the angiotensin 1 receptor (AT1R). Further, it stimulates RV hypertrophy and fibrosis in experimental chronic RV pressure-overload models.[82,83] In experimental models with RV failure, recombinant ACE2 improved RV function and reduced RV hypertrophy and fibrosis.[84,85] Chronic RV pressure overload resulted in angiotensin 2 receptors uncoupling in an RV hypertrophy rabbit model, and the RAAS signaling impairments led to severe cardiac contractility performance, although it is reversed by the ACE inhibitor ramipril.[86] Further studies should reveal the applicability of drugs intervening in the RAAS system in experimental models of chronic RV pressure overload.

SUMMARY

Remarkable progress has been achieved in the past decade in understanding the genetic, embryologic, cellular, molecular, and biomechanical processes driving the pathophysiology of acute and chronic RHF and the pulmonary circuit. As mentioned in the official American Thoracic Society research statement on the current state of knowledge regarding right ventricular function in the research setting, there exist major areas in need of further exploration and a need for the application of well-designed preclinical models that translate to human studies and correlate with the genetic, molecular, and metabolic pathways associated with RV dysfunction and RHF.[87] Future translational research involving human RV specimens needs to investigate the mechanisms elucidated by the animal models of acute and chronic RHF pathophysiology discussed earlier to determine the extent to which these preclinical models simulate human disease processes. Further studies are needed to correlate physiologic and clinical studies on RV-arterial functional adaptations to PH with invasive hemodynamics in different clinical scenarios. In addition, much work is needed to explore the different phenotypes of CRHF from the different World Health Organization subgroups of PH and should investigate the hemodynamic, imaging, and cardiopulmonary exercise testing predictors of functional capacity and survival. The state of knowledge regarding RV function and failure has significantly progressed, especially with regard to the molecular and metabolic pathways, although much work remains to correlate these insights to patient care and development of novel RV-targeted therapies.

ACKNOWLEDGMENTS

The authors acknowledge funding from the Roswell and Ann Vaughan Fund to A. Guha and the American Heart Association, United States (19TPA34880039 and 18IPA34170497) to R.A. Thandavarayan. The authors thank Pranalisree Rajarajan, seventh grader, Bob Lanier Middle School, Houston, for assisting with the artwork.

DISCLOSURE

The authors have no commercial or financial conflicts of interest or disclosures.

REFERENCES

1. Samson N, Paulin R. Epigenetics, inflammation and metabolism in right heart failure associated with pulmonary hypertension. Pulm Circ 2017;7(3):572–87.
2. Sanz J, Sanchez-Quintana D, Bossone E, et al. Anatomy, function, and dysfunction of the right ventricle: JACC state-of-the-art review. J Am Coll Cardiol 2019;73(12):1463–82.
3. Waskova-Arnostova P, Elsnicova B, Kasparova D, et al. Right-to-left ventricular differences in the expression of mitochondrial hexokinase and phosphorylation of Akt. Cell Physiol Biochem 2013; 31(1):66–79.
4. Brown SB, Raina A, Katz D, et al. Longitudinal shortening accounts for the majority of right ventricular contraction and improves after pulmonary vasodilator therapy in normal subjects and patients with pulmonary arterial hypertension. Chest 2011; 140(1):27–33.
5. Tello K, Axmann J, Ghofrani HA, et al. Relevance of the TAPSE/PASP ratio in pulmonary arterial hypertension. Int J Cardiol 2018;266:229–35.
6. Lewis GD, Ngo D, Hemnes AR, et al. Metabolic profiling of right ventricular-pulmonary vascular function reveals circulating biomarkers of pulmonary hypertension. J Am Coll Cardiol 2016;67(2):174–89.
7. Maggioni AP, Dahlström U, Filippatos G, et al. EURObservational Research programme: the heart failure pilot survey (ESC-HF Pilot). Eur J Heart Fail 2010;12(10):1076–84.
8. Logeart D, Isnard R, Resche-Rigon M, et al. Current aspects of the spectrum of acute heart failure syndromes in a real-life setting: the OFICA study. Eur J Heart Fail 2013;15(4):465–76.
9. Ventetuolo CE, Klinger JR. Management of acute right ventricular failure in the intensive care unit. Ann Am Thorac Soc 2014;11(5):811–22.
10. Goldhaber SZ, Elliott CG. Acute pulmonary embolism: part I: epidemiology, pathophysiology, and diagnosis. Circulation 2003;108(22):2726–9.
11. Smulders YM. Pathophysiology and treatment of haemodynamic instability in acute pulmonary

embolism: the pivotal role of pulmonary vasocon-striction. Cardiovasc Res 2000;48(1):23–33.

12. McIntyre KM, Sasahara AA. The hemodynamic response to pulmonary embolism in patients without prior cardiopulmonary disease. Am J Cardiol 1971; 28(3):288–94.

13. Konstantinides SV, Barco S, Lankeit M, et al. Management of pulmonary embolism: an update. J Am Coll Cardiol 2016;67(8):976–90.

14. Bowers TR, O'Neill WW, Pica M, et al. Patterns of coronary compromise resulting in acute right ventricular ischemic dysfunction. Circulation 2002; 106(9):1104–9.

15. Konstam MA, Kiernan MS, Bernstein D, et al. Evaluation and management of right-sided heart failure: a scientific statement from the American Heart Association. Circulation 2018;137(20):e578–622.

16. Goldstein JA, Barzilai B, Rosamond TL, et al. Determinants of hemodynamic compromise with severe right ventricular infarction. Circulation 1990;82(2):359–68.

17. Goldstein JA, Harada A, Yagi Y, et al. Hemodynamic importance of systolic ventricular interaction, augmented right atrial contractility and atrioventricular synchrony in acute right ventricular dysfunction. J Am Coll Cardiol 1990;16(1):181–9.

18. Mehta SR, Eikelboom JW, Natarajan MK, et al. Impact of right ventricular involvement on mortality and morbidity in patients with inferior myocardial infarction. J Am Coll Cardiol 2001;37(1):37–43.

19. Maughan WL, Kallman CH, Shoukas A. The effect of right ventricular filling on the pressure-volume relationship of ejecting canine left ventricle. Circ Res 1981;49(2):382–8.

20. Bartelds B, Borgdorff MA, Smit-Van Oosten A, et al. Differential responses of the right ventricle to abnormal loading conditions in mice: pressure vs. volume load. Eur J Heart Fail 2011;13(12): 1275–82.

21. Urabe Y, Hamada Y, Spinale FG, et al. Cardiocyte contractile performance in experimental biventricular volume-overload hypertrophy. Am J Physiol 1993;264(5 Pt 2):H1615–23.

22. Malinowski M, Proudfoot AG, Eberhart L, et al. Large animal model of acute right ventricular failure with functional tricuspid regurgitation. Int J Cardiol 2018;264:124–9.

23. Zagorski J, Sanapareddy N, Gellar MA, et al. Transcriptional profile of right ventricular tissue during acute pulmonary embolism in rats. Physiol Genomics 2008;34(1):101–11.

24. Reddy S, Bernstein D. Molecular mechanisms of right ventricular failure. Circulation 2015;132(18): 1734–42.

25. Watts JA, Zagorski J, Gellar MA, et al. Cardiac inflammation contributes to right ventricular dysfunction following experimental pulmonary embolism in rats. J Mol Cell Cardiol 2006;41(2):296–307.

26. Mani SK, Shiraishi H, Balasubramanian S, et al. In vivo administration of calpeptin attenuates calpain activation and cardiomyocyte loss in pressure-overloaded feline myocardium. Am J Physiol Heart Circ Physiol 2008;295(1):H314–26.

27. Boulate D, Arthur Ataam J, Connolly AJ, et al. Early development of right ventricular ischemic lesions in a novel large animal model of acute right heart failure in chronic thromboembolic pulmonary hypertension. J Card Fail 2017;23(12):876–86.

28. Shah AS, Atkins BZ, Hata JA, et al. Early effects of right ventricular volume overload on ventricular performance and beta-adrenergic signaling. J Thorac Cardiovasc Surg 2000;120(2):342–9.

29. Reddy S, Zhao M, Hu DQ, et al. Physiologic and molecular characterization of a murine model of right ventricular volume overload. Am J Physiol Heart Circ Physiol 2013;304(10):H1314–27.

30. Shults NV, Kanovka SS, Ten Eyck JE, et al. Ultrastructural changes of the right ventricular myocytes in pulmonary arterial hypertension. J Am Heart Assoc 2019;8(5):e011227.

31. Schmuck EG, Hacker TA, Schreier DA, et al. Beneficial effects of mesenchymal stem cell delivery via a novel cardiac bioscaffold on right ventricles of pulmonary arterial hypertensive rats. Am J Physiol Heart Circ Physiol 2019;316(5):H1005–13.

32. da Silva Goncalves Bos D, Van Der Bruggen CEE, Kurakula K, et al. Contribution of impaired parasympathetic activity to right ventricular dysfunction and pulmonary vascular remodeling in pulmonary arterial hypertension. Circulation 2018;137(9):910–24.

33. Urashima T, Zhao M, Wagner R, et al. Molecular and physiological characterization of RV remodeling in a murine model of pulmonary stenosis. Am J Physiol Heart Circ Physiol 2008;295(3):H1351–68.

34. Kang IS, Redington AN, Benson LN, et al. Differential regurgitation in branch pulmonary arteries after repair of tetralogy of Fallot: a phase-contrast cine magnetic resonance study. Circulation 2003; 107(23):2938–43.

35. Nollert G, Fischlein T, Bouterwek S, et al. Long-term survival in patients with repair of tetralogy of Fallot: 36-year follow-up of 490 survivors of the first year after surgical repair. J Am Coll Cardiol 1997;30(5): 1374–83.

36. Miranda-Silva D, Goncalves-Rodrigues P, Almeida-Coelho J, et al. Characterization of biventricular alterations in myocardial (reverse) remodelling in aortic banding-induced chronic pressure overload. Sci Rep 2019;9(1):2956.

37. Ryan JJ, Huston J, Kutty S, et al. Right ventricular adaptation and failure in pulmonary arterial hypertension. Can J Cardiol 2015;31(4):391–406.

38. Zhou X, Ferrara F, Contaldi C, et al. Right ventricular size and function in chronic heart failure: not to be forgotten. Heart Fail Clin 2019;15(2):205–17.

39. Vonk-Noordegraaf A, Haddad F, Chin KM, et al. Right heart adaptation to pulmonary arterial hypertension: physiology and pathobiology. J Am Coll Cardiol 2013;62(25 Suppl):D22–33.

40. Haddad F, Doyle R, Murphy DJ, et al. Right ventricular function in cardiovascular disease, part II: pathophysiology, clinical importance, and management of right ventricular failure. Circulation 2008;117(13): 1717–31.

41. Bhatt AB, Foster E, Kuehl K, et al. Congenital heart disease in the older adult: a scientific statement from the American Heart Association. Circulation 2015;131(21):1884–931.

42. Yerebakan C, Sandica E, Prietz S, et al. Autologous umbilical cord blood mononuclear cell transplantation preserves right ventricular function in a novel model of chronic right ventricular volume overload. Cell Transplant 2009;18(8):855–68.

43. Marino TA, Kent RL, Uboh CE, et al. Structural analysis of pressure versus volume overload hypertrophy of cat right ventricle. Am J Physiol 1985;249(2 Pt 2):H371–9.

44. Rungatscher A, Hallstrom S, Linardi D, et al. S-nitroso human serum albumin attenuates pulmonary hypertension, improves right ventricular-arterial coupling, and reduces oxidative stress in a chronic right ventricle volume overload model. J Heart Lung Transplant 2015;34(3):479–88.

45. Oosterhof T, Tulevski II, Vliegen HW, et al. Effects of volume and/or pressure overload secondary to congenital heart disease (tetralogy of fallot or pulmonary stenosis) on right ventricular function using cardiovascular magnetic resonance and B-type natriuretic peptide levels. Am J Cardiol 2006;97(7):1051–5.

46. Bowen ME, Selzman CH, McKellar SH. Right ventricular involution: big changes in small hearts. J Surg Res 2019;243:255–64.

47. Budas GR, Boehm M, Kojonazarov B, et al. ASK1 inhibition halts disease progression in preclinical models of pulmonary arterial hypertension. Am J Respir Crit Care Med 2018;197(3):373–85.

48. Clapham KR, Singh I, Capuano IS, et al. MEF2 and the right ventricle: from development to disease. Front Cardiovasc Med 2019;6:29.

49. Kojonazarov B, Novoyatleva T, Boehm M, et al. p38 MAPK inhibition improves heart function in pressure-loaded right ventricular hypertrophy. Am J Respir Cell Mol Biol 2017;57(5):603–14.

50. Rain S, Handoko ML, Vonk Noordegraaf A, et al. Pressure-overload-induced right heart failure. Pflugers Arch 2014;466(6):1055–63.

51. Vonk Noordegraaf A, Westerhof BE, Westerhof N. The relationship between the right ventricle and its load in pulmonary hypertension. J Am Coll Cardiol 2017;69(2):236–43.

52. Rain S, Handoko ML, Trip P, et al. Right ventricular diastolic impairment in patients with pulmonary arterial hypertension. Circulation 2013;128(18): 2016–25, 2011–2010.

53. van Wolferen SA, Marcus JT, Boonstra A, et al. Prognostic value of right ventricular mass, volume, and function in idiopathic pulmonary arterial hypertension. Eur Heart J 2007;28(10):1250–7.

54. Voelkel NF, Gomez-Arroyo J, Abbate A, et al. Pathobiology of pulmonary arterial hypertension and right ventricular failure. Eur Respir J 2012;40(6):1555–65.

55. Ikeda S, Satoh K, Kikuchi N, et al. Crucial role of rhokinase in pressure overload-induced right ventricular hypertrophy and dysfunction in mice. Arterioscler Thromb Vasc Biol 2014;34(6):1260–71.

56. Avazmohammadi R, Hill M, Simon M, et al. Transmural remodeling of right ventricular myocardium in response to pulmonary arterial hypertension. APL Bioeng 2017;1(1) [pii:016105].

57. Mikhael M, Makar C, Wissa A, et al. Oxidative stress and its implications in the right ventricular remodeling secondary to pulmonary hypertension. Front Physiol 2019;10:1233.

58. Ryan JJ, Archer SL. The right ventricle in pulmonary arterial hypertension: disorders of metabolism, angiogenesis and adrenergic signaling in right ventricular failure. Circ Res 2014;115(1):176–88.

59. Bogaard HJ, Abe K, Vonk Noordegraaf A, et al. The right ventricle under pressure: cellular and molecular mechanisms of right-heart failure in pulmonary hypertension. Chest 2009;135(3):794–804.

60. Simon MA, Pinsky MR. Right ventricular dysfunction and failure in chronic pressure overload. Cardiol Res Pract 2011;2011:568095.

61. Trac D, Maxwell JT, Brown ME, et al. Aggregation of child cardiac progenitor cells into spheres activates notch signaling and improves treatment of right ventricular heart failure. Circ Res 2019;124(4):526–38.

62. Omura J, Satoh K, Kikuchi N, et al. ADAMTS8 promotes the development of pulmonary arterial hypertension and right ventricular failure: a possible novel therapeutic target. Circ Res 2019;125(10):884–906.

63. Ren X, Johns RA, Gao WD. EXPRESS: right heart in pulmonary hypertension: from adaptation to failure. Pulm Circ 2019. https://doi.org/10.1177/ 2045894019845611. 2045894019845611.

64. Kolb TM, Peabody J, Baddoura P, et al. Right ventricular angiogenesis is an early adaptive response to chronic hypoxia-induced pulmonary hypertension. Microcirculation 2015;22(8):724–36.

65. Agarwal U, Smith AW, French KM, et al. Age-dependent effect of pediatric cardiac progenitor cells after juvenile heart failure. Stem Cells Transl Med 2016; 5(7):883–92.

66. Hassoun PM. The right ventricle in scleroderma (2013 Grover Conference Series). Pulm Circ 2015; 5(1):3–14.

67. Mendes-Ferreira P, Santos-Ribeiro D, Adao R, et al. Distinct right ventricle remodeling in response to

pressure overload in the rat. Am J Physiol Heart Circ Physiol 2016;311(1):H85–95.

68. Rain S, Andersen S, Najafi A, et al. Right ventricular myocardial stiffness in experimental pulmonary arterial hypertension: relative contribution of fibrosis and myofibril stiffness. Circ Heart Fail 2016;9(7) [pii: e002636].

69. Boehm M, Novoyatleva T, Kojonazarov B, et al. Nitric oxide synthase 2 induction promotes right ventricular fibrosis. Am J Respir Cell Mol Biol 2019;60(3): 346–56.

70. Andersen S, Birkmose Axelsen J, Ringgaard S, et al. Pressure overload induced right ventricular remodeling is not attenuated by the anti-fibrotic agent pirfenidone. Pulm Circ 2019;9(2). 2045894019848659.

71. Borgdorff MA, Koop AM, Bloks VW, et al. Clinical symptoms of right ventricular failure in experimental chronic pressure load are associated with progressive diastolic dysfunction. J Mol Cell Cardiol 2015; 79:244–53.

72. Koop AMC, Hagdorn QAJ, Bossers GPL, et al. Right ventricular pressure overload alters cardiac lipid composition. Int J Cardiol 2019;287:96–105.

73. Hemnes AR, Brittain EL, Trammell AW, et al. Evidence for right ventricular lipotoxicity in heritable pulmonary arterial hypertension. Am J Respir Crit Care Med 2014;189(3):325–34.

74. van der Bruggen CE, Happe CM, Dorfmuller P, et al. Bone morphogenetic protein receptor type 2 mutation in pulmonary arterial hypertension: a view on the right ventricle. Circulation 2016;133(18): 1747–60.

75. Adrogue JV, Sharma S, Ngumbela K, et al. Acclimatization to chronic hypobaric hypoxia is associated with a differential transcriptional profile between the right and left ventricle. Mol Cell Biochem 2005; 278(1–2):71–8.

76. Piao L, Sidhu VK, Fang YH, et al. FOXO1-mediated upregulation of pyruvate dehydrogenase kinase-4 (PDK4) decreases glucose oxidation and impairs right ventricular function in pulmonary hypertension: therapeutic benefits of dichloroacetate. J Mol Med (Berl) 2013;91(3):333–46.

77. Sutendra G, Dromparis P, Paulin R, et al. A metabolic remodeling in right ventricular hypertrophy is associated with decreased angiogenesis and a transition from a compensated to a decompensated state in pulmonary hypertension. J Mol Med (Berl) 2013; 91(11):1315–27.

78. Lundgrin EL, Park MM, Sharp J, et al. Fasting 2-deoxy-2-[18F]fluoro-D-glucose positron emission tomography to detect metabolic changes in pulmonary arterial hypertension hearts over 1 year. Ann Am Thorac Soc 2013;10(1):1–9.

79. Emanuel R, Chichra A, Patel N, et al. Neurohormonal modulation as therapeutic avenue for right ventricular dysfunction in pulmonary artery hypertension: till the dawn, waiting. Ann Transl Med 2018;6(15):301.

80. Groeneveldt JA, de Man FS, Westerhof BE. The right treatment for the right ventricle. Curr Opin Pulm Med 2019;25(5):410–7.

81. Zelt JGE, Chaudhary KR, Cadete VJ, et al. Medical therapy for heart failure associated with pulmonary hypertension. Circ Res 2019;124(11):1551–67.

82. Maron BA, Leopold JA. Emerging concepts in the molecular basis of pulmonary arterial hypertension: part II: neurohormonal signaling contributes to the pulmonary vascular and right ventricular pathophenotype of pulmonary arterial hypertension. Circulation 2015;131(23):2079–91.

83. Te Riet L, van Esch JH, Roks AJ, et al. Hypertension: renin-angiotensin-aldosterone system alterations. Circ Res 2015;116(6):960–75.

84. Johnson JA, West J, Maynard KB, et al. ACE2 improves right ventricular function in a pressure overload model. PLoS One 2011;6(6):e20828.

85. Hemnes AR, Rathinasabapathy A, Austin EA, et al. A potential therapeutic role for angiotensin-converting enzyme 2 in human pulmonary arterial hypertension. Eur Respir J 2018;51(6) [pii:1702638].

86. Rouleau JL, Kapuku G, Pelletier S, et al. Cardioprotective effects of ramipril and losartan in right ventricular pressure overload in the rabbit: importance of kinins and influence on angiotensin II type 1 receptor signaling pathway. Circulation 2001;104(8): 939–44.

87. Lahm T, Douglas IS, Archer SL, et al. Assessment of right ventricular function in the research setting: knowledge gaps and pathways forward. an official American Thoracic Society Research Statement. Am J Respir Crit Care Med 2018;198(4):e15–43.

Right Heart Failure
A Hemodynamic Review

Milad C. El Hajj, MD[a], Michael C. Viray, MD[b], Ryan J. Tedford, MD[b],*

KEYWORDS

- Right ventricle • Right ventricular function • Right ventricular afterload • Right ventricular reserve
- Hemodynamics • Pressure-volume relationships • Multibeat • Single beat

KEY POINTS

- The anatomy of the right ventricle and its physiologic response to changes in load are important determinants of contractility and overall function.
- Direct measurement of intracardiac pressures with right heart catheterization is the most common method of determining right ventricular (RV) preload and afterload, two determinants of RV function.
- The gold standard for assessment of RV function requires pressure-volume relations.
- Simplified methods to calculate right ventricle–pulmonary artery coupling have been proposed but require further validation.

INTRODUCTION

The symptomatic and prognostic relevance of the right ventricle in a myriad of conditions, including pulmonary arterial hypertension (PAH), left heart failure, and after implantation of left ventricular assist devices (LVADs), has renewed interest in the right ventricle as more than a mere conduit for transmitting blood to the lungs. Accordingly, there has been growing interest in proper and accurate assessment of right ventricular (RV) function. Because right heart failure is typically a consequence of increased afterload, a careful study of functional interactions between the right ventricle and pulmonary vascular system is warranted. Traditional hemodynamics by right heart catheterization (RHC) is routinely used to draw inferences on RV function, preload, and afterload. However, more robust methods for characterizing function, load, ventricular-vascular coupling, and diastole are available and can more accurately interpret hemodynamics in patients with RV failure. This article reviews traditional and gold-standard hemodynamic assessments of the right ventricle in health and disease.

TRADITIONAL HEMODYNAMICS

Direct measurement of intracardiac pressures during RHC remains the most common method of determining RV preload and afterload, two determinants of RV function.[1] A comprehensive hemodynamic assessment comprises routinely measuring right atrial pressure (RAP), pulmonary artery (PA) pressures, PA wedge pressure (PAWP), and cardiac output (CO). From these measurements, parameters such as PA pulsatility index (PAPi), RV stroke volume (SV), and RV stroke work index (RVSWI) are calculated.

The accuracy of pressure measurements may be affected by several external factors, including zeroing and proper leveling of the transducer. To ensure accuracy of hemodynamic measurements, pressure lines must be properly flushed and equipment properly calibrated. With the patient lying supine, the pressure transducer should be set to zero

a Department of Medicine, Internal Medicine, Medical University of South Carolina, 96 Jonathan Lucas Street, Suite 807, Charleston, SC 29425-8900, USA; b Department of Medicine, Division of Cardiology, Medical University of South Carolina, 30 Courtenay Drive, MSC592/BM215, Charleston, SC 29425-6230, USA
* Corresponding author.
E-mail address: tedfordr@musc.edu
Twitter: @MiladElHajjMD (M.C.E.H.); @MichaelCViray1 (M.C.V.); @RyanTedfordMD (R.J.T.)

Cardiol Clin 38 (2020) 161–173
https://doi.org/10.1016/j.ccl.2020.01.001

level at the midchest at the level of the left atrium (halfway between the anterior sternum and table surface).[2,3]

RAP is a surrogate of central venous pressure but is also affected by right atrial compliance, tricuspid valve function, and RV compliance. In patients with advanced heart failure, an increased RAP is associated with an increased all-cause mortality.[4] Also, in the subset of patients who are deemed eligible for mechanical circulatory support (LVAD), a high preoperative RAP and RAP/PAWP is associated with an increased risk of postoperative RV failure.[5,6] In addition, coupling the ratio of systolic PA pressure (PAP) to SV (ie, PA elastance), a marker of total RV afterload, with RAP may help identify patients at risk for severe right heart failure post-LVAD.[7]

A paradoxic inspiratory increase in RAP (Kussmaul sign) can also be observed during RHC. It is attributed to an increase in venous return into a noncompliant or constricted right ventricle and is a marker of intrinsic RV dysfunction and adverse right heart–pulmonary vascular interaction.[8] Kussmaul physiology is common in patients with advanced heart failure and, in the subset of patients referred for heart transplant, is associated with worse prognosis.[9]

PAWP is obtained by inflating the PA catheter balloon until it obstructs blood flow in the distal PA and is an estimate of LA pressure in the absence of mitral stenosis. It is measured at end-diastole as the mean of the a wave in patients in sinus rhythm and 130 to 160 milliseconds after the onset of QRS and before the v wave in patients in atrial fibrillation. Current guidelines recommend obtaining a PAWP saturation when the PAWP is increased (PAWP>15 mm Hg) or when the accuracy of PAWP is in question. The PAWP saturation should be greater than or equal to 90% or within 5% of the systemic oxygen saturation.[3,10] Although PAWP is a measure of left-sided filling pressures, it is helpful in differentiating the cause of RV failure (cardiomyopathic, pressure-overloaded vs volume-overloaded RV).

Under normal conditions, the CO of the RV in adults closely approximates the CO of the left ventricle, albeit with less myocardial work.[11] Therefore, the CO measured during RHC indirectly reflects RV function in the absence of significant valvular regurgitation. The Fick principle, based on conservation of mass, assumes that oxygen uptake in the lungs is entirely transferred in the blood and therefore CO can be calculated knowing oxygen consumption, the difference in oxygen content between arterial and venous blood, and the hemoglobin concentration of blood:

$$\text{Cardiac output (CO)} = \frac{\text{Oxygen Consumption (VO}_2)}{(\text{Arterial} - \text{Venous})\text{O2} \times \text{Hgb conc} \times 1.36 \times 10}$$

Because it requires measurement of the individual's oxygen consumption (V_{O_2}), the direct Fick method is rarely used in clinical practice. Therefore, current methods of assessing CO by invasive hemodynamics include the estimated Fick method and the thermodilution (TD) method. The major drawback of the estimated Fick method is its reliance on V_{O_2} estimation. Narang and colleagues[12] showed that estimation of resting V_{O_2} by all 3 commonly used formula are inaccurate, especially in obese individuals with body mass index greater than or equal to 40 kg/m^2.[12]

The TD method is based on the principle of conservation of energy and involves the injection of an indicator (saline is most commonly used) into the proximal port of a fluid-filled catheter and then measuring the temperature of blood in the PA beyond the pulmonary valve. The transient decrease in the temperature of blood as it travels from the right atrium to the PA produces a distinct TD curve that is generated by plotting the temperature of the PA versus time. A computer-generated CO is calculated based on the area under the TD curve.[13] Although there traditionally has been concern about inaccuracies of TD in the setting of low CO or tricuspid regurgitation (TR), more recent studies show that the overall agreement between CO measured by TD and direct Fick is not diminished in low-CO states and not affected by the severity of TR.[14,15] In a large national cohort and a second validation cohort of patients, there was a modest correlation between TD and estimated Fick measured COs ($r = 0.65$). In addition, CO estimates measured by TD were superior to estimated Fick for predicting all-cause mortality.[16] Considering these recent studies, guidelines recommend using TD CO in the absence of direct Fick measurement unless an intracardiac shunt is present.

Hemodynamic measures of RV afterload, which include pulmonary vascular resistance (PVR), compliance, and pulmonary effective arterial elastance (Ea), can also be calculated from RHC data and these are discussed in more detail later. Although load significantly affects RV function, it is important to remember that these parameters are not markers of RV function. RV SV can be calculated by dividing the CO by heart rate. Although clinically relevant, the marked load dependence of the RV precludes the ability of SV to define intrinsic RV contractility. RVSWI is a derived hemodynamic parameter calculated using the formula, RVSWI = 0.0136 × SV index × (mean PAP – RAP). It represents the effective work of the RV during a cardiac cycle. Some studies have shown that a low RVSWI is a predictor of RV failure after LVAD implantation.[17] However, much like SV, RVSWI is also load dependent.

PA pulsatility index (PAPi) is another hemodynamic metric calculated by dividing PA pulsatility (systolic PAP – diastolic PAP) by the RAP. Some small studies have shown PAPi to have prognostic ability in advanced heart failure[18] as well as postoperative RV dysfunction after LVAD implantation.[19,20] Despite its promise, the PAPi has several limitations that should be considered. First, pulmonary pulse pressure is affected not only by SV but also by compliance of the pulmonary circulation. As such, it is highly dependent on left atrial pressure. In addition, because RAP is in the denominator of the PAPi equation, very small changes in RAP can result in large changes in PAPi. The prognostic relevance of PAPi, particularly to predict RV failure after LVAD implantation, has been questioned in larger cohort studies.[7,21]

RIGHT VENTRICULAR SYSTOLIC FUNCTION

Just as in the left ventricle, RV function is determined by preload (venous return), afterload (imposed from the pulmonary circulation), and contractility. It is traditionally assessed via noninvasive imaging, most commonly by echocardiography. Tricuspid annular plane systolic excursion (TAPSE) and RV fractional area change (FAC) are easily obtainable by two-dimensional (2D) echocardiography and have both been shown to predict mortality in PAH[22] and left heart disease.[23] The triangular shape of the RV limits the use of simple geometric models and 2D echocardiography to derive reproducible volumetric data. Quantification of RV ejection fraction (RVEF) by cardiac MRI has accordingly emerged as the reference standard for RV function and volume because of its fidelity and reproducibility. More recently, real-time 3D echocardiography is being increasingly used to quantitate RV function and has been validated against cardiac MRI–derived volumetry.[24] However, just like SV, RVEF, FAC, and TAPSE are all afterload dependent, even in the chronic setting,[25] and are therefore not true measures of contractility (defined as the intrinsic ability of the ventricular myocardium to stiffen). The gold standard for assessing contractility independent of load is through the simultaneous assessment of pressure and volume, allowing for construction of the pressure-volume (PV) loop.

The use of PV relationships to determine global ventricular function was first shown in the left ventricle by Suga and colleagues,[26] who found that the ventricle stiffens (and relaxes) along a predictable time course throughout the cardiac cycle, suggesting that cardiac contraction could be modeled as a time-varying volume elastance. By generating multiple PV loops during variably loaded cardiac contractions (multibeat method), a straight line could be drawn to connect PV points synchronized in time. This technique became known as the isochrone method, in which the isochrone, or slope of each regression line, was the time-varying elastance, or E(t). These isochrones intersected the volume axis at a similar point (Vo), such that

$$E(t) = P(t)/[V(t) - Vo(t)]$$

where *E(t)* is the slope, *Vo(t)* is the volume intercept of the regression line at time t; *P* is the instantaneous intraventricular pressure, and *V* is the instantaneous intraventricular volume.

The maximal value of the time-varying elastance (Emax), or the maximal ratio of ventricular pressure to volume during the cardiac cycle (maximal P/[V-Vo]), was the isochrone with the highest slope. Suga and colleagues[26,27] found that Emax varied with changes in contractility by norepinephrine and isoproterenol challenge but remained constant with changes in preload, afterload, and heart rate. However, the time to reach end-systole for each individual loop was later found to vary by load,[28] prompting investigators to replace the isochrone technique with a method that would determine the maximal ratio of pressure and volume by connecting end-systolic beats regardless of timing.[29] Thus, the end-systolic pressure (ESP)–volume relationship (ESPVR) was derived, its slope being the end-systolic elastance (Ees; **Fig. 1**A).[27]

The first RV PV loop was performed in an isolated canine heart by Maughan and Weisfeldt,[30] and was later reproduced in normal human subjects.[31] The RV PV loop is triangular because of the absence of isovolumic periods of contraction and relaxation, reflecting the low impedance of the normal pulmonary vascular circuit. In keeping with the shape of the RV PV loop, a lesser change in ESP generates a greater change in end-systolic volume (ESV), making the right ventricle more sensitive to afterload than the LV.[32,33] As the afterload increases, as seen in pulmonary hypertension (PH), RV pressure no longer declines throughout ejection,[34] and the shape of the RV loop changes, becoming more rectangular in mild PH, resembling the LV loop, and eventually becoming trapezoidal in severe PH (**Fig. 2**).[35–37]

Unlike the LV, RV end-ejection (under normal pressure conditions) continues well after the onset

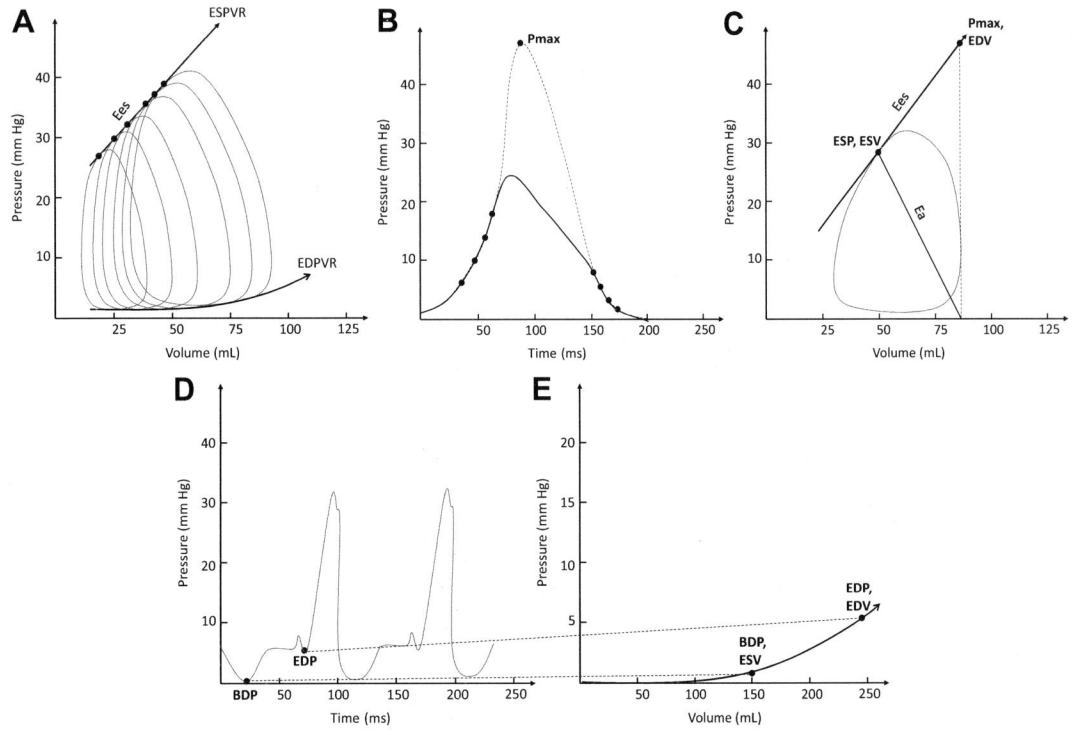

Fig. 1. Single-beat and multibeat estimates of ESPVR and end-diastolic PV relationships (EDPVR). (*A*) PV loops during preload reduction. ESPVR is derived by connecting end-systolic points, its slope is the Ees. EDPVR, which is curvilinear, is defined by fitting end-diastolic points. (*B, C*) Single-beat estimation of ESPVR using Brimioulle and colleagues'[40] method. Peak isovolumic pressure (Pmax) was extrapolated by fitting a sine curve to the isovolumetric portions of the RV pressure tracing. (*C*) A straight line is used to connect Pmax to the RV PV diagram to form the ESPVR line, its slope is Ees. A line connecting the end-systolic point to end-diastole is also drawn, its slope Ea. (*D, E*) Single-beat estimation of EDPVR. (*D*) End-diastolic volume (EDV) is combined with end-diastolic pressure (EDP), and end-systolic volume (ESV) is combined with beginning-diastolic pressure (BDP). (*E*) Fitting of a nonlinear exponential curve through the derived points using the formula $P = \alpha(e^{V\beta} - 1)$.

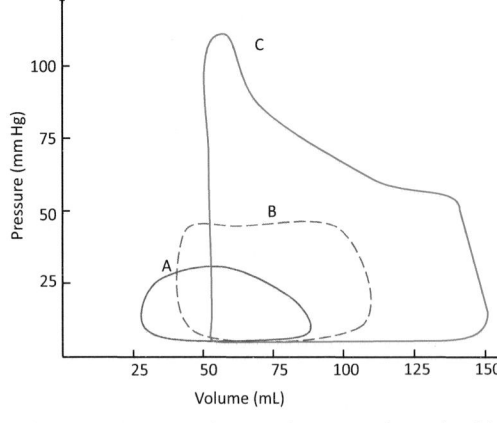

Fig. 2. Sample RV PV loops. The RV PV loop (A; *blue line*) is normally triangular but takes on a more rectangular shape with mild PH, similar to the tradition LV loop (B; *dotted blue line*). With development of more severe PH, pressure increases throughout ejection and the loop takes on a more trapezoidal shape (C; *red line*).

of RV peak pressure,[30] and thus Emax no longer occurs at end-ejection. Nonetheless, Dell'italia and Walsh[38] found that the RV Ees is generally an acceptable approximation for maximum elastance (Emax), even in normal right ventricles.[38,39] Ees is the current reference measure of the global contractile force of the RV myocardium,[40] which has the capacity to increase contractility up to 5-fold in patients with PAH.[41] Ees has been successfully measured in human right ventricles using the multibeat method.[36,42–45] Most recently, this methodology has been shown to predict time to clinical worsening in PAH,[45,46] even in patients with preserved RVEF.

In efforts to simplify the approach and requirement for load alteration, single-beat methods to estimate Ees have been developed to measure Ees in the left ventricle[47–49] and were then reproduced in the right ventricle.[40] Brimioulle and colleagues'[40] method relies on extrapolating a peak isovolumic pressure (Pmax) by fitting a sine curve to the isovolumetric portions of the RV pressure tracing (**Fig. 1B**). This PV point (Pmax, end-diastolic volume [EDV]) is connected to the end-systolic PV point (ESP, ESV) to derive ESPVR and determine Ees and Vo (**Fig. 1C**), such that

$$Ees = (Pmax - ESP)/SV$$

Thus far, this single-beat approach has not been successful in predicting prognosis in PH[50,51] and there are conflicting data on correlation between single-beat and multibeat approaches in humans.[45,46,52] What is clear is that the selection of points during the isovolumetric periods is critical and can yield vastly different Pmax values, perhaps limiting the reproducibility and clinical applicability of this approach. Bellofiore and colleagues[53] have developed new methodology based on the second derivative of the isovolumetric periods, which may lead to improved fidelity. However, the prognostic value of this method has not been tested.

Other measurements of systolic chamber function have been developed but are principally limited to research because of their complexity. The relationship between stroke work and preload, termed preload recruitable stroke work (PRSW),[54] is an index of contractility thought to be even more load insensitive than Ees.[55] A single-beat version of PRSW has also been developed.[52] The maximal rate of pressure increase during isovolumic contraction (dP/dtmax) to EDV relationship[56] has fallen out of favor because of its preload and heart rate dependence.

Technical Considerations

In order to simultaneously measure pressure and volume, a conductance catheter is used. The catheter contains several ring-shaped electrodes along its length, and the tip of the catheter is positioned in the RV apex. By continuously measuring electrical conductivity between the proximal and distal electrodes of the catheter, changes in volume can be derived. Despite the trabeculated nature of the RV, this technique seems to measure volumes accurately, even in situations of an absent tricuspid value.[57] The catheter is volume calibrated with cardiac MRI or hypertonic saline. Preload alteration is performed by partial balloon occlusion of the inferior vena cava (IVC),[43] manual external compression of the IVC,[42] or Valsalva maneuver.[36,58]

RIGHT VENTRICULAR AFTERLOAD

The right ventricle must overcome the afterload imposed on it by the pulmonary circulation in order to eject blood. RV afterload can be described as maximum wall tension, which is directly proportional to intracavitary pressure and internal ventricular diameter and inversely proportional to ventricular wall thickness as determined by Laplace's law for spheres. Given the nonspherical shape of the RV, regional wall stress may vary widely.[59] Furthermore, the ventricular diameter at end-systole is minimal and RV wall thickness is relatively constant. RV afterload can therefore be estimated as RV wall stress during systolic ejection and can be estimated by the summation of the resistive and pulsatile components of blood flow,[60] which include (1) mean resistance (mean pulmonary resistance, proximal stiffness of pulmonary conduit arteries), (2) compliance (blood storage capacity of the vascular system), (3) reflected waves (pulsatility of blood flow), and (4) inertness of blood.

PA input impedance, as described by Milnor and colleagues,[61] is the most comprehensive method to assess RV vascular load. However, pulmonary impedance is difficult to both measure and interpret because it requires Fourier transformation of simultaneous measures of pressure and flow and is reported in the frequency domain rather than the time domain. Therefore, a more practical mode, based on electric circuits, was developed. This 3-element Windkessel model accounts for resistance, compliance, and characteristic impedance (ratio of blood mass inertia to the proximal vessel compliance).[62] Clinically, the most widely used parameters to describe resistive (steady) and pulsatile load of the pulmonary circulation are PVR and pulmonary arterial compliance (PAC).

PVR represents resistive load in the Windkessel model and depends on the diameter of distal arteries and arterioles. In most circumstances, PVR accounts for about 75% of total RV afterload.[63] PVR can be calculated from RHC data using the following equation:

$$PVR = (mPAP - PAWP)/CO$$

where *mPAP* is mean PAP. PAC is a measure of arterial distensibility and accounts for pulsatile load, which is the capacity of all arteries and arterioles to accumulate blood in systole and release it in diastole. Several methods have been proposed to measure PAC. The pulse pressure method uses a 2-element Windkessel model (flow and resistance as inputs) to estimate the compliance value that best predicts systolic and diastolic pressures.[64] However, the simplest method to estimate PAC is the ratio of SV to PA pulse pressure, and correlates reasonably well with the 2-element Windkessel model.[65] Pulsatile load accounts for approximately 25% of the total RV afterload in absence of left heart failure.[66]

The relationship between resistive and pulsatile load is represented by the product of PVR and PAC, the diastolic decay constant of PAP (resistance-compliance time). The normal pulmonary circulation is a low-pressure and high-compliance system. In patients with suspected or confirmed PH and normal PAWP, resistance and compliance in the pulmonary circulation show an inverse hyperbolic relationship,[67,68] and the RC time is relatively constant. The constant RC implies that the proximal vasculature contributes little to the overall compliance in the pulmonary circulation because the smaller distal vessels account for both resistance and compliance. A notable exception to this relationship occurs when left atrial pressures are increased, with the RC time declining with higher PAWP.[67] Thus, as PAWP increases, net RV afterload increases by increasing pulsatile relative to resistive load.[67] It is therefore not surprising that PAC has been shown to be a superior prognostic marker to PVR in patients with left heart failure.[69–71]

In addition, Ea, first described by Sunagawa and colleagues[62] in 1983, is a lumped parameter that accounts for all components of load on the heart, including mean resistance, compliance, characteristic impedance, and systolic and diastolic time intervals, such that

$$E_a = R_T / \left[t_s + \tau \left(1 - e^{-t_d/\tau}\right)\right]$$

where R_T is the total mean resistance, t_s and t_d are the systolic and diastolic time periods respectively, and τ is the diastolic pressure decay time constant.[62] Ea, like Ees, is measured in units of elastance. Ea can be more easily derived from steady-state PV loops as ESP divided by SV,[72] which approximated Ea Windkessel in pig models.[73,74] In PH, ESP is best approximated by systolic PAP (sPAP),[50,75] and, in normotensive subjects, mPAP better approximates ESP.[76,77] This metric has been shown to have superior prognostic value compared with precapillary parameters such as PVR in the setting of left heart disease.[78,79]

RIGHT VENTRICULAR–PULMONARY ARTERY COUPLING

Ees and Ea are matched in the healthy human right ventricle to provide optimal mechanical efficiency in the transfer of blood to the pulmonary circulation. This hemodynamic assessment of the cardiopulmonary unit is known as RV–pulmonary arterial (PA) coupling and represents the adequacy of homeometric adaptation to overcome the afterload it must eject against. RV-PA coupling is considered the gold standard to assess ventricular

function, and, perhaps most importantly, can be useful to detect RV dysfunction well before overt decline in RVEF.[36,50] Optimal coupling takes place when there is maximal transference of potential energy from the ventricle to the circulation.[80] The optimal Ees/Ea ratio for ejection in the normal right ventricle is 1.5 to 2.[36,81] In PH, the Ees/Ea ratio decreases[36,37,42]; acute increases in afterload lead to out-of-proportion increase in Ea compared with Ees, and subsequent loss of RV-PA coupling (a ratio between 0.7 and 1.0).[81,82] This uncoupling phenomenon indicates decreased mechanical efficiency and increased oxygen consumption in order to maintain adequate RV output. Despite its proven utility in basic and clinical research, assessment of RV-PA coupling through multibeat PV assessment is not routine clinical practice given its complexity.

RIGHT VENTRICULAR COUPLING AND RIGHT VENTRICULAR RESERVE

RV contractile reserve, or the capacity of the ventricle to increase contractility at a given level of loading, is determined using exercise or pharmacologic stress tests (typically an infusion of dobutamine).[83] Emerging data suggest that RV reserve is associated with resting RV-PA coupling and thus may present a less invasive surrogate of the gold standard. Guihaire and colleagues[84] found that the degree of RV contractile reserve impairment during dobutamine infusion correlated with RV-PA uncoupling at rest in a pig model of PAH. More recently, Hsu and colleagues[42] showed that, compared with patients with idiopathic PAH, patients with systemic sclerosis–associated PAH could not augment contractility during submaximal exercise (blunted homeometric adaptation) and subsequently witnessed substantial increases in RV EDV (heterometric adaptation). Although SV was preserved, RVEF decreased because of progressive dilatation, suggesting RV dilatation and RVEF with stress may be used as a surrogate for RV-PA coupling.

RV reserve has been shown to have both diagnostic and prognostic value in several conditions (**Table 1**). It may be particularly useful to detect so-called hidden RV failure. Sharma and colleagues[85] found evidence of reduced RV reserve in subjects with PAH, even when resting RV function seemed normal. In a cohort of subjects with left heart failure and reduced ejection fraction, Guazzi and colleagues[86] found that impaired RV reserve more closely associated with functional capacity compared with resting measures. Similar findings have been observed in heart failure with preserved ejection fraction;.[87,88] In addition,

Table 1
Studies assessing right ventricular reserve

Author	Study Type	Population	Diagnostic Modality	Parameters Used to Assess RV Reserve	Findings
Gorcsan et al,[101] 1996	Single-center prospective cohort	HFrEF (n = 13)	High-fidelity pressure with dobutamine	Δ Ees and Emax	Prognostic
Deswarte et al,[92] 2010	Dual-center prospective cohort	LVAD candidates (n = 14)	DSE	Δ PASP and TAPSE	Prognostic
Grünig et al,[90] 2013	Multicenter, multinational prospective cohort	PAH or inoperable CTEPH (n = 124)	ESE	Δ PASP	Prognostic
Blumberg et al,[102] 2013	Single-center prospective cohort	PAH or inoperable CTEPH (n = 36)	RHC	Peak CI	Diagnostic and prognostic
Sharma et al,[85] 2015	Single-center prospective cohort	PAH (n = 17) Age-matched controls (n = 18)	DSE	Δ TAPSE and s'	Diagnostic
Guihaire et al,[84] 2015	Animal study (piglets)	Surgical PH (n = 13) Sham (n = 6)	P-V loops with dobutamine	Δ RV SVI	Diagnostic
Claessen et al,[103] 2015	Single-center prospective cohort	CTEPH (n = 15) Post-PEA resting mPAP $\le$ 25 mm Hg (n = 7) Controls (n = 15)	Exercise CMR	peak exercise RV EF	Diagnostic
Matsumoto et al,[89] 2015	Single-center prospective cohort	DCM (n = 104)	Speckle-tracking strain DSE	Δ RV free wall GLS	Prognostic
Spruijt et al,[104] 2015	Single-center prospective cohort	PH (n = 16) Control (n = 7)	iCPET	Δ Ees/Ea	Prognostic
Guazzi et al,[86] 2016	Single-center prospective cohort	HFrEF (n = 97) stratified by varying rest and peak exercise TAPSE	ESE	TAPSE/PASP	Diagnostic
Hsu et al,[42] 2016	Single-center prospective cohort	IPAH (n = 9) SSc-PAH (n = 15)	Exercise or atrial-paced CMR, P-V catheterization	Δ Ees/Ea and Δ RV EDV	Diagnostic
Borlaug et al,[87] 2016	Single-center prospective cohort	HFpEF (n = 50) Controls (n = 24)	ESE and iCPET	Δ Biventricular mechanics (s' and e')	Diagnostic

(continued on next page)

Table 1
(continued)

Author	Study Type	Population	Diagnostic Modality	Parameters Used to Assess RV Reserve	Findings
D'Alto et al,[105] 2017	Single-center prospective cohort	Healthy subjects (n = 90)	ESE	Δ TAPSE, s', TAPSE/PASP, SV, and PASP	Diagnostic
D'Andrea et al,[106] 2017	Single-center prospective cohort	HCM (n = 45) Age-matched and sex-matched controls (n = 45)	Speckle-tracking strain ESE	Δ TAPSE, RV Sm peak velocity, RV ESP area, and regional and GLS	Diagnostic
DeFaria Yeh et al,[91] 2018	Single-center retrospective cohort	ACHD (n = 147)	FPRV	RV EF at peak exercise, Δ RV EF	Diagnostic and prognostic
Obokata et al,[88] 2019	Single-center prospective cohort	HFpEF (n = 38) Controls (n = 20)	iCPET	Δ RV mechanics (s' and e')	Diagnostic
Claeys et al,[107] 2019	Single-center prospective cohort	CTEPH (n = 25) CTED (n = 14) Controls (n-13)	Exercise CMR, iCPET	Exercise mPAP/ESV and Δ RVEF	Diagnostic

Abbreviations: ACHD, adults with congenital heart disease; CI, cardiac index; CMR, cardiac MRI; CTED, chronic thromboembolic disease; CTEPH, chronic thromboembolic PH; DCM, dilated cardiomyopathy; DSE, dobutamine stress echocardiography; e', tricuspid annular diastolic velocity; EF, ejection fraction; ESE, exercise stress echo; FPRV, first-pass radionuclide ventriculography; GLS, global longitudinal strain; HCM, hypertrophic cardiomyopathy; HFpEF, heart failure with preserved ejection fraction; HFrEF, heart failure with reduced ejection fraction; iCPET, invasive cardiopulmonary exercise stress testing; IPAH, idiopathic pulmonary arterial hypertension; PAC, pulmonary arterial compliance; PASP, PA systolic pressure; PEA, pulmonary endarterectomy; s', tricuspid annular systolic velocity; Sm, systolic mitral; SSc, systemic sclerosis; SVI, SV index.

multiple recent studies have highlighted the prognostic value of RV reserve, including left heart failure with preserved[87,88] and reduced EF,[89] PAH,[90] and congenital heart disease.[91] Using RV reserve to risk stratify patients before implantation of ventricular assist devices has also been investigated.[92]

RIGHT VENTRICULAR DIASTOLIC FUNCTION

RV diastolic function is an area of renewed interest in PH and heart failure. In response to pressure overload, changes in RV diastolic function may precede changes in contractility.[93,94] The end-diastolic PV relationship (EDPVR) is the gold-standard assessment of RV stiffness and has been described using multibeat and single-beat assessments. The EDPVR reflects the net effect of all facets of myocardial material properties, chamber structural properties, and extracellular matrix.[95] During load alternation, end-diastolic pressure and volume points are determined for each loop. EDPVR is intrinsically nonlinear, such that the slope is shallower at low ventricular volumes and steep at higher volume ranges (**Fig. 1**D). The dependence of diastolic stiffness on volume is thought to be caused by matrix biomechanics; at higher volumes, slack lengths of collagen fibers and titin molecules are exceeded, thus more strongly resisting stretch.[96] A variety of curve fits have been applied to EDPVR[95] in the left ventricle; however, accurate fitting can be difficult. RV diastolic stiffness derived by both single-beat and multibeat methods closely correlated in an open-chest rat model of PAH ($r^2 = 0.94$).[97] Rain and colleagues[97] constructed a single-beat PV loop in patients with PAH by using 3 points: (beginning-diastolic pressure, ESV), (end-diastolic pressure, EDV), and (0,0). RV diastolic stiffness was estimated using an exponential fit, such that

$$P = \alpha\,(e^{V\beta} - 1)$$

where α is a curve fitting constant, β is a diastolic stiffness constant, and V is volume (**Fig. 1**E). This method has been adopted by other investigators to describe RV diastolic stiffness,[50,98,99] but it has not been compared with the multibeat methodology. Rain and colleagues[97] have shown that RV diastolic stiffness is significantly increased in PAH and associated with disease severity. The same group suggested that assessing the relationship between diastolic stiffness and RV wall thickness may help identify patients at higher risk of maladaptive remodeling and death.[98] Diastolic dysfunction in PAH seems more myofibril mediated rather than being related to fibrosis.[100] More studies are needed in order to further elucidate

the role of RV diastolic stiffness and potentially identify therapeutic targets.

SUMMARY

The right ventricle plays an important role in prognosis in a myriad of cardiovascular syndromes. The physiologic response of the right ventricle to load is an important determinant of contractility and function. Understanding of RV function remains incomplete and more research is needed for accurate and early detection of RV failure. The gold standard for assessment of RV function is multibeat PV analysis, although its clinical application is limited because of technical difficulty and invasiveness. Simplified methods to estimate ventricular-arterial coupling have been proposed but require further validation with multibeat assessments and clinical end points. Among those, assessment of RV reserve seems most promising.

DISCLOSURE

M.C. El Hajj has no conflicts of interest to disclose. M. Viray has no conflicts of interest to disclose. R.J. Tedford serves as a consultant to Merck, Actelion, Arena Pharmaceuticals, Abiomed, Medtronic and United Therapeutics.

REFERENCES

1. Sayer GT, Semigran MJ. Right ventricular performance in chronic congestive heart failure. Cardiol Clin 2012;30(2):271–82.
2. Rosenkranz S, Preston IR. Right heart catheterisation: best practice and pitfalls in pulmonary hypertension. Eur Respir Rev 2015;24(138):642–52.
3. Vachiery JL, Tedford RJ, Rosenkranz S, et al. Pulmonary hypertension due to left heart disease. Eur Respir J 2019;53(1). https://doi.org/10.1183/13993003.01897-2018.
4. Damman K, van Deursen VM, Navis G, et al. Increased central venous pressure is associated with impaired renal function and mortality in a broad spectrum of patients with cardiovascular disease. J Am Coll Cardiol 2009;53(7):582–8.
5. Dandel M, Potapov E, Krabatsch T, et al. Load dependency of right ventricular performance is a major factor to be considered in decision making before ventricular assist device implantation. Circulation 2013;128(11 Suppl 1):S14–23.
6. Lampert BC, Teuteberg JJ. Right ventricular failure after left ventricular assist devices. J Heart Lung Transplant 2015;34(9):1123–30.
7. Muslem R, Ong CS, Tomashitis B, et al. Pulmonary arterial elastance and INTERMACS-defined right heart failure following left ventricular assist device. Circ Heart Fail 2019;12(8):e005923.

8. Meyer TE, Sareli P, Marcus RH, et al. Mechanism underlying Kussmaul's sign in chronic constrictive pericarditis. Am J Cardiol 1989;64(16):1069–72.

9. Nadir AM, Beadle R, Lim HS. Kussmaul physiology in patients with heart failure. Circ Heart Fail 2014; 7(3):440–7.

10. Ramu B, Houston BA, Tedford RJ. Pulmonary vascular disease: hemodynamic assessment and treatment selection-focus on group II pulmonary hypertension. Curr Heart Fail Rep 2018;15(2): 81–93.

11. Sheehan F, Redington A. The right ventricle: anatomy, physiology and clinical imaging. Heart 2008; 94(11):1510–5.

12. Narang N, Thibodeau JT, Levine BD, et al. Inaccuracy of estimated resting oxygen uptake in the clinical setting. Circulation 2014;129(2):203–10.

13. Fegler G. Measurement of cardiac output in anaesthetized animals by a thermodilution method. Q J Exp Physiol Cogn Med Sci 1954;39(3):153–64.

14. Hoeper MM, Maier R, Tongers J, et al. Determination of cardiac output by the Fick method, thermodilution, and acetylene rebreathing in pulmonary hypertension. Am J Respir Crit Care Med 1999; 160(2):535–41.

15. Khirfan G, Ahmed MK, Almaaitah S, et al. Comparison of different methods to estimate cardiac index in pulmonary arterial hypertension. Circulation 2019;140(8):705–7.

16. Opotowsky AR, Hess E, Maron BA, et al. Thermodilution vs estimated Fick cardiac output measurement in clinical practice: an analysis of mortality from the veterans affairs clinical assessment, reporting, and tracking (VA CART) program and Vanderbilt University. JAMA Cardiol 2017;2(10): 1090–9.

17. Bellavia D, Iacovoni A, Scardulla C, et al. Prediction of right ventricular failure after ventricular assist device implant: systematic review and meta-analysis of observational studies. Eur J Heart Fail 2017; 19(7):926–46.

18. Kochav SM, Flores RJ, Truby LK, et al. Prognostic impact of pulmonary artery pulsatility index (PAPi) in patients with advanced heart failure: insights from the ESCAPE trial. J Card Fail 2018;24(7): 453–9.

19. Morine KJ, Kiernan MS, Pham DT, et al. Pulmonary artery pulsatility index is associated with right ventricular failure after left ventricular assist device surgery. J Card Fail 2016;22(2):110–6.

20. Kang G, Ha R, Banerjee D. Pulmonary artery pulsatility index predicts right ventricular failure after left ventricular assist device implantation. J Heart Lung Transplant 2016;35(1):67–73.

21. Soliman OII, Akin S, Muslem R, et al. Derivation and validation of a novel right-sided heart failure model after implantation of continuous flow left ventricular assist devices: the EUROMACS (European Registry for patients with mechanical circulatory support) right-sided heart failure risk score. Circulation 2018;137(9):891–906.

22. Grapsa J, Pereira Nunes MC, Tan TC, et al. Echocardiographic and hemodynamic predictors of survival in precapillary pulmonary hypertension: seven-year follow-up. Circ Cardiovasc Imaging 2015;8(6). https://doi.org/10.1161/CIRCIMAGING. 114.002107.

23. Damy T, Kallvikbacka-Bennett A, Goode K, et al. Prevalence of, associations with, and prognostic value of tricuspid annular plane systolic excursion (TAPSE) among out-patients referred for the evaluation of heart failure. J Card Fail 2012;18(3): 216–25.

24. Maffessanti F, Mirea O, Tamborini G, et al. Three-dimensional echocardiography of the mitral valve: lessons learned. Curr Cardiol Rep 2013;15(7):377.

25. Newman JH, Brittain EL, Robbins IM, et al. Effect of acute arteriolar vasodilation on capacitance and resistance in pulmonary arterial hypertension. Chest 2015;147(4):1080–5.

26. Suga H, Sagawa K, Shoukas AA. Load independence of the instantaneous pressure-volume ratio of the canine left ventricle and effects of epinephrine and heart rate on the ratio. Circ Res 1973; 32(3):314–22.

27. Suga H, Sagawa K. Instantaneous pressure-volume relationships and their ratio in the excised, supported canine left ventricle. Circ Res 1974; 35(1):117–26.

28. Kass DA, Maughan WL. From 'Emax' to pressure-volume relations: a broader view. Circulation 1988;77(6):1203–12.

29. Kono A, Maughan WL, Sunagawa K, et al. The use of left ventricular end-ejection pressure and peak pressure in the estimation of the end-systolic pressure-volume relationship. Circulation 1984;70(6): 1057–65.

30. Maughan WL, Shoukas AA, Sagawa K, et al. Instantaneous pressure-volume relationship of the canine right ventricle. Circ Res 1979;44(3):309–15.

31. Redington AN, Gray HH, Hodson ME, et al. Characterisation of the normal right ventricular pressure-volume relation by biplane angiography and simultaneous micromanometer pressure measurements. Br Heart J 1988;59(1):23–30.

32. Konstam MA, Cohen SR, Salem DN, et al. Comparison of left and right ventricular end-systolic pressure-volume relations in congestive heart failure. J Am Coll Cardiol 1985;5(6):1326–34.

33. Haddad F, Hunt SA, Rosenthal DN, et al. Right ventricular function in cardiovascular disease, part I. Circulation 2008;117(11):1436–48.

34. Redington AN, Rigby ML, Shinebourne EA, et al. Changes in the pressure-volume relation of the

right ventricle when its loading conditions are modified. Br Heart J 1990;63(1):45–9.

35. Ryan JJ, Tedford RJ. Diagnosing and treating the failing right heart. Curr Opin Cardiol 2015;30(3).

36. Tedford RJ, Mudd JO, Girgis RE, et al. Right ventricular dysfunction in systemic sclerosis associated pulmonary arterial hypertension. Circ Heart Fail 2013;6(5):953–63.

37. McCabe C, White PA, Hoole SP, et al. Right ventricular dysfunction in chronic thromboembolic obstruction of the pulmonary artery: a pressure-volume study using the conductance catheter. J Appl Physiol (1985) 2014;116(4):355–63.

38. Dell'italia LJ, Walsh RA. Application of a time varying elastance model to right ventricular performance in man. Cardiovasc Res 1988;22(12):864–74.

39. Dell'Italia LJ. The right ventricle: anatomy, physiology, and clinical importance. Curr Probl Cardiol 1991;16(10):653–720.

40. Brimioulle S, Wauthy P, Ewalenko P, et al. Single-beat estimation of right ventricular end-systolic pressure-volume relationship. Am J Physiol Heart Circ Physiol 2003;284(5):H1625–30.

41. Spruijt OA, Bogaard HJ, Vonk-Noordegraaf A. Assessment of right ventricular responses to therapy in pulmonary hypertension. Drug Discov Today 2014;19(8):1246–50.

42. Hsu S, Houston BA, Tampakakis E, et al. Right ventricular functional reserve in pulmonary arterial hypertension. Circulation 2016;133(24):2413–22.

43. Latus H, Binder W, Kerst G, et al. Right ventricular–pulmonary arterial coupling in patients after repair of tetralogy of Fallot. J Thorac Cardiovasc Surg 2013;146(6):1366–72.

44. Rommel KP, von Roeder M, Oberueck C, et al. Load-independent systolic and diastolic right ventricular function in heart failure with preserved ejection fraction as assessed by resting and handgrip exercise pressure-volume loops. Circ Heart Fail 2018;11(2):e004121.

45. Tello K, Wan J, Dalmer A, et al. Validation of the tricuspid annular plane systolic excursion/systolic pulmonary artery pressure ratio for the assessment of right ventricular-arterial coupling in severe pulmonary hypertension. Circ Cardiovasc Imaging 2019;12(9):e009047.

46. Damico RL, Hsu S, Houston BA, et al. Multi-beat right ventricular pulmonary arterial coupling predicts clinical worsening in PAH [abstract]. 13th PVRI Annual World Congress on PVD. Barcelona (Spain), February 4-5, 2019.

47. Sunagawa K, Yamada A, Senda Y, et al. Estimation of the hydromotive source pressure from ejecting beats of the left ventricle. IEEE Trans Biomed Eng 1980;27(6):299–305.

48. Takeuchi M, Igarashi Y, Tomimoto S, et al. Single-beat estimation of the slope of the end-systolic pressure-volume relation in the human left ventricle. Circulation 1991;83(1):202–12.

49. Senzaki H, Chen C-H, Kass DA. Single-beat estimation of end-systolic pressure-volume relation in humans: a new method with the potential for noninvasive application. Circulation 1996;94(10):2497–506.

50. Vanderpool RR, Pinsky MR, Naeije R, et al. RV-pulmonary arterial coupling predicts outcome in patients referred for pulmonary hypertension. Heart 2015;101(1):37–43.

51. Brewis MJ, Bellofiore A, Vanderpool RR, et al. Imaging right ventricular function to predict outcome in pulmonary arterial hypertension. Int J Cardiol 2016;218:206–11.

52. Inuzuka R, Hsu S, Tedford RJ, et al. Single-beat estimation of right ventricular contractility and its coupling to pulmonary arterial load in patients with pulmonary hypertension. J Am Heart Assoc 2018;7(10). https://doi.org/10.1161/JAHA.117. 007929.

53. Bellofiore A, Vanderpool R, Brewis MJ, et al. A novel single-beat approach to assess right ventricular systolic function. J Appl Physiol (1985) 2018;124(2):283–90.

54. Glower DD, Spratt JA, Snow ND, et al. Linearity of the Frank-Starling relationship in the intact heart: the concept of preload recruitable stroke work. Circulation 1985;71(5):994–1009.

55. Karunanithi MK, Michniewicz J, Copeland SE, et al. Right ventricular preload recruitable stroke work, end-systolic pressure-volume, and dP/dtmax-end-diastolic volume relations compared as indexes of right ventricular contractile performance in conscious dogs. Circ Res 1992;70(6):1169–79.

56. Little WC. The left ventricular dP/dtmax-end-diastolic volume relation in closed-chest dogs. Circ Res 1985;56(6):808–15.

57. White PA, Bishop AJ, Conroy B, et al. The determination of volume of right ventricular casts using a conductance catheter. Eur Heart J 1995;16(10): 1425–9.

58. Wang Z, Yuan L-J, Cao T-S, et al. Simultaneous beat-by-beat investigation of the effects of the Valsalva maneuver on left and right ventricular filling and the Possible mechanism. PLoS One 2013; 8(1):e53917.

59. Simon MA, Deible C, Mathier MA, et al. Phenotyping the right ventricle in patients with pulmonary hypertension. Clin Transl Sci 2009;2(4):294–9.

60. Tedford RJ. Determinants of right ventricular afterload (2013 Grover Conference series). Pulm Circ 2014;4(2):211–9.

61. Milnor WR, Conti CR, Lewis KB, et al. Pulmonary arterial pulse wave velocity and impedance in man. Circ Res 1969;25(6):637–49.

62. Sunagawa K, Maughan WL, Burkhoff D, et al. Left ventricular interaction with arterial load studied in

isolated canine ventricle. Am J Physiol Heart Circ Physiol 1983;245(5):H773–80.

63. Saouti N, Westerhof N, Helderman F, et al. Right ventricular oscillatory power is a constant fraction of total power irrespective of pulmonary artery pressure. Am J Respir Crit Care Med 2010; 182(10):1315–20.

64. Stergiopulos N, Segers P, Westerhof N. Use of pulse pressure method for estimating total arterial compliance in vivo. Am J Physiol Heart Circ Physiol 1999;276(2):H424–8.

65. Chemla D, Hebert JL, Coirault C, et al. Total arterial compliance estimated by stroke volume-to-aortic pulse pressure ratio in humans. Am J Physiol 1998;274(2):H500–5.

66. Vonk-Noordegraaf A, Haddad F, Chin KM, et al. Right heart adaptation to pulmonary arterial hypertension: physiology and pathobiology. Updates in Pulmonary Hypertension. J Am Coll Cardiol 2013; 62(25, Supplement):D22–33.

67. Tedford RJ, Hassoun PM, Mathai SC, et al. Pulmonary capillary wedge pressure augments right ventricular pulsatile loading/clinical perspective. Circulation 2012;125(2):289–97.

68. Lankhaar JW, Westerhof N, Faes TJ, et al. Pulmonary vascular resistance and compliance stay inversely related during treatment of pulmonary hypertension. Eur Heart J 2008;29(13):1688–95.

69. Wong YY, Westerhof N, Ruiter G, et al. Systolic pulmonary artery pressure and heart rate are main determinants of oxygen consumption in the right ventricular myocardium of patients with idiopathic pulmonary arterial hypertension. Eur J Heart Fail 2011;13(12):1290–5.

70. Aschauer S, Kammerlander AA, Zotter-Tufaro C, et al. The right heart in heart failure with preserved ejection fraction: insights from cardiac magnetic resonance imaging and invasive haemodynamics. Eur J Heart Fail 2016;18(1):71–80.

71. Al-Naamani N, Preston IR, Paulus JK, et al. Pulmonary arterial capacitance is an important predictor of mortality in heart failure with a preserved ejection fraction. JACC Heart Fail 2015;3(6):467–74.

72. Kelly RP, Ting CT, Yang TM, et al. Effective arterial elastance as index of arterial vascular load in humans. Circulation 1992;86(2):513–21.

73. Morimont P, Lambermont B, Ghuysen A, et al. Effective arterial elastance as an index of pulmonary vascular load. Am J Physiol Heart Circ Physiol 2008;294(6):H2736–42.

74. Ghuysen A, Lambermont B, Kolh P, et al. Alteration of right ventricular-pulmonary vascular coupling in a porcine model of progressive pressure overloading. Shock 2008;29(2):197–204.

75. Tedford RJ, Kelemen BW, Mathai SC, et al. Abstract 11450: comparison of simplified (Single-beat) estimates to measured right ventricular end-systolic elastance and RV-pulmonary vascular coupling in patients with pulmonary hypertension. Circulation 2014;130(Suppl 2). A11450-A50.

76. Chemla D, Hebert JL, Coirault C, et al. Matching dicrotic notch and mean pulmonary artery pressures: implications for effective arterial elastance. Am J Physiol 1996;271(4 Pt 2):H1287–95.

77. Vonk Noordegraaf A, Westerhof BE, Westerhof N. The relationship between the right ventricle and its load in pulmonary hypertension. J Am Coll Cardiol 2017;69(2):236–43.

78. Tampakakis E, Shah SJ, Borlaug BA, et al. Pulmonary effective arterial elastance as a measure of right ventricular afterload and its prognostic value in pulmonary hypertension due to left heart disease. Circ Heart Fail 2018;11(4):e004436.

79. Vanderpool RR, Saul M, Nouraie M, et al. Association between hemodynamic markers of pulmonary hypertension and outcomes in heart failure with preserved ejection fraction. JAMA Cardiol 2018; 3(4):298–306.

80. Burkhoff D, Sagawa K. Ventricular efficiency predicted by an analytical model. Am J Physiol 1986; 250(6 Pt 2):R1021–7.

81. Fourie PR, Coetzee AR, Bolliger CT. Pulmonary artery compliance: its role in right ventricular-arterial coupling. Cardiovasc Res 1992;26(9):839–44.

82. Tello K, Dalmer A, Axmann J, et al. Reserve of right ventricular-arterial coupling in the setting of chronic overload. Circ Heart Fail 2019;12(1):e005512.

83. Haddad F, Kudelko K, Mercier O, et al. Pulmonary hypertension associated with left heart disease: characteristics, emerging concepts, and treatment strategies. Prog Cardiovasc Dis 2011;54(2): 154–67.

84. Guihaire J, Haddad F, Noly P, et al. Right ventricular reserve in a piglet model of chronic pulmonary hypertension. Eur Respir J 2015;45(3):709–17.

85. Sharma T, Lau EMT, Choudhary P, et al. Dobutamine stress for evaluation of right ventricular reserve in pulmonary arterial hypertension. Eur Respir J 2015;45(3):700–8.

86. Guazzi M, Villani S, Generati G, et al. Right ventricular contractile reserve and pulmonary circulation uncoupling during exercise challenge in heart failure: pathophysiology and clinical phenotypes. JACC Heart Fail 2016;4(8):625–35.

87. Borlaug BA, Kane GC, Melenovsky V, et al. Abnormal right ventricular-pulmonary artery coupling with exercise in heart failure with preserved ejection fraction. Eur Heart J 2016;37(43): 3293–302.

88. Obokata M, Kane GC, Reddy YNV, et al. The neurohormonal basis of pulmonary hypertension in heart failure with preserved ejection fraction. Eur Heart J 2019. https://doi.org/10.1093/eurheartj/ehz626.

89. Matsumoto K, Tanaka H, Onishi A, et al. Bi-ventricular contractile reserve offers an incremental prognostic value for patients with dilated cardiomyopathy. Eur Heart J Cardiovasc Imaging 2015;16(11):1213–23.

90. Grünig E, Tiede H, Enyimayew EO, et al. Assessment and prognostic relevance of right ventricular contractile reserve in patients with severe pulmonary hypertension. Circulation 2013;128:2005–15.

91. DeFaria Yeh D, Stefanescu Schmidt AC, Eisman AS, et al. Impaired right ventricular reserve predicts adverse cardiac outcomes in adults with congenital right heart disease. Heart 2018; 104(24):2044–50.

92. Deswarte G, Kirsch M, Lesault PF, et al. Right ventricular reserve and outcome after continuous-flow left ventricular assist device implantation. J Heart Lung Transplant 2010;29(10):1196–8.

93. Gaynor SL, Maniar HS, Bloch JB, et al. Right atrial and ventricular adaptation to chronic right ventricular pressure overload. Circulation 2005;112(9 suppl):I-212-I--218.

94. Alaa M, Abdellatif M, Tavares-Silva M, et al. Right ventricular end-diastolic stiffness heralds right ventricular failure in monocrotaline-induced pulmonary hypertension. Am J Physiol Heart Circ Physiol 2016;311(4):H1004–13.

95. Burkhoff D, Mirsky I, Suga H. Assessment of systolic and diastolic ventricular properties via pressure-volume analysis: a guide for clinical, translational, and basic researchers. Am J Physiol Heart Circ Physiol 2005;289(2):H501–12.

96. Labeit S, Kolmerer B. Titins: giant proteins in charge of muscle ultrastructure and elasticity. Science 1995;270(5234):293–6.

97. Rain S, Handoko ML, Trip P, et al. Right ventricular diastolic impairment in patients with pulmonary arterial hypertension. Circulation 2013;128(18): 2016–25, 1-10.

98. Trip P, Rain S, Handoko ML, et al. Clinical relevance of right ventricular diastolic stiffness in pulmonary hypertension. Eur Respir J 2015;45(6):1603–12.

99. Vanderpool RR, Desai AA, Knapp SM, et al. How prostacyclin therapy improves right ventricular function in pulmonary arterial hypertension. Eur Respir J 2017;50(2). https://doi.org/10.1183/13993003. 00764-2017.

100. Rain S, Andersen S, Najafi A, et al. Right ventricular myocardial stiffness in experimental pulmonary arterial hypertension: relative contribution of fibrosis and myofibril stiffness. Circ Heart Fail 2016;9(7). https:// doi.org/10.1161/CIRCHEARTFAILURE.115.002636.

101. Gorcsan J, Murali S, Counihan PJ, et al. Right ventricular performance and contractile reserve in patients with severe heart failure: assessment by pressure-area relations and association with outcome. Circulation 1996;94(12): 3190–7.

102. Blumberg FC, Arzt M, Lange T, et al. Impact of right ventricular reserve on exercise capacity and survival in patients with pulmonary hypertension. Eur J Heart Fail 2013;15(7):771–5.

103. Claessen G, La Gerche A, Dymarkowski S, et al. Pulmonary vascular and right ventricular reserve in patients with normalized resting hemodynamics after pulmonary endarterectomy. J Am Heart Assoc 2015;4(3):e001602.

104. Spruijt OA, de Man FS, Groepenhoff H, et al. The effects of exercise on right ventricular contractility and right ventricular-arterial coupling in pulmonary hypertension. Am J Respir Crit Care Med 2015; 191(9):1050–7.

105. D'Alto M, Pavelescu A, Argiento P, et al. Echocardiographic assessment of right ventricular contractile reserve in healthy subjects. Echocardiography 2017;34(1):61–8.

106. D'Andrea A, Limongelli G, Baldini L, et al. Exercise speckle-tracking strain imaging demonstrates impaired right ventricular contractile reserve in hypertrophic cardiomyopathy. Int J Cardiol 2017;227: 209–16.

107. Claeys M, Claessen G, La Gerche A, et al. Impaired cardiac reserve and abnormal vascular load limit exercise capacity in chronic thromboembolic disease. JACC Cardiovasc Imaging 2019; 12(8 Pt 1):1444–56.

Right Heart Failure
Causes and Clinical Epidemiology

Hasan Ashraf, MD*, Julie L. Rosenthal, MD

KEYWORDS

- Right heart failure • Right ventricular dysfunction • Epidemiology • Cause

KEY POINTS

- Right heart failure is a complex and diverse syndrome with unique causes and pathophysiology, each of which have distinct criteria for diagnosis and management.
- Right heart failure is an independent predictor of mortality.
- Improvements in imaging have led to better understanding of the pathophysiology of right heart failure, transformed the way it is diagnosed, and have thereby informed epidemiologic studies.

 Video content accompanies this article at http://www.cardiology.theclinics.com.

INTRODUCTION

The right ventricle (RV) has historically been an overlooked component of the heart, as it has been perceived as a nonessential component of the myocardial pump and merely as a conduit for the pulmonary circulation. However, in recent years, the RV has experienced a resurgence in interest, owing in part to growing interest in emerging treatments for pulmonary hypertension (PH) as well as studies that have established the prognostic value of RV failure and right heart failure (RHF) independently from the left ventricle (LV). Isolated RV dysfunction (RVD) and RHF have also been increasingly established as distinct entities that contribute to growing cardiovascular morbidity and mortality.

This article is one among a larger series that reviews some of the salient features of RHF. In preparing this article, an extensive literature review was conducted through September 2019. Studies included in the review were limited to English language studies, reviews, and guidelines and were included based on the strength of the studies and their relevance to the current work.

DEFINITION AND CLASSIFICATION

Multiple definitions of RHF have been proposed, but most have not gained widespread acceptance[1,2] (**Table 1**). Accordingly, major society guidelines are largely silent regarding RHF, and neither the American College of Cardiology Foundation (ACCF)/American Heart Association (AHA) 2013 heart failure (HF) guidelines nor the 2017 focused update address RHF.[3,4] The European Society of Cardiology (ESC) is similarly quiet on RHF in its most recent guidelines published in 2016, although the 2008 iteration does categorize RHF as one of the 5 cardinal manifestations of HF. Neverthless, a formal definition is not provided.[5,6]

In 2014, the International Right Heart Failure Foundation Scientific Working Group published a position document in an attempt to further a common language and uniform definition of RHF. RHF was defined as a "clinical syndrome due to an alteration of structure and/or function of the right heart circulatory system that leads to suboptimal delivery of blood flow (high or low) to the pulmonary circulation and/or elevated venous pressures at rest or with exercise."[7] This definition is contrasted with RV failure, which is just "one

Department of Cardiovascular Diseases, Mayo Clinic, 13737 North 92nd Street, Scottsdale, AZ 85260, USA
* Corresponding author.
E-mail address: ashraf.hasan@mayo.edu

Cardiol Clin 38 (2020) 175–183
https://doi.org/10.1016/j.ccl.2020.01.008
0733-8651/20/© 2020 Elsevier Inc. All rights reserved.

Table 1
Definitions of right heart failure and right ventricular dysfunction

General Definitions and Descriptions	
2008 European Society of Cardiology Heart Failure Guidelines	A common clinical manifestation of HF characterized by breathlessness, fatigue, evidence of RV dysfunction, raised JVP, peripheral edema, hepatomegaly, and gut congestion
2014 International Right Heart Failure Foundation Scientific Working Group	A clinical syndrome caused by an alteration of structure and/or function of the right heart circulatory system that leads to suboptimal delivery of blood flow (high or low) to the pulmonary circulation and/or increased venous pressures at rest or with exercise
2018 American Heart Association Scientific Statement	A clinical syndrome with signs and symptoms of HF resulting from abnormal RV structure or function, caused by the inability of the RV to support optimal circulation in the presence of adequate preload
Specific Definitions and Descriptions	
2014 Interagency Registry for Mechanically Assisted Circulatory Support definition of RHF in setting of LVAD	Increased right atrial pressure >16 mm Hg, measured directly by right heart catheterization or indirectly by jugular venous distension or dilated inferior vena cava, plus clinical or laboratory evidence of venous congestion
2014 International Society for Heart and Lung Transplantation definition of primary graft dysfunction with isolated RV involvement	Graft dysfunction of primary cause with diagnosis made within 24 h of implantation and either (1) and (2), or (3) alone: (1) RAP>15 mm Hg, PCWP<15 mm Hg, CI < 2.0 L/min/m²; and (2) TPG<15 mm Hg and/or SPAP<50 mm Hg; or (3) need for RVAD
2018 6th World Symposium on Pulmonary Hypertension	A clinical syndrome characterized by decreased right ventricular function that leads to insufficient blood flow and/or increased filling pressures at rest or during physiologically demanding conditions such as exercise, developmental growth, or pregnancy

Abbreviations: CI, cardiac index; JVP, jugular venous pulsations; LVAD, left ventricular assist device; PCWP, pulmonary capillary wedge pressure; RAP, right atrial pressure; RVAD, right ventricular assist device; SPAP, systolic pulmonary artery pressure; TPG, transpulmonary pressure gradient.

component of a pathophysiological entity that can result" in RHF. The advantages of this definition include its breadth and inclusivity.

Because most of the studies discussed here include varied definitions of RHF and RVD, this article consistently uses the term RHF to refer to the clinical syndrome of HF with the concomitant right ventricular structural and physiologic changes, and RVD to refer solely to pathologic structural changes in the RV.

EPIDEMIOLOGY OF RIGHT HEART FAILURE AND DYSFUNCTION

A predominant presentation with the clinical symptoms consistent with RHF was present in 2.2% of all acute decompensated HF admissions in the European CHARITEM registry. However, RHF in as much as a fifth of these patients was secondary to acute LV failure.[8] In addition, in the ESC-HF Long-term Registry, 4.5% of Egyptian patients and 3.0% of non-Egyptian patients who were hospitalized with acute decompensated HF presented primarily with RHF.[9] The origin of the difference in prevalence has been attributed to a higher incidence of rheumatic valvular heart disease and pulmonary hypertension (PH) from schistosomiasis.

In a cohort of 259 Asian patients hospitalized for acute decompensated HF, RVD (tricuspid annular planar systolic excursion [TAPSE] ≤16 mm) was present in 53.7% of patients.[10] In addition, RVD was a stronger predictor of longer hospitalization duration than clinical symptoms, blood pressure, and pulmonary artery pressure.

Several studies have evaluated the prevalence of RVD using primarily echocardiographic parameters in HF with preserved ejection fraction (HFpEF). Shah and colleagues[11] evaluated RVD in a large cohort of 673 patients with HFpEF, in whom RVD was present in 4% of the patients if a fractional area change (FAC) cutoff of less than 35% was used, 11% if FAC was less than 40%, and 31% if the FAC cutoff was increased to less than 45%. In other, smaller studies the prevalence of RVD using FAC (with cutoffs ranging from <35% to <45%) was greater, ranging from 28% to 33%.[12] Studies using TAPSE to define RVD (ranging from <15 to <16 mm) show a prevalence of 40% to 49% in patients with HFpEF.[13] The higher prevalence of RVD using TAPSE suggests that longitudinal function is a more sensitive marker of RVD than the two-dimensional FAC.

The prevalence and severity of RVD correlates with LV systolic function. One study directly comparing 100 patients with HF with reduced ejection fraction (HFrEF) and HFpEF found that the prevalence of RVD in this population was 50% in the HFpEF cohort and 73% in the HFrEF cohort, with the prevalence of RVD increasing with worse LV systolic function.[14] In addition, the severity of RVD also was worse with lower LV ejection fraction (LVEF), and those with HFpEF had a milder degree of RVD compared with those with HFrEF.[13]

The prevalence of RVD in individuals with left HF is greater in nonischemic compared with ischemic cardiomyopathies. This finding may be a result of a higher frequency or primary RV myocardial dysfunction in patients with genetically predisposed nonischemic cardiomyopathies. In some studies, this difference can be striking, as in a series of 153 patients with nonischemic and ischemic cardiomyopathy all with LVEF less than 45%, in which RVD (RV ejection fraction [RVEF] <35% determined by invasive ventriculography) was present in 16% of ischemic patients and 65% of nonischemic patients.[15]

Prognosis

HFrEF complicated by RVD is associated with a 2.4-fold increased risk of mortality compared with patients without RVD. Importantly, although a lower LVEF has been associated with worse RVD, RVD is predictive of all-cause mortality and cardiac transplant independently of LV systolic dysfunction.[16]

Cardiac imaging can assist greatly in evaluation of right heart anatomy and function. There is a substantial body of evidence showing that RV size and function provide excellent prognostic potential. Echocardiographic parameters that evaluate the right heart include right atrium (RA) and RV chamber size, TAPSE, tricuspid annular velocity (S′), and three-dimensional assessment of RVEF. Apart from functional data, many of these echocardiographic parameters additionally provide prognostic information. TAPSE is easily calculated, highly reproducible, and has been studied in patients with PH, congenital heart disease, HFpEF, and HFrEF. In addition, RVD using TAPSE (<1.8 cm) has been associated with as high as a 4-fold increased risk of death when compared with patients with normal TAPSE independent of other echocardiographic parameters.[17]

CAUSES: ACUTE

Multiple classification schemes can be used to describe the causes of RHF and RVD, including acute versus chronic and pathophysiologic and mechanistic causes. Acute RHF can include both acute de novo and acute on chronic, of which some of the common causes are presented later.

Right Ventricular Myocardial Infarction

Acute right ventricular myocardial infarction (RVMI) usually occurs in the context of occlusion of the proximal right coronary artery (RCA), resulting in depressed RV systolic function. Isolated RVMI is an uncommon occurrence, because it usually occurs in conjunction with an infarct of the inferior LV wall. Of all inferior acute ST-elevation myocardial infarctions (STEMIs), RV involvement occurs in 30% to 50% of cases.[18] Out of this population, 25% to 50% of patients present with hemodynamic compromise. RVMI only comprised 5% of all patients with myocardial infarction (MI)–induced cardiogenic shock in the SHOCK trial[19] (**Fig. 1**J–M).

The prognosis of RVMI is more favorable than that of an LV myocardial infarction, with improvement and even resolution of RV function in most patients with RVMI.[20,21] In a small Mayo Clinic series characterizing inferior MI, 82% of patients had recovery of RV function after revascularization with thrombolysis, and there was only a mortality of 3.5% of patients at 1 year.[22] However, a more recent study did show greater (18%) 1-year mortality in patients with RVMI and isolated RCA involvement. Recovery of RV function has also been described in individuals in whom revascularization was unsuccessful or not attempted.[23]

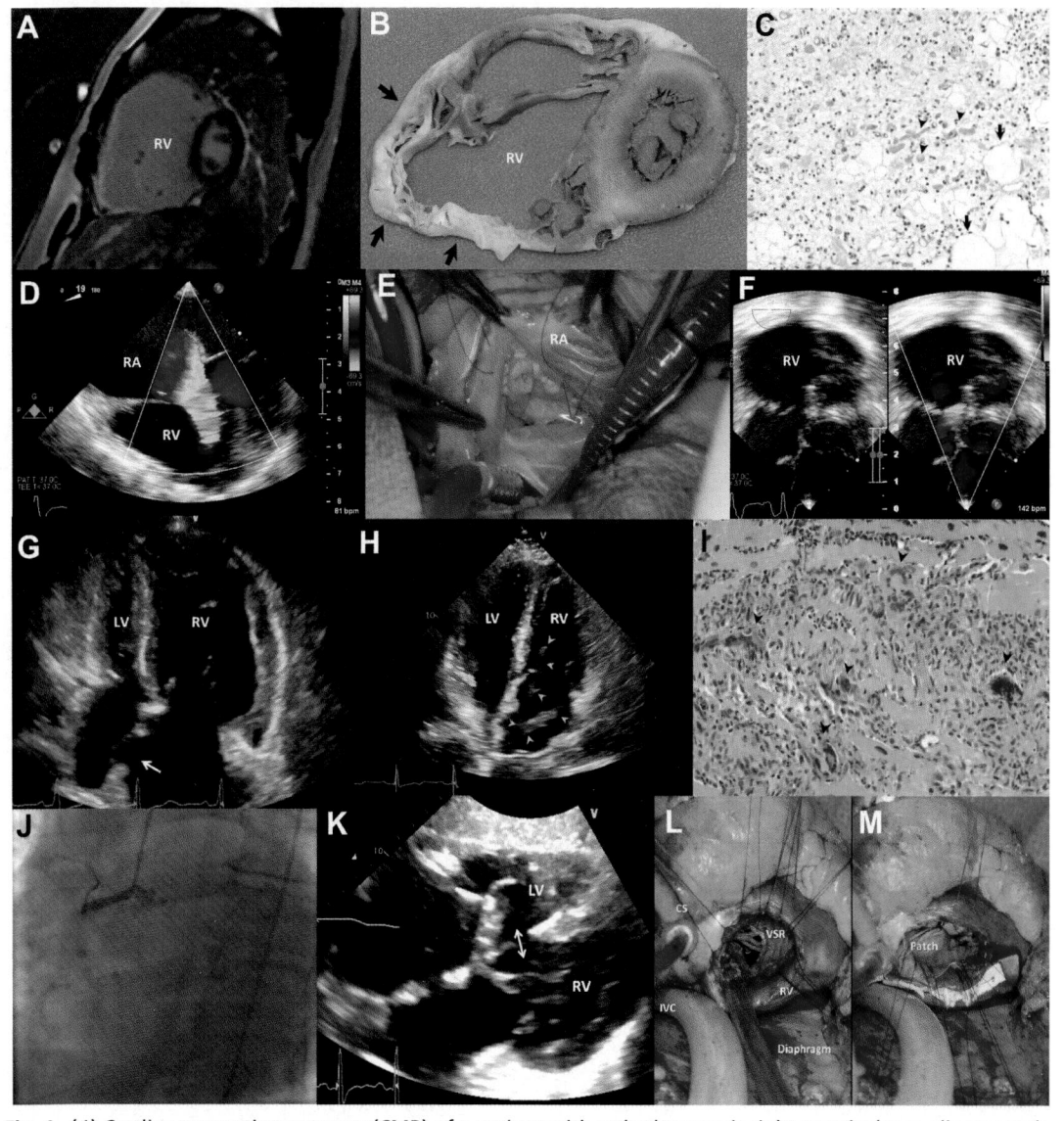

Fig. 1. (*A*) Cardiac magnetic resonance (CMR) of a patient with arrhythmogenic right ventricular cardiomyopathy (ARVC) showing a severely dilated RV and delayed gadolinium enhancement along a thinned RV. (*B*) Gross specimen obtained after heart transplant shows extensive fibrofatty replacement of the RV myocytes with thinning of the free wall (*arrows*), as highlighted in the CMR image. (*C*) Microscopic examination of this ARVC heart shows fibrosis and fatty replacement (*arrows*) and a paucity of cardiomyocytes (*arrowheads*). (*D*) Transesophageal echocardiography (TEE) image of Ebstein anomaly. There is a sail-like anterior leaflet with multiple areas of tethering of the septal and inferior leaflets resulting in severe malcoaptation and torrential tricuspid regurgitation (TR) by color Doppler and atrialization of the RV. (*E*) Intraoperative image of the repaired tricuspid valve after cone-shaped reconstruction. (*F*) Intraoperative TEE after cone reconstruction of the tricuspid valve with mild residual central TR. (*G*) Mayo apical 4-chamber image of severe pulmonary arterial hypertension with interventricular septal flattening and RA bowing into the left atrium (*arrow*), suggestive of right-sided pressure and volume overload. (*H*) Mayo apical 4-chamber view of a severely enlarged RA with reduced systolic function in the setting of a massive acute pulmonary embolism (*arrowheads*) that extends from the RA to the RV. Catheter-directed mechanical thrombectomy revealed a 13-cm serpiginous thrombus. (*I*) Histopathologic examination of a giant cell myocarditis obtained from a right ventricular endomyocardial biopsy. Giant cells (*arrowheads*) can be identified by their prominent multinucleated morphology. (*J*) Coronary angiogram of a patient who presented with Killip class IV STEMI of the RCA. (*K*) Subcostal transthoracic echocardiogram of the RCA STEMI with dilatation of the RV and a large ventricular septal rupture (VSR, *double-headed arrow*) at the basal inferior septum. (*L*) Intraoperative image of the basilar VSR. (*M*) Intraoperative image of the basilar VSR after patch repair. CS, coronary sinus; IVC, inferior vena cava. (Histopathologic images *courtesy* of Dr. Brandon T. Larsen and Dr. Henry D. Tazelaar.)

Primary Graft Dysfunction

Primary graft dysfunction (PGD) is a common occurrence during the early post–cardiac transplant period. Of patients undergoing heart transplant, 31% developed some form of PGD in a small study of 325 patients, although this number varies based on the definition of PGD used (see **Table 1**). Isolated RV involvement (primary graft dysfunction with isolated RV involvement [PGD-RV]) is present in 5% of patients undergoing heart transplant.[24] The mechanisms of PGD in general and PGD-RV specifically are multifactorial. A validated scoring system used as a predictor of PGD is the RADIAL score, with 6 factors that form the acronym: right atrial pressure greater than 10 mm Hg, age of the recipient greater than 60 years, diabetes, inotropic support dependence, age of donor greater than 30 years, and length of ischemia time greater than 240 minutes.[25]

Acute Right Heart Failure After Left Ventricular Assist Device Implantation

Most patients with advanced LV failure undergoing long-term left ventricular assist device (LVAD) implantation have some form of RVD as well, and so it is unsurprising that LVAD patients can develop acute right HF (ARHF) in the post-LVAD implant setting. ARHF after LVAD implantation is thought to be from increased blood return to a dysfunctional RV, subsequent RV dilation, and decrease in RV stroke volume. ARHF has been described in 10% to 40% of patients post-LVAD.[2,26] ARHF in post-LVAD patients is associated with worse outcomes, with a 1-year mortality of 29% versus just 11% without ARHF. It is also associated with prolonged length of stay and worse survival even after cardiac transplant.

Predicting which patients will develop ARHF in this population is an area of clinical interest because it can improve selection of candidates for LVAD implantation. As a consequence, risk

models and scores have been developed to prognosticate ARHF in LVAD patients. Hemodynamic parameters such as RA pressure, RA/pulmonary capillary wedge ratio, RV stroke-work index, and pulmonary artery pulsatility index can also help predict ARHF.[27]

Pulmonary Embolism

The mechanism of ARHF in a setting of acute pulmonary embolism (PE) is similar to that in chronic pressure overload states but lacks the chronic compensatory response that reduces wall stress in a high afterload state. Echocardiographic features of RVD are present in 25% to 60% of patients with PE and portend a poorer prognosis as independent risk factors, and mortality can be 2.4 to 3.5 times greater than in those without RVD[28] (**Fig. 1**H, Video 1). The presence of RVD on echocardiography may warrant more aggressive treatment of PE, although outcomes in this setting remain an ongoing area of investigation.

CAUSES: CHRONIC

Causes of chronic RHF are broadly place into 1 of 3 mechanistic classifications: primary RV myocardial disease, PH (including left heart disease), and right-sided valvular heart disease (**Table 2**). Evaluation for causes of RHF should therefore always include a hemodynamic assessment of the right heart, including pulmonary artery pressures, right-sided valve morphology and function, and RV structure and function.

MYOCARDIAL DISORDERS
Arrhythmogenic Right Ventricular Cardiomyopathy/Dysplasia

Arrhythmogenic right ventricular cardiomyopathy (ARVC) is a heritable primary myocardial disorder that affects primarily the RV.[29] ARVC is characterized by loss of RV myocardium with inflammatory

---

Table 2
Causes of chronic right heart failure

Primary Myocardial Disease	PH	Right-Sided Valvular Disease
RV cardiomyopathy	Pulmonary arterial hypertension	Tricuspid regurgitation
Restrictive cardiomyopathy	Congenital heart disease	Ebstein anomaly
Myocarditis	Left ventricular systolic dysfunction	Pulmonary regurgitation
ARVC	Left ventricular diastolic dysfunction	Pulmonary stenosis
	Left sided valvular disease	Tricuspid stenosis
	Chronic thromboembolic PH	
	Chronic lung disease	

Abbreviation: ARVC, arrhythmogenic right ventricular cardiomyopathy.

changes leading to myocyte death and replacement by fibrous and fatty tissue leading to RVD and dysrhythmias (**Fig. 1**A–C). The molecular mechanism of ARVC most commonly involves mutations in the genes encoding desmosomal proteins, which leads to disruption of the intercellular junction and myocyte detachment, particularly under conditions of mechanical stress.[30,31]

ARVC presents between the ages of 20 and 40 years most commonly, with a median age of 29 years.[32] Sudden cardiac death is occasionally the initial presentation. The prevalence of ARVC is estimated to be 1 in 2000 persons in the general population.[33] There is a higher prevalence of ARVC in men than in women, and a positive family history is identified in more than 50% of patients.[34] ARVC has a more malignant course in men, possibly from sex hormone involvement or sex-based variations in the intensity or amount of exercise.[35]

Myocarditis

Myocarditis is an inflammatory myocardial disease that has a variety of infectious, autoimmune, idiopathic, toxic, and familial causes. Severe diffuse inflammation can eventually lead to dilated cardiomyopathy, and the underlying pathologic cause cannot always be identified. Myocarditis can present as either diffuse or focal involvement, and the clinical presentation may be acute fulminant, subacute, or chronic. Cardiac imaging, including cardiac magnetic resonance and endomyocardial biopsy, can assist in diagnosis (**Fig. 1**I).

Involvement of the RV may portend poorer prognosis in that it reflects a greater burden of inflammation or an increased afterload caused by LV dysfunction.[36] Right heart involvement may be the strongest predictor of death or transplant in myocarditis.[37]

Peripartum Cardiomyopathy

Peripartum cardiomyopathy (PPCM) is a cause of HF that affects women during the later stages of pregnancy or during the early puerperium period. The ESC Working Group's current definition of PPCM defines PPCM as a HF with an LVEF of less than 45% that develops near the end of pregnancy or within 5 months after delivery without any other identifiable cause of HF.[38] The incidence of PPCM in the United States is around 1 in 968 to 4000, although in a Haitian cohort it was as high as 1 in 300 to 400.[39,40] The rate of hospitalizations in pregnant patients for PPCM was 0.18 per 1000 deliveries.[41] RVD (RV FAC <35%) is found in 38% of patients with PPCM, and worse RV FAC is highly prognostic for worse clinical outcome and less myocardial (both RV and LV) recovery.[42]

PULMONARY HYPERTENSION

PH describes a broad group of disorders characterized by increased pulmonary artery pressure (mean pulmonary artery pressure $\geq$20 mm Hg at rest).[43] Chronic PH increases RV afterload, resulting in compensatory remodeling of the RV and eventually RHF (**Fig. 1**G). The World Health Organization classification scheme groups PH into 5 groups based on cause.

Among the general population, European registries put the prevalence of pulmonary arterial hypertension (PAH) at 5 to 52 cases per million adults.[44] In a multicenter study of 674 patients with PAH, idiopathic PAH accounted for 39.2% of cases, familial 3.9%, connective tissue disease 15.3%, congenital heart disease 11.3%, portal hypertension 10.4%, and human immunodeficiency virus–associated PAH 6.2% of cases.[45] Schistosomiasis remains the most common cause of PAH worldwide.[46]

Despite the growing number of pulmonary vasodilatory drugs, PAH continues to have a high morbidity and mortality. In the REVEAL registry, the 1-year and 5-year survival of patients with PAH was 85% and 57% respectively.[47] Risk stratification of patients in the COMPERA registry based in Europe into 3 risk strata based on various risk factors revealed a 1-year survival of 97.8% for the low-risk cohort, 90.1% for the intermediate cohort, and 78.8% in the highest-risk cohort.[48]

PH can also be caused by LV systolic or diastolic dysfunction as well as valvular heart disease. The prevalence of PH is 68% in HFrEF and 54% in HFpEF. Combined postcapillary and precapillary PH is present in 12% of patients with HF, with a similar prevalence in HFrEF and HFpEF. PH caused by chronic lung disease and/or hypoxemia is typically mild to moderate; fewer than 5% of patients have severe PH. PH is present in 25% to 90% of patients with chronic obstructive pulmonary disease, and 20% of patients with obstructive sleep apnea also have PH.[49,50]

CONGENITAL HEART DISEASE

Congenital heart disease (CHD) is discussed here as a separate entity given its unique epidemiology and management, although mechanistically it usually overlaps with the other 3 causes. CHD occurs during embryogenesis and results in the abnormal formation of the walls of the heart, valves, and/or blood vessels. The birth prevalence of CHD according to US Centers for Disease Control and

Prevention data is slightly less than 1% of all births, with the most common causes of noncyanotic CHD being ventricular septal defect (VSD) and secundum atrial septal defect (ASD), and tetralogy of Fallot (TOF) as the most common cyanotic CHD. Clinical evaluation and assessment of CHD has been galvanized by the evolution of imaging techniques, invasive hemodynamic evaluation, and both surgical and nonsurgical interventions, which has led to a growing adult congenital population (**Fig. 1**D–F).

CHD is often associated with RVD and RHF as a result of volume or pressure overload from intracardiac shunting, right-sided valvular lesions, or a systemic RV physiology. Pressure overload usually results from PH, whereas volume overload results from chronic intracardiac shunting such as with ASD and VSD. Uncorrected large, nonrestrictive shunts can lead to PH, and subsequent increased right-sided pressures result in reversal of the shunt and the Eisenmenger syndrome.

Some of the most complex forms of CHD present with single-ventricle physiology, which can present with varying levels of severity. The most severe forms include absence of the LV (such as hypoplastic left heart), in which palliative interventions are essential. Expectedly, RHF in this population can present in a patient's 20s, and the incidence of HF in single-ventricle physiology is higher than in those with a normal systemic LV.[51]

An exceedingly rare cause of RHF is Uhl anomaly, which is characterized by absent RV myocytes and direct apposition of the endocardium with the epicardium. The dysfunctional RV eventually results in RHF and arrhythmias.

VALVULAR HEART DISEASE

A mild amount of tricuspid regurgitation (TR) is present in 80% to 90% of individuals, but moderate to severe TR affects more than 1 million people in the United States.[52] Primary valvular TR can be caused by direct valve injury, endocarditis, Ebstein anomaly, rheumatic valve disease, connective tissue disorders, tumors, or myxomatous degeneration associated with tricuspid valve prolapse. In a study of 242 patients with severe TR, only 10% had primary TR.[53] Secondary TR is usually caused by dilatation of the RA and RV and is much more frequently found in patients with RHF. The severity of TR is associated with the prognosis in patients with RHF, with a 1-year survival of 64% in patients with severe TR.

Pulmonary valve disease can include either pulmonary stenosis (PS) or pulmonary regurgitation (PR). The former is encountered in CHD as part of TOF or other complex CHDs. Some estimates put the prevalence of PS as high as 10% of all patients with CHD. However, in isolated cases of congenital PS, RHF is not common.[54] In contrast, PR is seen as a late complication of TOF repair or after balloon valvuloplasty and can lead to RV dilatation and dysfunction.[55]

SUMMARY

RHF occurs in a wide range of clinical conditions and populations, and is consistently associated with increased morbidity and mortality. Following review of current literature, it is even more apparent that there is a lack of consensus on what either right ventricular dysfunction or RHF entail. RHF often gets relegated to a secondary position behind left HF, which has led to amorphous and heterogeneous definitions in epidemiologic studies. Nevertheless, emerging studies have contributed to a growing body of data highlighting the importance of the right heart, which will continue to expand and evolve the approach to combatting RHF.

DISCLOSURE

None of the authors have any financial conflicts to disclose.

SUPPLEMENTARY DATA

Supplementary data to this article can be found online at https://doi.org/10.1016/j.ccl.2020.01.008.

REFERENCES

1. Galiè N, McLaughlin VV, Rubin LJ, et al. An overview of the 6th World Symposium on pulmonary hypertension. Eur Respir J 2019;53(1) [pii:1802148].
2. Lampert BC, Teuteberg JJ. Right ventricular failure after left ventricular assist devices. J Heart Lung Transplant 2015;34:1123–30.
3. Yancy CW, Jessup M, Bozkurt B, et al, American College of Cardiology Foundation, American Heart Association Task Force on Practice Guidelines. 2013 ACCF/AHA guideline for the management of heart failure: a report of the American College of Cardiology Foundation/American heart association Task Force on practice guidelines. J Am Coll Cardiol 2013;62(16):e147–239.
4. Yancy CW, Jessup M, Bozkurt B. 2017 ACC/AHA/HFSA focused update of the 2013 ACCF/AHA guideline for the management of heart failure: a report of the American College of Cardiology/American heart association Task Force on clinical practice guidelines and the heart failure society of America. Circulation 2017;136(6):e137–61.

5. Ponikowski P, Voors AA, Anker SD, et al. 2016 ESC Guidelines for the diagnosis and treatment of acute and chronic heart failure: the Task Force for the diagnosis and treatment of acute and chronic heart failure of the European Society of Cardiology (ESC). Developed with the special contribution of the Heart Failure Association (HFA) of the ESC. Eur J Heart Fail 2016;18(8):891–975.

6. Dickstein K, Cohen-Solal A, Filippatos G, et al. ESC guidelines for the diagnosis and treatment of acute and chronic heart failure 2008: the Task Force for the diagnosis and treatment of acute and chronic heart failure 2008 of the European Society of Cardiology. Developed in collaboration with the Heart Failure Association of the ESC (HFA) and endorsed by the European Society of Intensive Care Medicine (ESICM). Eur J Heart Fail 2008;10(10):933–89.

7. Mehra MR, Park MH, Landzberg MJ, et al. Right heart failure: toward a common language. Pulm Circ 2013;3:963–7.

8. Mockel M, Searle J, Muller R, et al. Chief complaints in medical emergencies: do they relate to underlying disease and outcome? The Charité Emergency Medicine Study (CHARITEM). Eur J Emerg Med 2013;20(2):103–8.

9. Hassanein M, Abdelhamid M, Ibrahim B, et al. Clinical characteristics and management of hospitalized and ambulatory patients with heart failure-results from ESC heart failure long-term registry-Egyptian cohort. ESC Heart Fail 2015;2(3):159–67.

10. Yamin PP, Raharjo SB, Putri VK, et al. Right ventricular dysfunction as predictor of longer hospital stay in patients with acute decompensated heart failure: a prospective study in Indonesian population. Cardiovasc Ultrasound 2016;14(1):25.

11. Shah AM, Shah SJ, Anand IS, et al. Cardiac structure and function in heart failure with preserved ejection fraction: baseline findings from the echocardiographic study of the treatment of preserved cardiac function heart failure with an aldosterone antagonist trial. Circ Heart Fail 2014;7(1):104–15.

12. Melenovsky V, Hwang SJ, Lin G, et al. Right heart dysfunction in heart failure with preserved ejection fraction. Eur Heart J 2014;35:3452–62.

13. Puwanant S, Priester TC, Mookadam F, et al. Right ventricular function in patients with preserved and reduced ejection fraction heart failure. Eur J Echocardiogr 2009;10:733–7.

14. Cenkerova K, Dubrava J, Pokorna V, et al. Right ventricular systolic dysfunction and its prognostic value in heart failure with preserved ejection fraction. Acta Cardiol 2015;70(4):387–93.

15. La Vecchia L, Zanolla L, Varotto L, et al. Reduced right ventricular ejection fraction as a marker for idiopathic dilated cardiomyopathy compared with ischemic left ventricular dysfunction. Am Heart J 2001;142:181–9.

16. Gulati A, Ismail TF, Jabbour A, et al. The prevalence and prognostic significance of right ventricular systolic dysfunction in nonischemic dilated cardiomyopathy. Circulation 2013;128(15):1623–33.

17. Forfia PR, Fisher MR, Mathai SC, et al. Tricuspid annular displacement predicts survival in pulmonary hypertension. Am J Respir Crit Care Med 2006; 174(9):1034–41.

18. Andersen HR, Falk E, Nielsen D. Right ventricular infarction: frequency, size and topography in coronary heart disease: a prospective study comprising 107 consecutive autopsies from a coronary care unit. J Am Coll Cardiol 1987;10(6):1223–32.

19. Jacobs AK, Leopold JA, Bates E, et al. Cardiogenic shock caused by right ventricular infarction: a report from the SHOCK registry. J Am Coll Cardiol 2003;41: 1273–9.

20. Bush LR, Buja LM, Samowitz W, et al. Recovery of left ventricular segmental function after long-term reperfusion following temporary coronary occlusion in conscious dogs. Comparison of 2- and 4-hour occlusions. Circ Res 1983;53(2):248–63.

21. Bowers TR, O'Neill WW, Grines C, et al. Effect of reperfusion on biventricular function and survival after right ventricular infarction. N Engl J Med 1998; 338(14):933–40.

22. Berger PB, Ruocco NA Jr, Ryan TJ, et al. Frequency and significance of right ventricular dysfunction during inferior wall left ventricular myocardial infarction treated with thrombolytic therapy (results from the thrombolysis in myocardial infarction [TIMI] II trial). The TIMI Research Group. Am J Cardiol 1993; 71(13):1148–52.

23. Lim ST, Marcovitz P, Pica M, et al. Right ventricular performance at rest and during stress with chronic proximal occlusion of the right coronary artery. Am J Cardiol 2003;92(10):1203–6.

24. Nicoara A, Ruffin D, Cooter M, et al. Primary graft dysfunction after heart transplantation: incidence, trends, and associated risk factors. Am J Transplant 2018;18(6):1461–70.

25. Segovia J, Cosío MD, Barceló JM, et al. RADIAL: a novel primary graft failure risk score in heart transplantation. J Heart Lung Transplant 2011;30(6):644–51.

26. Kormos RL, Teuteberg JJ, Pagani FD, et al, HeartMate II Clinical Investigators. Right ventricular failure in patients with the HeartMate II continuous-flow left ventricular assist device: incidence, risk factors, and effect on outcomes. J Thorac Cardiovasc Surg 2010; 139(5):1316–24.

27. Fitzpatrick JR 3rd, Frederick JR, Hsu VM, et al. Risk score derived from pre-operative data analysis predicts the need for biventricular mechanical circulatory support. J Heart Lung Transplant 2008;27(12): 1286–92.

28. Coutance G, Cauderlier E, Ehtisham J, et al. The prognostic value of markers of right ventricular dysfunction in pulmonary embolism: a meta-analysis. Crit Care 2011;15:R103.

29. Corrado D, Basso C, Thiene G, et al. Spectrum of clinicopathologic manifestations of arrhythmogenic right ventricular cardiomyopathy/dysplasia: a multicenter study. J Am Coll Cardiol 1997;30:1512–20.

30. Rampazzo A, Nava A, Malacrida S, et al. Mutation in human desmoplakin domain binding to plakoglobin causes a dominant form of arrhythmogenic right ventricular cardiomyopathy. Am J Hum Genet 2002;71:1200–6.

31. Pilichou K, Nava A, Basso C, et al. Mutations in desmoglein-2 gene are associated with arrhythmogenic right ventricular cardiomyopathy. Circulation 2006;113:1171–9.

32. Groeneweg JA, Bhonsale A, James CA, et al. Clinical presentation, long-term follow-up, and outcomes of 1001 arrhythmogenic right ventricular dysplasia/cardiomyopathy patients and family members. Circ Cardiovasc Genet 2015;8:437–46.

33. Peters S, Trümmel M, Meyners W. Prevalence of right ventricular dysplasia-cardiomyopathy in a non-referral hospital. Int J Cardiol 2004;97:499–501.

34. Corrado D, Thiene G. Arrhythmogenic right ventricular cardiomyopathy/dysplasia: clinical impact of molecular genetic studies. Circulation 2006;113: 1634–7.

35. James CA, Bhonsale A, Tichnell C, et al. Exercise increases age-related penetrance and arrhythmic risk in arrhythmogenic right ventricular dysplasia/cardiomyopathy-associated desmosomal mutation carriers. J Am Coll Cardiol 2013;62:1290–7.

36. Caforio AL, Calabrese F, Angelini A, et al. A prospective study of biopsy-proven myocarditis: prognostic relevance of clinical and aetiopathogenetic features at diagnosis. Eur Heart J 2007;28(11): 1326–33.

37. Caforio AL, Calabrese F, Angelini A, et al. A prospective study of biopsy-proven myocarditis: prognostic relevance of clinical and aetiopathogenetic features at diagnosis. Eur Heart J 2007;28: 1326–33.

38. Sliwa K, Hilfiker-Kleiner D, Petrie MC, et al, Heart Failure Association of the European Society of Cardiology Working Group on Peripartum Cardiomyopathy. Current state of knowledge on aetiology, diagnosis, management, and therapy of peripartum cardiomyopathy: a position statement from the Heart Failure Association of the European Society of Cardiology Working Group on peripartum cardiomyopathy. Eur J Heart Fail 2010;12(8): 767–78.

39. Fett JD, Carraway RD, Dowell DL, et al. Peripartum cardiomyopathy in the hospital Albert Schweitzer District of Haiti. Am J Obstet Gynecol 2002;186: 1005–10.

40. Fett JD, Christie LG, Carraway RD, et al. Unrecognized peripartum cardiomyopathy in Haitian women. Int J Gynaecol Obstet 2005;90:161–6.

41. Kuklina EV, Callaghan WM. Cardiomyopathy and other myocardial disorders among hospitalizations for pregnancy in the United States: 2004–2006. Obstet Gynecol 2010;115:93–100.

42. Blauwet LA, Delgado-Montero A, Ryo K, et al, IPAC Investigators*. Right ventricular function in peripartum cardiomyopathy at presentation is associated with subsequent left ventricular recovery and clinical outcomes. Circ Heart Fail 2016;9(5) [pii:e002756].

43. Simonneau G, Montani D, Celermajer DS, et al. Haemodynamic definitions and updated clinical classification of pulmonary hypertension. Eur Respir J 2019;53(1) [pii:1801913].

44. Peacock AJ, Murphy NF, McMurray JJ, et al. An epidemiological study of pulmonary arterial hypertension. Eur Respir J 2007;30(1):104–9.

45. Humbert M, Sitbon O, Chaouat A, et al. Pulmonary arterial hypertension in France: results from a national registry. Am J Respir Crit Care Med 2006;173(9):1023–30.

46. de Cleva R, Herman P, Pugliese V, et al. Prevalence of pulmonary hypertension in patients with hepatosplenic mansonic schistosomiasis—prospective study. Hepatogastroenterology 2003;50(54):2028–30.

47. Benza RL, Miller DP, Barst RJ, et al. An evaluation of long-term survival from time of diagnosis in pulmonary arterial hypertension from the REVEAL Registry. Chest 2012;142:448–56.

48. Hoeper MM, Kramer T, Pan Z, et al. Mortality in pulmonary arterial hypertension: prediction by the 2015 European pulmonary hypertension guidelines risk stratification model. Eur Respir J 2017;50(2) [pii: 1700740].

49. Arcasoy SM, Christie JD, Ferrari VA. Echocardiographic assessment of pulmonary hypertension in patients with advanced lung disease. Am J Respir Crit Care Med 2003;167(5):735–40.

50. Minai OA, Ricaurte B, Kaw R. Frequency and impact of pulmonary hypertension in patients with obstructive sleep apnea syndrome. Am J Cardiol 2009;104:1300–6.

51. Julsrud PR, Weigel TJ, Van Son JA, et al. Influence of ventricular morphology on outcome after the Fontan procedure. Am J Cardiol 2000;86:319–23.

52. Taramasso M, Vanermen H, Maisano F, et al. The growing clinical importance of secondary tricuspid regurgitation. J Am Coll Cardiol 2012;59:703–10.

53. Mutlak D, Lessick J, Reisner SA, et al. Echocardiography-based spectrum of severe tricuspid regurgitation: the frequency of apparently idiopathic tricuspid regurgitation. J Am Soc Echocardiogr 2007;20(4):405–8.

54. Hayes CJ, Gersony WM, Driscoll DJ, et al. Second natural history study of congenital heart defects: results of treatment of patients with pulmonary valvar stenosis. Circulation 1993;87(suppl):I28–37.

55. Wald RM, Valente AM, Marelli A. Heart failure in adult congenital heart disease: emerging concepts with a focus on tetralogy of Fallot. Trends Cardiovasc Med 2015;25:422–32.

Right Heart Failure and Cardiorenal Syndrome

Thida Tabucanon, MD, MSc[a], Wai Hong Wilson Tang, MD[a,b],*

KEYWORDS

- Cardiorenal syndrome • Right heart failure • Systemic venous congestion • Diuretics

KEY POINTS

- The physiologic definition of cardiorenal syndrome refers to cardiorenal dysregulation as therapy for congestive symptoms and is limited by decline in renal function.
- Right heart failure contributes to the traditional concept of "forward failure" by providing inadequate preload to maintain cardiac output, thereby creating arterial underfilling and impaired renal perfusion.
- Systemic venous congestion as a result of "backward failure" has gained better recognition as an important contributor to increased renal venous pressure, renal interstitial pressure, and increased intra-abdominal pressure as part of splanchnic congestion.
- Current diagnostic strategies, besides bedside assessment, include novel serum or urine biomarkers, renal ultrasonography, and intra-abdominal pressure measurements.
- Effective relief of congestion and maintenance of circulatory organ perfusion remain the primary treatment goals along with the lack of targeted specific therapy improvement in right ventricular reserve.

INTRODUCTION

Heart failure (HF) and renal dysfunction are common coexisting problems in clinical practice. There are bidirectional interrelationships between the heart and kidney, and it has been stated that the kidney is the most important organ related to acute HF (AHF). Acute or chronic dysfunction of one organ induces acute or chronic dysfunction of the other, described as cardiorenal syndrome (CRS).[1,2] In addition, renal dysfunction in HF may lead to reduced diuretic efficiency, diuretic resistance, and worsening of congestion, followed by further deteriorated renal function, which become a vicious cycle. Renal dysfunction also is a strong independent predictor for short-term and long-term outcomes in patients with AHF.[3–9] Traditionally, the causes of CRS have been attributed to renal hypoperfusion, resulting from low cardiac output and over-diuresis. In the past decades, however, data have increasingly demonstrated more of a correlation between venous congestion and CRS, rather than low cardiac output, linking the failing right heart to CRS. Right HF (RHF) and CRS both have complex and intertwining pathophysiologies that may involve various organs and systems beyond isolated dysfunction of the heart and/or kidneys. This review focuses on pathophysiology intersections between RHF and cardiocentric phenotypes of CRS (type 1 and type 2) as well as considerations of therapeutic management.

DEFINITION AND CLASSIFICATION OF CARDIORENAL SYNDROME

The Working Group of the National Heart, Lung, and Blood Institute in 2004 first described CRS

[a] Kaufman Center for Heart Failure Treatment and Recovery, Heart, Vascular, and Thoracic Institute, Cleveland Clinic, Cleveland, OH, USA; [b] Department of Cardiovascular Medicine, Cleveland Clinic, 9500 Euclid Avenue, Desk J3-4, Cleveland, OH 44195, USA
* Corresponding author. Department of Cardiovascular Medicine, Cleveland Clinic, 9500 Euclid Avenue, Desk J3-4, Cleveland, OH 44195.
E-mail address: TANGW@ccf.org

Cardiol Clin 38 (2020) 185–202
https://doi.org/10.1016/j.ccl.2020.01.004

as the result of interaction between the kidney and other circulatory compartments that increase circulating volume and symptoms of HF and disease progression.[10] The most extreme progression of cardiorenal dysregulation leads to the condition, CRS, and therapy for congestive symptoms is limited by decline in renal function. This physiologic concept is in stark contrast with classification schemes proposed by Ronco and colleagues[1] and the Acute Dialysis Quality Initiative (ADQI)[2] that described the primary organ dysfunction (heart or kidney) and time course (acute or chronic), with an additional subtype for a systemic condition affecting both organs simultaneously (**Table 1**). Although useful to clarify more precisely the clinical presentation of CRS, the overlap between the Ronco/ADQI subtypes and frequent evolution of one subtype to another could be challenging and has limited such a classification scheme to guide therapeutic management. Furthermore, there are limited quantifications of cardiac and renal functional assessments to determine these subtypes, rendering them largely descriptive and academic in clinical applications.

TRADITIONAL CONCEPT OF IMPAIRED FORWARD PERFUSION IN CARDIORENAL SYNDROME

Traditionally, RHF often has been characterized by the inability of the right ventricle (RV) to generate enough stroke volume, thereby resulting in systemic venous congestion, underfilling of the left ventricle (LV), and, in the most advanced cases, cardiogenic shock. Acute RHF can occur because of abruptly increased RV afterload (pulmonary embolus, hypoxia, and acidemia) or decreased RV contractility (RV ischemia, myocarditis, and postcardiotomy shock). Each condition represents a unique hemodynamic challenge for the RV. In addition, the failing right heart can be a downstream manifestation of a primary insult (eg, pulmonary hypertension or tricuspid valve dysfunction due to pacemaker lead interference), even though the downstream disturbances of the cardiorenal interactions likely are similar.

Historically, impairment in forward flow (cardiac output) leading to decreased renal arterial perfusion and neurohormonal activation has been considered a key event in CRS.[11,12] It, therefore, is logical that the RV as the primary contributor to adequate preload directly contributes to CRS. Original descriptions of CRS postulated that renal blood flow could be preserved until the cardiac index fell below 1.5 L/min/m²,[12] which often is described as *prerenal*. Arterial underfilling, secondary to low cardiac output and increased peripheral vascular resistance, may activate the renin-angiotensin-aldosterone system (RAAS), sympathetic nervous system (SNS), and release of arginine vasopressin, resulting in water and sodium retention and worsening HF.[11]

CLINICAL EVIDENCE OF SYSTEMIC VENOUS CONGESTION AND IMPAIRED RENAL FUNCTION

Over the past decade, there has been increasing evidence that worsening renal function (WRF) in the setting of CRS may not be adequately explained solely due to arterial underfilling.[4,13–16] The Acute Decompensated Heart Failure National Registry observed the same incidence rate of renal

Table 1
Types of cardiorenal syndrome

Type of Cardiorenal Syndrome	Definition	Conditions
Type 1: acute CRS	Acute worsening of heart function leading to kidney injury and/or dysfunction	AHF, acute cardiogenic shock
Type 2: chronic CRS	Chronic abnormalities in heart function leading to progressive and permanent CKD	Chronic HF
Type 3: acute renocardiac syndrome	AKI causing acute heart dysfunction	Acute glomerulonephritis/AKI cause AHF
Type 4: chronic renocardiac syndrome	CKD leading to chronic heart disease and CKD progression	CKD cause cardiac hypertrophy, decreased cardiac function
Type 5: secondary CRS	Systemic diseases leading to heart and kidney damage/dysfunction	Diabetes, sepsis, septic shock

dysfunction in AHF with reduced and preserved systolic function,[17] indicating that impairment of forward flow is not likely the primary culprit in the large majority of patients experiencing CRS. Meanwhile, WRF after treatment occurs more often in the setting of HF with preserved ejection fraction than those with severely reduced ejection fraction.[18] It, therefore, is important to recognize that the occurrence of WRF in the setting of impaired perfusion (cardiogenic or distributive shock leading to intravascular depletion that often is a detrimental consequence) can be significantly different from that in the setting of systemic venous congestion. The latter often leads to increased venous pressure and increases the backward pressure into the intra-abdominal organs that can be reversed with effective decongestion. Signs and symptoms of congestion, such as the presence of elevated jugular venous pressure, orthopnea, ascites, and edema, were independently related to the reduced estimated glomerular filtration rate (eGFR) and were associated with increased mortality.[19] In patients with predominant RHF, systemic venous congestion assessed by inferior vena cava diameter was an independent determinant of eGFR,[20] and reduction of inferior vena cava size after treatment was associated with improvement of eGFR. This is supported by the study of noninvasive and invasive measurements of venous congestion that showed correlation between high central venous pressure (CVP) with baseline renal impairment[4,15,16,21] and WRF in AHF[14] and WRF less frequently in patients with CVP less than 8 mm Hg after intensive medical therapy.[14] Moreover, high CVP also was an independent predictor for cardiac rehospitalization[22] and all-cause mortality.[4,15] Finally, in patients who had congestion confirmed by echocardiography, relief of venous congestion showed significant renal function improvement in HF with RV dysfunction.[23] **Table 2** is a summary of studies that showed an association between venous congestion and renal dysfunction. It is important to recognize that WRF in the setting of aggressive diuresis also can lead to hemoconcentration that is not necessarily worsening and can indicate an effective therapeutic response with effective relief of systemic venous congestion.

PATHOPHYSIOLOGY OF RIGHT HEART FAILURE AND CARDIORENAL SYNDROME

As discussed previously, the overarching pathophysiology of CRS in RHF is complex through a variety of mechanisms due to the complex interrelationship between the heart and kidney, as shown in **Fig. 1**. Systemic venous congestion develops in the context of RHF—often the final pathway of many cardiovascular diseases—can be found in either isolated RV failure or biventricular failure. The consequences of venous congestion on various organs (backward congestion) play a pivotal role in the pathophysiology of CRS and have both local and systemic effects. Local venous congestion effects the kidneys and splanchnic organs and leads to renal and splanchnic congestion. Also, venous congestion produces systemic vascular congestion. Therefore, the effects of venous congestion resulting in mechanical, biological and immune responses, which contribute to CRS development.

Several mechanisms have been postulated to explain the effect of venous congestion and renal dysfunction involving various organs, not only the heart and kidneys, which originally were called CRS. Elevated renal venous pressure obliterated renal tubules by distending renal venules,[24] reducing renal perfusion pressure (RPP), and increasing renal interstitial pressure by fluid extravasation, leading to a hypoxic state of renal parenchyma, tubular dysfunction. It also activated the RAAS[25–29] and SNS,[30] activated vascular inflammation by endothelial cell dysfunction,[31] and contributed to other abdominal organs (ie, splanchnic venous and intestinal congestion) and lymphatic congestion.[32] These mechanisms are not mutually exclusive, and a large majority of them have been difficult to assess at the bedside. These mechanisms are discussed further as they relate to the pathophysiology of RHF and CRS.

Renal Congestion

Effect of the pressure
Backward pressure from systemic venous into renal veins can generate increased renal venous pressure that can directly impair a wide range of kidney functions.[33] Studies demonstrated that increased renal venous pressure showed a relationship with reduction in urine flow and alteration in glomerular and tubular function. Furthermore, renal blood flow decreased by increased venous pressure more than an equivalent decrease in arterial pressure.[34] It was previously postulated that increased renal venous pressure leads to renal parenchymal congestion within the nondistensible renal capsule (so-called renal tamponade), resulting in increased interstitial pressure that affects the entire capillary bed and tubules.[35,36] Experimental models have demonstrated the effects of increased renal venous pressures on changes in filtration fraction, flow from baroreceptor, intrinsic vascular reflex

Table 2
Summary of studies linking venous congestion and renal dysfunction in heart failure

Author, Reference, Year	Objectives	Study Population and Study Design	Results	Conclusion
Nohria et al,[4] 2008	To evaluate correlation between hemodynamic parameters using pulmonary artery catheter and renal function	Prospective RCT of 433 patients with AHF	RAP correlated with serum Cr	Renal dysfunction or WRF does not related to poor forward flow alone
Mullens et al,[14] 2009	To determine whether venous congestion, rather than low CO, is associated primarily with WRF in ADHF	Prospective observational study of 145 ADHF treated with PAC guided	WRF associated with high CVP with 75% of patients with baseline CVP >24 mm Hg developed WRF	Venous congestion is more important factor driving WRF
Damman et al,[15] 2009	To investigate the relationship between increased CVP, renal function, and mortality	Retrospective study of 2557 CVD patients with RHC	CVP >6 mm Hg showed steep declined in eGFR	Increased CVP is associated with impaired renal function
Damman et al,[19] 2010	To investigate the relationship between signs and symptoms of congestion, renal impairment and outcomes	Double-blind RCT of 2647 HF NYHA class III/VI	Signs and symptoms of congestion were independently related to low eGFR and increase in mortality	Signs and symptoms of congestion are associated with renal impairment and independent determinants of prognosis
Guglin et al,[16] 2011	To assess correlation of congestion and renal function	Retrospective study of 178 patients with HF and who underwent RHC	Serum Cr correlated with CVP, PCWP, and RPP but not with CI or LVEF	Renal dysfunction correlated with venous congestion and low RPP
Testani et al,[23] 2010	To assess diuresis in RV dysfunction and resulting in reduced venous congestion and improving in renal function	Prospective study of 141 patients with HF with congestion assessed by echocardiography	RV dysfunction had more frequent venous congestion and lower incidence of WRF	Relief of venous congestion in RV dysfunction likely leads to improved renal function

Abbreviations: ADHF, acute decompensated heart failure; AHF, acute heart failure; CI, cardiac index; Cr, creatinine; CO, cardiac output; CVP, central venous pressure; eGFR, estimated glomerular filtration rate; LVEF, left ventricular ejection fraction; NYHA, New York Heart Association; PAC, pulmonary arterial catheter; PCWP, pulmonary capillary wedge pressure; RAP, right atrial pressure; RCT, randomized control trial; RHC, right heart catheterization; RPP, renal perfusion pressure; RV, right ventricle; WRF, worsening renal function.

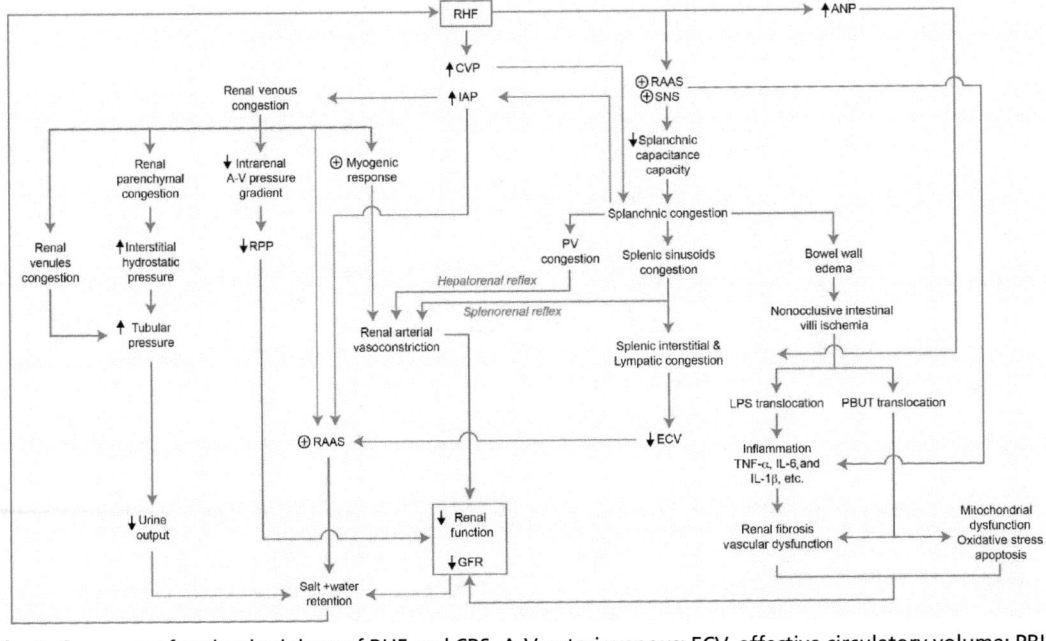

Fig. 1. Summary of pathophysiology of RHF and CRS. A-V, arteriovenous; ECV, effective circulatory volume; PBUT, protein-bound uremic toxins; PV, portal vein.

response (myogenic response), tubuloglomerular feedback (TGF), RAAS, and SNS.[37]

Clinically, renal venous congestion secondary to increased systemic pressure often is reflected by high CVP and may lead to decreased intrarenal arteriovenous gradient and, theoretically, decreased RPP. It is a gradient between aortic and renal venous pressure that is equal to mean arterial pressure (MAP) minus CVP. Studies in AHF patients, however, showed incongruous results that demonstrated the similarity in RPP (estimated by MAP − CVP) in those with and without WRF during AHF hospitalization.[14] These observations may imply that mechanisms of WRF may be related more directly to venous congestion. Meanwhile, in animal experimental studies, an increased renal venous pressure retards urine flow equal to the decrease in arterial pressure.[24,38] Therefore, congested renal venules and increased interstitial hydrostatic pressure may compress renal tubules and obstruct the urine flow.[24,39] Moreover, increased renal interstitial pressure may decrease renal blood flow even in the presence of furosemide (to block TGF), renal decapsulation (local sympathetic inhibition), or systemic inhibition of SNS (using phentolamine).[40] In a human study, abdominal compression led to increased intraabdominal and renal venous pressure and was associated with a fall in urine output.[41] Regarding filtration function, stepwise increase in renal venous pressure, particularly during volume expansion, showed decrease of GFR,[42–46] which

is explained by increased renal venous pressure, resulting in increased tubular pressure,[43] which opposes filtration and net ultrafiltration pressure.[39] As early as 1913, the experimental study of chronic passive renal congestion in dogs created by selective banding of the unilateral renal vein showed effect on renal excretory function.[47] Conversely, reduction in venous pressure demonstrated reversibility of impaired natriuresis/aquaresis and GFR.[42,45]

Neural reflex and neurohormonal mechanism
Myogenic response is an autoregulatory mechanism in mammalian kidney and is the intrinsic capability of the renal vasculature, particularly in the small-diameter vessels, in response to an increase in wall tension, which results in smooth muscle cell contraction by increased intracellular calcium and activation of myosin light chain kinase.[48] Rise in renal venous pressure by a partially obstructed renal vein, resulting in vasoconstriction, has been studied in animal models and showed a strong effect on arterial microcirculation by triggered sympathetic vasoconstrictive neural responses[49] that were both extrarenal and intrarenal mechanisms.[50] Surgical or pharmacologic sympathectomy partially prevents the effects of venous congestion.[50] In addition, stimulation of mechanoreceptors in an intrarenal vein by venous pressure enhanced local sympathetic renal nerve activation, resulting in intrarenal arterial vasoconstriction and decreased GFR.[51,52]

Experimental studies have demonstrated increase in both intra-abdominal pressure (IAP) and renal venous pressure, affecting an increase in plasma renin activity and aldosterone level.[53–55] These effects seem not to be affecting by hemodynamic effect which showed no significant changes in hemodynamic parameters such as cardiac index.[46] An animal study as early as 1949 showed elevated renal venous pressure can significantly diminish sodium and water excretion but with modest elevations in renal venous pressure and slight changes in renal plasma flow, GFR, and filtration fraction.[45] These effects of congestion impinging on renal sodium excretion lead to a vicious cycle of salt and water retention and more renal congestion.[56]

Splanchnic Congestion

Studies of the interaction between splanchnic congestion and CRS have demonstrated that they might be a strong contributor to development of renal dysfunction in HF. The splanchnic veins have a function as a blood reservoir and actively function in regulation for cardiac preload during changes in volume status,[57] which is regulated by passive (transmural pressure changes) or active (SNS regulation) mechanisms.[57–59] Furthermore, splanchnic veins have high capability to pool additional blood volume, which contributed up to 66% of total additional volume.[58] Maladaptation of splanchnic capacitance function in HF, however, has been demonstrated,[60] which raised speculation that incremental capacity of splanchnic capacitance is limited and, thereby, could be the result of long-standing venous congestion and neurohormonal activation in advanced HF[61] and might be a significant factor in CRS development.

Liver and spleen are crucial visceral organs in the splanchnic circulation and contain approximately a quarter of total blood volume in the human body.[58,62] Studies in splanchnic compartment and CRS showed correlation between major visceral organs and kidney by local reflex systems. The first reflex system is hepatorenal reflex, which is regulated by receptors in intrahepatic circulation and affecting to kidney function by neurally mediated.[63,64] This occurs through (1) chronic splanchnic congestion, resulting in portal vein distension and stretch of the venous wall, which leads to renal vasoconstriction,[65] and (2) increased intrahepatic adenosine by portal vasoconstriction activated by SNS mediated α-adrenergic receptor and release to circulation. This results in renal vasoconstriction and sodium retention by activation TGF.[66,67] The splenorenal reflex is the second local reflex system which activated by raised intrasplenic

venous pressure and resulting in neurally medicated renal vasoconstriction.[68,69] Conversely, interruption of either afferent or efferent reflex pathway results in elimination of both hepatorenal and splenorenal reflexes.[64,69] Furthermore, splenic congestion leads to interstitial edema by intrasplenic fluid extravasation from splenic sinusoids, which are freely permeable for plasma protein. Thus, intravascular hydrostatic pressure becomes a main determinant for fluid transport. Fluid extravasation from splenic sinusoids to lymphatic circulation and interstitial tissue, respectively, lead to perception of decreased effective circulatory volume and exacerbate neurohormonal activation, creating a vicious cycle of sodium and water retention.[32] Atrial natriuretic peptide (ANP) might be another contributor to promote reduction in central plasma volume. Infusion of ANP in rats resulted in hemoconcentration and reduction in plasma volume, which are not entirely accounted for by excretion of urine.[70] This effect was explained as ANP having effects on splanchnic hemodynamics, including increased intrasplenic pressure and increased intrasplenic fluid extravasation.[71]

Dysfunction of intestinal endothelial cells secondary to bowel edema due to backward congestion and consequences in alteration of gut microbiota have been demonstrated and speculated to be a contributor to development of CRS in RHF. Intestinal villi have a unique microcirculation, and the tips of intestinal villi are the most susceptible to anoxic damage.[72] Splanchnic congestion, coexisting with low perfusion and sympathetic activation, leads to increased risk of nonocclusive ischemia of intestinal villi.[73] In addition, increased intestinal wall thickness and edema have been observed in patients with HF and have been shown to have a direct correlation with increased paracellular intestinal permeability[74] which is secondary to hypoxia, hypoperfusion, and endotoxin production by intestinal gram-negative bacteria.[74,75] These structural and functional alterations of gut barrier result in translocation of gut microbiota and their components into host circulation, including lipopolysaccharides (LPSs) and protein-bound uremic toxins produced by gut microbiota, which contribute to renal dysfunction.[76–78] LPSs, found in the outer membrane of gram-negative bacteria, further promote mucosal barrier function deterioration and systemic inflammatory processes.[79] LPSs and proinflammatory cytokines levels were found to be higher in patients with edematous chronic HF than in nonedematous and healthy volunteers. Also, reduction could be demonstrated after diuretic treatment.[80] Inflammation activation is discussed later.

Although evaluation of splanchnic congestion is not clinically available unless there are detectable ascites, increased IAP might be used and reflects splanchnic congestion. As reported in the study, increased IAP ($\geq$8 mm Hg) was found in 60% of patients admitted with advanced HF,[81] and ascites were found in a small number, which suggested splanchnic congestion could contribute to increased IAP.[32] Furthermore, increased IAP was associated with impaired renal function, and changes in IAP were strong predictors of change in renal function compared with hemodynamic parameters.[41,81] IAP may contribute to renal dysfunction by increased renal parenchyma, renal venous and intraglomerular pressures, and decreased RPP reflected by reduced GFR.[41,46,55,81–83] Moreover, increased IAP also was associated with RAAS activation, which showed increased plasma renin activity and aldosterone level.[55] Reduction in IAP by ultrafiltration or paracentesis has corresponded with improvement in renal function in some patients.[84]

INFLAMMATION AND CARDIORENAL SYNDROME

There are increasing data that inflammation could be related to pathogenesis of CRS. Production of proinflammatory cytokines as a consequence of HF could be from neurohormonal activation; venous congestion, including either local congestion, such as splanchnic congestion and intrarenal venous congestion; or systemic venous congestion. Elevated cytokines in HF have been demonstrated, such as tumor necrotic factor α (TNF-α), interleukin (IL)-6, and IL-1,[85,86] and correlate with poor clinical outcomes.[87–89] These cytokines have direct biological effects on both structural and functional damage to various end organs, including the heart, vasculature, and kidney.[90] Studies have shown that inflammation results in depressed cardiac function, vascular dysfunction, renal fibrosis, and progressive renal dysfunction.[91–97] Finally, inflammation may increase vascular permeability and promote absorption of proinflammatory endotoxins from the bowel.[90] Hence, a vicious cycle develops, leading to increased congestion due to end organ damage and more inflammation activation.

Inflammation Consequences of Neurohormonal Activation

Increased activity of RAAS and SNS in HF leading to chronic inflammation has been demonstrated. Angiotensin II (AII) increases TNF-α biosynthesis in myocardium, which is mediated through the angiotensin 1 receptor.[98] The animal study with AII-treated rats showed increased renal tissue expression of TNF-α (glomeruli, mainly at endothelium of tubules and vasculature), activated nuclear factor κB, and systemic infusion of AII-induced renal synthesis of IL-6, and monocyte chemoattractant protein-1 coexisting with glomerular and interstitial inflammatory cells in kidney.[99,100] Chronic blockage of angiotensin 1 receptor supports the role of AII inflammatory responses, which showed reduction in circulating proinflammatory cytokines, such as TNF-α.[101] SNS also promoted inflammatory responses, which was demonstrated in the animal study when isoproterenol infusion increased expression of TNF-α, IL-6, and IL-1β in myocardium cells and cardiac blood vessels,[102] and β-adrenergic blocker administration decreases those effects.[102]

Inflammatory Consequences of Venous Congestion

Venous and tissue congestion may promote inflammatory responses by various mechanisms.[90] Mesenteric venous congestion leads to bowel wall edema and increased vascular permeability and gram-negative bacterial translocation through the endothelial cells of the intestinal villi; thereby, endotoxin release has been proposed.[103] Endotoxins, such as LPSs, which is elevated in HF,[104] promotes the secretion of proinflammatory cytokines through the effect on human monocyte and macrophage function, such as TNF-α, the IL-1 family, IL-6, IL-8, the IL-10 family, the IL-12 family, IL-15, and transforming growth factor β.[105] LPSs and cytokine levels have shown to be increased in edematous chronic HF.[80] According to a cohort study in chronic HF, more elevated LPS levels in patients with peripheral edema were demonstrated, and these levels showed a reduction after acute diuretic treatment.[80] In addition, supporting data showed higher endotoxin levels in the hepatic vein compared with the LV in AHF, which suggests bacterial or endotoxin translocation from bowel to the blood stream.[106]

Besides bacterial and endotoxin translocation, hemodynamic stimulation by intravascular volume expansion can promote vascular inflammation and endothelial cell activation through cytokine secretion itself[31,90] and alter other bioactive molecules, such as nitric oxide and prostacyclin function.[107] Regarding inflammation, both in vitro and in vivo studies have shown evidence of activation of vascular endothelial cells and increased production of a variety of vasoactive mediators, including inflammatory cytokines after biomechanical stress, including TNF-α and IL-6.[108–110] A specific study of fluid load in normal dogs created venous congestion accompanied by vascular endothelial activation of inflammation and oxidative stress.[111] Moreover, in a human study, peripheral congestion was created through applied pressure using a tourniquet on the arms of healthy subjects, which caused release of inflammatory markers, IL-6 and endothelin-1.[112]

Hence, evidence of systemic inflammation in HF has been increasing and is postulated to contribute to CRS development, which could be secondary to neurohormonal and sympathetic activation, and vascular and tissue congestion. Inflammation leads to end organ damage, causing progressive fluid accumulation; thereby, further inflammatory activation occurs.

EFFECTS OF RIGHT VENTRICULAR VOLUME OVERLOAD

RF dysfunction and dilation in RHF secondary to increased RV filling pressure lead to ventricular interdependence, which result in leftward shift of interventricular septum and altered LV geometry.[113] Hence, reducing LV distensibility, preload, and cardiac output, thereby reducing renal arterial pressure, might be another therapeutic options in CRS management.[15,113,114] This often is seen in isolated RHF, as in advanced pulmonary arterial hypertension.

NOVEL DIAGNOSTIC STRATEGIES FOR CONGESTION AND CARDIORENAL SYNDROME
Serum and Urine Biomarkers

Biomarkers provide a wide spectrum of prevention, early diagnosis, treatment, and outcomes of organ injury, including in the heart and kidney.[115] There are various biomarkers for renal and cardiac injury, which provide different roles in diagnosis and prognosis in acute kidney injury (AKI), HF, and CRS.[116,117] B-type natriuretic peptide (BNP), a cardiac biomarker, is a marker of myocardial stretch and has both diagnostic and prognostic roles in HF and CRS.[116] In HF with impaired renal function, including CRS, there are higher BNP levels compared with patients with normal renal function, which could be attributed to impaired renal excretion, volume overload by impaired renal function, and cardiomyopathy associated with renal dysfunction.[118–120] In CRS, there is elevation of other cardiac biomarkers, such as cardiac troponin[120,121] and galactin-3.[122] High levels of glactin-3 and cardiac troponin were associated with higher mortality in HF.[121,122]

Besides cardiac biomarkers, which are directly associated with congestion, renal biomarkers also have value for both diagnosis and prognosis in CRS. Neutrophil gelatinase-associated lipocalin (NGAL) is a large lysosomal enzyme originating in the proximal tubular cell; detection of urine NGAL indicates proximal tubular injury.[123] Elevated NGAL was observed in HF with renal dysfunction,[120] and elevated serum and urine levels of NGAL could be a useful predictor for dialysis and death in AKI, including CRS.[124] Serial measurement of NGAL in AHF is an accurate predictor of WRF,[125] although a majority of patients with CRS have relatively low urine NGAL levels because significant intrinsic kidney injuries are relatively uncommon. AKI biomarkers, such as NGAL, are not readily available for clinical use.

Cystatin C (CysC) is a renal biomarker present in all nucleated cells with a constant production rate. It is freely filtrated, completely reabsorbed, and not secreted by renal tubules.[117] CysC is dramatically better than creatinine for measuring GFR, because CysC is not determined primarily by muscle mass.[126] The studied use of CysC calculation for GFR and reclassified chronic kidney disease (CKD) stage showed stronger correlation and more linear correlation to death along with all eGFR.[127] Combined CysC and others biomarkers, such as N-terminal pro-BNP and cardiac troponin T, had additive prognostic value for adverse events in AHF.[128] Albuminuria in HF without concomitant comorbidity, such as renal dysfunction, hypertension, and diabetes, might provide greater diagnostic power for CRS than by using eGFR alone.[129,130] Albuminuria also had a prognostic value in HF and is associated with increased mortality and increased admissions for HF independent of eGFR, diabetes, and hypertension.[129,131]

It is important to recognize that few cardiac or renal biomarkers are specific to RHF or CRS. Biomarker-guided strategies also have failed to uniformly provide incremental treatment benefits over standard of care, largely because the biomarkers, discussed previously, have not distinguished RHF as a unique contributor to CRS, and a majority of biomarkers have been developed with diagnosing a clinical condition in mind (eg, AKI or HF).

Renal Ultrasonography

Renal vein flow pattern using Doppler ultrasound is a noninvasive tool, which has been studied in several situations, including HF with renal venous congestion.[132–137] In HF, intrarenal venous flow patterns depend on right atrial pressure (RAP) and are strongly correlated with clinical outcomes.[136] Patterns of renal venous vein flow were stratified by RAP. Continuous renal vein flow patterns were correlated with normal RAP (RAP <8 mm Hg). A discontinuous renal flow pattern was associated with increased RAP, and a monophasic pattern had the highest RAP and poorest prognosis (<40% survival at 1 year).[136] The discontinuous pattern is explained by transmission of backward pressure from increased RAP to the renal vein, which results in increased pulsatility of flow pattern and reflects the response of renal vessels in increased intrarenal pressure within the encapsulated capsule[132] **(Fig. 2)**.

Moreover, renal flow pattern, rather than renal resistive index (RI), which is calculated from renal arterial waveform, was shown to have incremental prognostic value[136] that could reflect the more important role of renal venous congestion rather than renal hypoperfusion. Reversibility of renal flow pattern has not been demonstrated, however, by any current therapeutic options; hence, data are lacking to support the use of renal venous flow pattern to make the decision for decongestive therapeutic strategies. In addition, this tool

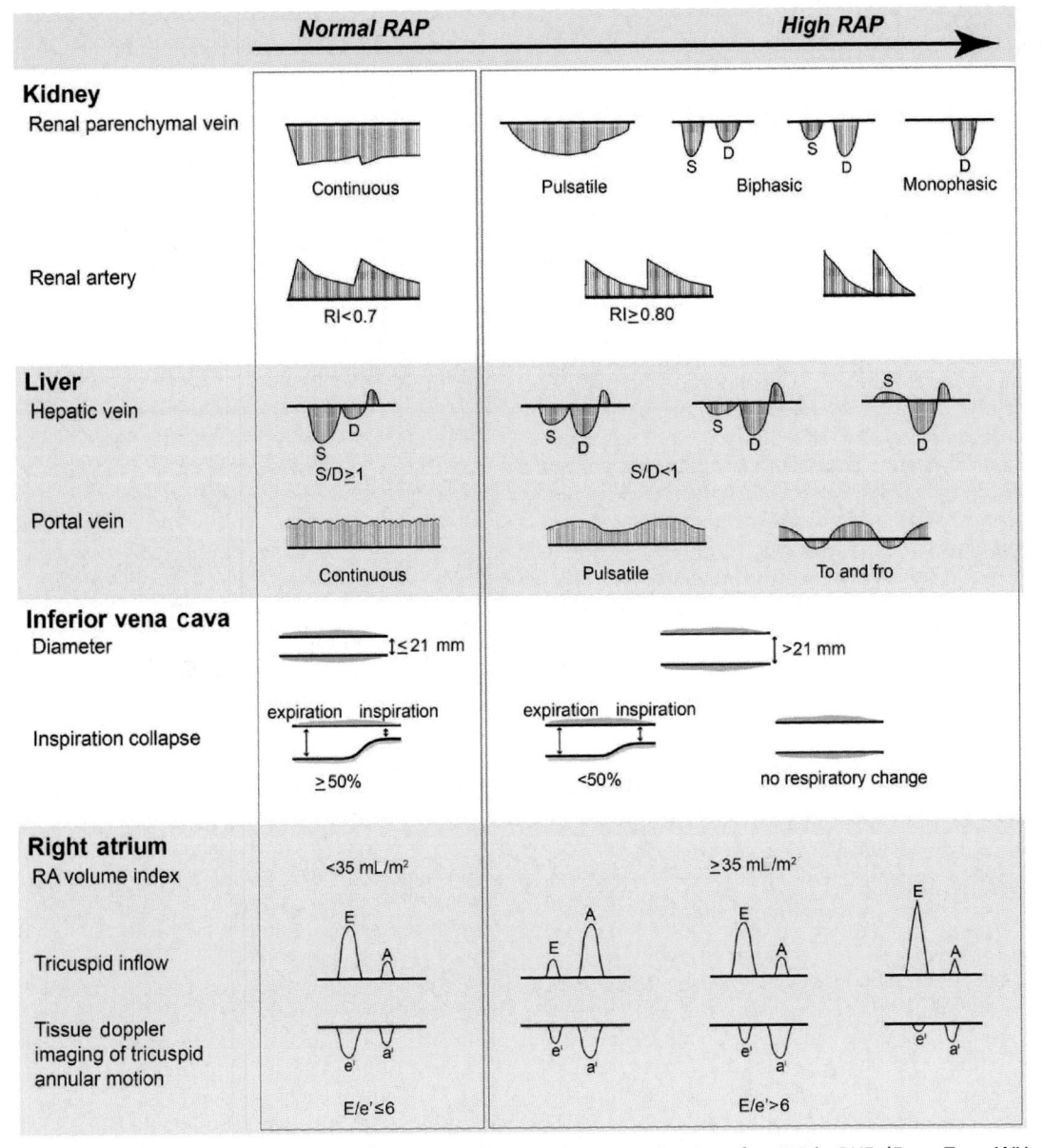

Fig. 2. Ultrasound profiles across the spectrum of elevated RAP as indications for CRS in RHF. (*From* Tang WH, Kitai T. Intrarenal Venous Flow: A Window Into the Congestive Kidney Failure Phenotype of Heart Failure? JACC Heart Fail. 2016;4(8):683-6; with permission.)

requires expertise to perform, technical feasibility, and validation for consistency of Doppler waveform sampling by operators and in a diverse group of patients.

Intra-abdominal Pressure via Indwelling Urine Catheter

Splanchnic congestion secondary to backward pressure in RHF can be evaluated by measure of IAP, as discussed previously. Measurements of IAP could be obtained by measuring intrabladder pressure using the intrabladder catheter connected to a transducer. Increased IAP is defined as elevated pressure greater than normal range of 5 mm Hg to 7 mm Hg.[81]

MEDICAL TREATMENT OPTIONS FOR RIGHT HEART FAILURE AND CARDIORENAL SYNDROME

Decongestion is the cornerstone in CRS treatment to reduce systemic venous congestion and return balance in hemodynamic, neurohormonal, and biological activation. Hence, improvement of RPP by reducing CVP, renal venous pressure, and RV volume overload thereby improve RV and LV performance.[138] Decongestion strategies include diuretics, ultrafiltration, and dialysis. Oral diuretic is the first-line strategy and has been used for years with natriuretic effect and volume reduction, leading to immediate relief of HF symptoms.[139] The most challenging management of decongestion in CRS is diuretic resistance due to several mechanisms, such as impaired renal function, reduced cardiac output leading to low delivery of diuretic to the site of action (kidney), inadequate dose of diuretic, and inadequate substrate (sodium and chloride) at the renal tubules.[138,140]

Loop Diuretics

Loop diuretics inhibit Na^+-K^+-$2Cl^-$ cotransporter at the thick ascending limb of the loop of Henle and are the most common diuretics used in clinical practice because they have a short peak of action (10–30 minutes and 1–1.5 hours for intravenous and administration oral administration, respectively).[141] Loop diuretics cause natriuresis, thereby causing net negative water and salt balance and reduced volume overload. The most commonly used loop diuretics are furosemide, torsemide, and bumetanide. Torsemide has greater and more consistent oral bioavailability (90%) than furosemide (10%–90%).[141–143] The oral bioavailability of furosemide can be improved when taken before a meal, because furosemide

has been shown to have a 30% reduction in oral bioavailability with food.[144] Intravenous or novel subcutaneous furosemide ensures 100% bioavailability.[145,146] Torsemide, with a longer half-life, however, leads to less frequent doses compared with furosemide.[142] Hence, torsemide is suggested as a more effective and well-tolerated diuretic in CHF compared with furosemide in several studies, including a meta-analysis.[147–149] Moreover, loop diuretics are protein-bound anions; greater than 90% bound to plasma proteins and are secreted in the proximal tubules to reach their site of action.[150] The ability of the diuretic to be protein-bound can have competition from exogenous anions, such as nonsteroidal anti-inflammatory drugs, and endogenous anions, such as bile acid and uremic toxin,[116,138] resulting in reduced diuretic efficacy. In addition, hypoalbuminemia, which is common in advanced HF, could contribute to decreased loop diuretic transportation to the site of action.[138]

Dose response to diuretic curve in HF shifts downward and to the right; therefore, a higher dose of diuretic is needed to achieve the same therapeutic effect in HF.[151] A single dose of furosemide elicits transient natriuresis.[152] Hence, increased frequency or continuous use of a loop diuretic could be considered. Continuous dosing of loop diuretics, however, showed no difference in symptom relief or change in renal function in the Diuretic Optimization Strategies Evaluation in Acute Heart Failure (DOSE-AHF) trial compared with a bolus strategy, whereas high doses were associated with greater diuresis, weight loss, and transient WRF.[153] A bolus dose of loop diuretic also showed no difference in mortality compared with continuous infusion. Continuous infusion is associated, however, with more hyponatremia, need for vasopressors, rehospitalization, and death at 6 months.[154] Starting with an intravenous diuretic dose, 2.5 times the daily oral equivalent diuretic dose, is reasonable, as advised in the DOSE-AHF trial.[138] On transition to oral therapy, the dosing frequency should depend on medication half-life, which is every 4 hours to 6 hours for furosemide and bumetanide and every 8 hours to 12 hours for torsemide.[155]

A stepwise pharmacologic strategy has been proposed and studied in post hoc analysis of 3 randomized controlled trials in AHF with CRS, including DOSE-AHF,[153] the Cardiorenal Rescue Study in Acute Decompensated Heart Failure,[156] and Renal Optimization Strategies Evaluation in Acute Heart Failure trial.[157] These studies showed superiority to standard decongestive therapy (including nonadjusted diuretic dose) without WRF and superiority to ultrafiltration in preservation of renal function at 96 hours.[158] The stepwise diuretic regimen is shown in **Table 3**. In the setting of significant venous congestion as a result of RHF, leading to progressive impedance of venous return from the kidneys, effective decongestion may improve RPP and, thereby, increase diuresis and natriuresis. On the other hand, excessive diuresis without adequate right heart reserve can reduce preload and impair cardiac output, leading to relative intravascular hypovolemia and decreased diuresis and natriuresis. Regardless, the rise in serum creatinine may or may not be indicative of intrinsic injury or damage to the kidneys, and the ultimate delicate balance can be impacted by the status of the right heart.

Diuretic Resistance

To date, the definition of diuretic resistance is not clear and no standard definition is available. It has been defined, however, as diminished or loss of diuretic response before the therapeutic goal of relief from edema has been achieved.[159] There are various metrics to measure either diuretic efficacy or resistance, including weight loss, net fluid loss, urine output per 40 mg of intravenous furosemide-equivalent doses, and natriuresis.[155] These measures account for loop diuretics, the most commonly used diuretics in volume overload, but do not account for other diuretics.[155] Moreover, there is no definite cutoff for those metrics for either diuretic resistance or efficacy. Diuretic efficacy in HF has been shown, however,

---

Table 3
Stepped diuretic strategy: treatment algorithm from Cardiorenal Rescue Study in Acute Decompensated Heart Failure

Daily using UO assessment
  UO >5 L/d: reduce current diuretic regimen if desired
  UO3-5 L/d: continue current diuretic regimen
  UO <3 L/d: see diuretic table

At 24-h assessment
  If persistent volume overload
  • Assess daily UO
  • Advance to the next step on diuretic table if UO <3 L/d

At 48-h assessment
  If persistent volume overload
  • Assess daily UO
  • Advance to the next step on diuretic table if UO <3 L/d and consider
    Dobutamine or dopamine at 2 μg/kg/min if SBP <110 mm Hg and LVEF <40% or RV systolic dysfunction
    Nitroglycerin or nesiritide if SBP >120 mm Hg and severe symptoms

At 72-96–h assessment
  If persistent volume overload
  • Assess daily UO
  • Advance to the next step on diuretic table if UO <3 L/d and consider
    Dobutamine or dopamine at 2 μg/kg/min if SBP <110 mm Hg and LVEF <40% or RV systolic dysfunction
    Nitroglycerin or nesiritide if SBP >120 mm Hg and severe symptoms
  • Hemodynamic guided IV therapy
  • LVAD
  • UF or dialysis

Diuretic table

Current loop diuretic dose ± thiazide	Suggested dose	
	Loop diuretic dose	Thiazide dose
≤80 mg	40 mg IV bolus + 5 mg/h	0
81–160 mg	80 mg IV bolus + 10 mg/h	5 mg metolazone QD
161–240 mg	80 mg IV bolus + 20 mg/h	5 mg metolazone BID
≥240 mg	80 mg IV bolus + 30 mg/h	5 mg metolazone BID

Abbreviations: LVAD, LV assist device; LVEF, LV ejection fraction; SBP, systolic blood pressure; UF, ultrafiltration; UO, urine output.
From https://biolincc.nhlbi.nih.gov/media/studies/carress/Protocol.pdf?link_time=2020-01-15_23:30:43.304569.

as a strong predictor for mortality and morbidity, including all-cause death, HF readmission, and renal-related readmission after correction with baseline eGFR.[140,160–165] This was attributed to GFR and diuretic efficacy represented in a different part of kidney function; whereas GFR is the glomerular function, diuretic efficacy is the tubular function.[155]

Braking phenomena, diminished diuretic-induced natriuresis by hemodynamic and neurohormonal responses, have been implied as contributors to diuretic resistance.[138] Hemodynamic braking develops when diuretic reduces extracellular fluid volume, thereby causing SNS and RAAS activation, which increases sodium reabsorption at proximal tubules.[166] Neurohormonal braking develops when diuretic increases urine sodium and activates TGF, causing renin production, thereby causing afferent arteriolar vasoconstriction, which indirectly reduces sodium filtration.[167] Nephron remodeling (distal tubular hypertrophy and hyperplasia) as a consequence of prolonged use of loop diuretic also is considered a determinant of diuretic efficacy.[168,169] In addition, furosemide-treatment in HF has demonstrated enhanced distal sodium transport more than proximal, which could attenuate the loop diuretic response.[170] Hence, addition of nonloop diuretics (ie, thiazide or potassium sparing diuretic), which is termed, *segmental nephron blockage*, may be reasonable and also might overcome the braking phenomenon and nephron remodeling, thereby augmenting natriuresis[171] without compromising GFR.[156] The evidence of this approach in CRS is still lacking, however, let alone in the setting of RHF. Moreover, renal dysfunction in the context of CRS reduces excretion of the diuretic into the tubular lumen and natriuresis in CKD is reduced by decreased sodium filtration.[172,173]

Other Medical Therapies

Vasoactive and inotropic drugs have been used extensively in clinical practice for significant RHF, although clinical trial evidence has been lacking (especially regarding preference of milrinone over other vasoactive drugs). Much of the literature is based on cardiocentric optimization of hemodynamic parameters in advanced HF patients. In the acute setting where pulmonary hypertension is a major contributor, selective pulmonary vasodilators have been used with success (eg, inhaled nitric oxide, prostacyclin, and iloprost), although there are few data to support the role of phosphodiesterase type 5 inhibitors for this indication.

SUMMARY

The heart and kidney have complex bidirectional interlinks, termed CRS type 1 and type 2, that represent the renal dysfunction secondary to acute and chronic heart problems, respectively. Contemporary data have shown more correlation of venous congestion and renal dysfunction in HF, which represents the significant influence from the right heart. Prevention of CRS should be the most important goal. This requires understanding of the pathophysiology of CRS, which involves several interfaces and is not limited to heart and kidney. Splanchnic organs play an important role in pathophysiology of CRS, such as pressure effect of venous congestion, inflammatory responses, and neurohormonal activation. Decongestion is still the mainstay strategy in HF with CRS and is clinically challenging including reduced diuretic efficiency and diuretic resistance. Dedicated diuretic strategy in CRS or diuretic resistance remain unclear, however, and further randomized trials are needed. In addition, clinical assessment of extracellular fluid status remains important to keep the balance between hypervolemia and dehydration.

REFERENCES

1. Ronco C, Haapio M, House AA, et al. Cardiorenal syndrome. J Am Coll Cardiol 2008;52(19):1527–39.
2. Ronco C, McCullough P, Anker SD, et al. Cardiorenal syndromes: report from the consensus conference of the acute dialysis quality initiative. Eur Heart J 2010;31(6):703–11.
3. Damman K, Valente MA, Voors AA, et al. Renal impairment, worsening renal function, and outcome in patients with heart failure: an updated meta-analysis. Eur Heart J 2014;35(7):455–69.
4. Nohria A, Hasselblad V, Stebbins A, et al. Cardiorenal interactions: insights from the ESCAPE trial. J Am Coll Cardiol 2008;51(13):1268–74.
5. Owan TE, Hodge DO, Herges RM, et al. Secular trends in renal dysfunction and outcomes in hospitalized heart failure patients. J Card Fail 2006; 12(4):257–62.
6. Forman DE, Butler J, Wang Y, et al. Incidence, predictors at admission, and impact of worsening renal function among patients hospitalized with heart failure. J Am Coll Cardiol 2004;43(1): 61–7.
7. Gottlieb SS, Abraham W, Butler J, et al. The prognostic importance of different definitions of worsening renal function in congestive heart failure. J Card Fail 2002;8(3):136–41.
8. Krumholz HM, Chen YT, Vaccarino V, et al. Correlates and impact on outcomes of worsening renal

function in patients > or =65 years of age with heart failure. Am J Cardiol 2000;85(9):1110–3.

9. Weinfeld MS, Chertow GM, Stevenson LW. Aggravated renal dysfunction during intensive therapy for advanced chronic heart failure. Am Heart J 1999;138(2 Pt 1):285–90.

10. National Heart Lung, and Blood Institute cardiorenal connections in heart failure and cardiovascular disease 2004. 2004. Available at: https://www.nhlbi.nih.gov/events/2004/cardio-renal-connections-heart-failure-and-cardiovascular-disease. Accessed August 19, 2019.

11. Schrier RW, Abraham WT. Hormones and hemodynamics in heart failure. N Engl J Med 1999;341(8):577–85.

12. Ljungman S, Laragh JH, Cody RJ. Role of the kidney in congestive heart failure. Relationship of cardiac index to kidney function. Drugs 1990;39(Suppl 4):10–21 [discussion: 2–4].

13. Hanberg JS, Sury K, Wilson FP, et al. Reduced cardiac index is not the dominant driver of renal dysfunction in heart failure. J Am Coll Cardiol 2016;67(19):2199–208.

14. Mullens W, Abrahams Z, Francis GS, et al. Importance of venous congestion for worsening of renal function in advanced decompensated heart failure. J Am Coll Cardiol 2009;53(7):589–96.

15. Damman K, van Deursen VM, Navis G, et al. Increased central venous pressure is associated with impaired renal function and mortality in a broad spectrum of patients with cardiovascular disease. J Am Coll Cardiol 2009;53(7):582–8.

16. Guglin M, Rivero A, Matar F, et al. Renal dysfunction in heart failure is due to congestion but not low output. Clin Cardiol 2011;34(2):113–6.

17. Adams KF Jr, Fonarow GC, Emerman CL, et al. Characteristics and outcomes of patients hospitalized for heart failure in the United States: rationale, design, and preliminary observations from the first 100,000 cases in the Acute Decompensated Heart Failure National Registry (ADHERE). Am Heart J 2005;149(2):209–16.

18. Sweitzer NK, Lopatin M, Yancy CW, et al. Comparison of clinical features and outcomes of patients hospitalized with heart failure and normal ejection fraction (> or =55%) versus those with mildly reduced (40% to 55%) and moderately to severely reduced (<40%) fractions. Am J Cardiol 2008;101(8):1151–6.

19. Damman K, Voors AA, Hillege HL, et al. Congestion in chronic systolic heart failure is related to renal dysfunction and increased mortality. Eur J Heart Fail 2010;12(9):974–82.

20. Tanaka M, Yoshida H, Furuhashi M, et al. Deterioration of renal function by chronic heart failure is associated with congestion and oxidative stress in the tubulointerstitium. Intern Med 2011;50(23):2877–87.

21. Damman K, Navis G, Smilde TD, et al. Decreased cardiac output, venous congestion and the association with renal impairment in patients with cardiac dysfunction. Eur J Heart Fail 2007;9(9):872–8.

22. Uthoff H, Thalhammer C, Potocki M, et al. Central venous pressure at emergency room presentation predicts cardiac rehospitalization in patients with decompensated heart failure. Eur J Heart Fail 2010;12(5):469–76.

23. Testani JM, Khera AV, St John Sutton MG, et al. Effect of right ventricular function and venous congestion on cardiorenal interactions during the treatment of decompensated heart failure. Am J Cardiol 2010;105(4):511–6.

24. Winton FR. The influence of venous pressure on the isolated mammalian kidney. J Physiol 1931;72(1):49–61.

25. Schrier RW, De Wardener HE. Tubular reabsorption of sodium ion: influence of factors other than aldosterone and glomerular filtration rate. 2. N Engl J Med 1971;285(23):1292–303.

26. Kastner PR, Hall JE, Guyton AC. Renal hemodynamic responses to increased renal venous pressure: role of angiotensin II. Am J Physiol 1982;243(3):F260–4.

27. Schrier RW. Blood urea nitrogen and serum creatinine: not married in heart failure. Circ Heart Fail 2008;1(1):2–5.

28. Komuro K, Seo Y, Yamamoto M, et al. Assessment of renal perfusion impairment in a rat model of acute renal congestion using contrast-enhanced ultrasonography. Heart Vessels 2018;33(4):434–40.

29. Ruggenenti P, Remuzzi G. Worsening kidney function in decompensated heart failure: treat the heart, don't mind the kidney. Eur Heart J 2011;32(20):2476–8.

30. Ross EA. Congestive renal failure: the pathophysiology and treatment of renal venous hypertension. J Card Fail 2012;18(12):930–8.

31. Ganda A, Onat D, Demmer RT, et al. Venous congestion and endothelial cell activation in acute decompensated heart failure. Curr Heart Fail Rep 2010;7(2):66–74.

32. Verbrugge FH, Dupont M, Steels P, et al. Abdominal contributions to cardiorenal dysfunction in congestive heart failure. J Am Coll Cardiol 2013;62(6):485–95.

33. Maxwell MH, Breed ES, Schwartz IL. Renal venous pressure in chronic congestive heart failure. J Clin Invest 1950;29(3):342–8.

34. Afsar B, Ortiz A, Covic A, et al. Focus on renal congestion in heart failure. Clin Kidney J 2016;9(1):39–47.

35. Gottschalk CW, Mylle M. Micropuncture study of pressures in proximal tubules and peritubular capillaries of the rat kidney and their relation to ureteral and renal venous pressures. Am J Physiol 1956;185(2):430–9.

36. Fiksen-Olsen MJ, Strick DM, Hawley H, et al. Renal effects of angiotensin II inhibition during increases in renal venous pressure. Hypertension 1992; 19(2 Suppl):I137–41.

37. Braam B, Cupples WA, Joles JA, et al. Systemic arterial and venous determinants of renal hemodynamics in congestive heart failure. Heart Fail Rev 2012;17(2):161–75.

38. Schirmer HK, Marshall RE, Jackson MP. The effect of altered renal venous pressure on urine flow and cortical metabolism. J Urol 1968;100(3):205–8.

39. Joles JA, Bongartz LG, Gaillard CA, et al. Renal venous congestion and renal function in congestive heart failure. J Am Coll Cardiol 2009;54(17): 1632 [author reply: 3].

40. Clausen G, Oien AH, Aukland K. Myogenic vasoconstriction in the rat kidney elicited by reducing perirenal pressure. Acta Physiol Scand 1992; 144(3):277–90.

41. Bradley SE, Bradley GP. The effect of increased intra-abdominal pressure on renal function in man. J Clin Invest 1947;26(5):1010–22.

42. Firth JD, Raine AE, Ledingham JG. Raised venous pressure: a direct cause of renal sodium retention in oedema? Lancet 1988;1(8593):1033–5.

43. Boberg U, Persson AE. Tubuloglomerular feedback during elevated renal venous pressure. Am J Physiol 1985;249(4 Pt 2):F524–31.

44. Burnett JC Jr, Knox FG. Renal interstitial pressure and sodium excretion during renal vein constriction. Am J Physiol 1980;238(4):F279–82.

45. Blake WD, Wegria R, Keating RP, et al. Effect of increased renal venous pressure on renal function. Am J Physiol 1949;157(1):1–13.

46. Doty JM, Saggi BH, Sugerman HJ, et al. Effect of increased renal venous pressure on renal function. J Trauma 1999;47(6):1000–3.

47. Rowntree LG, Fitz R, Geraghty JT. The effects of experimental chronic passive congestion on renal function. Arch Intern Med (Chic) 1913;11(2): 121–47.

48. Carmines PK, Inscho EW, Gensure RC. Arterial pressure effects on preglomerular microvasculature of juxtamedullary nephrons. Am J Physiol 1990;258(1 Pt 2):F94–102.

49. Abildgaard U, Henriksen O, Amtorp O. Sympathetic reflex-induced vasoconstriction during renal venous stasis elicited from the capsule in the dog kidney. Acta Physiol Scand 1985;123(1):1–8.

50. Abildgaard U, Amtorp O, Agerskov K, et al. Renal vascular adjustments to partial renal venous obstruction in dog kidney. Circ Res 1987;61(2): 194–202.

51. Dilley JR, Corradi A, Arendshorst WJ. Glomerular ultrafiltration dynamics during increased renal venous pressure. Am J Physiol 1983;244(6): F650–8.

52. Haddy FJ. Effect of elevation of intraluminal pressure on renal vascular resistance. Circ Res 1956; 4(6):659–63.

53. Kishimoto T, Maekawa M, Abe Y, et al. Intrarenal distribution of blood flow and renin release during renal venous pressure elevation. Kidney Int 1973; 4(4):259–66.

54. Gudmundsson FF, Gislason HG, Myking OL, et al. Hormonal changes related to reduced renal blood flow and low urine output under prolonged increased intra-abdominal pressure in pigs. Eur J Surg 2002;168(3):178–86.

55. Bloomfield GL, Blocher CR, Fakhry IF, et al. Elevated intra-abdominal pressure increases plasma renin activity and aldosterone levels. J Trauma 1997;42(6):997–1004 [discussion: 5].

56. Guazzi M, Gatto P, Giusti G, et al. Pathophysiology of cardiorenal syndrome in decompensated heart failure: role of lung-right heart-kidney interaction. Int J Cardiol 2013;169(6):379–84.

57. Fudim M, Hernandez AF, Felker GM. Role of volume redistribution in the congestion of heart failure. J Am Heart Assoc 2017;6(8) [pii:e006817].

58. Greenway CV, Lister GE. Capacitance effects and blood reservoir function in the splanchnic vascular bed during non-hypotensive haemorrhage and blood volume expansion in anaesthetized cats. J Physiol 1974;237(2):279–94.

59. Greenway CV. Role of splanchnic venous system in overall cardiovascular homeostasis. Fed Proc 1983;42(6):1678–84.

60. Rapaport E, Weisbart MH, Levine M. The splanchnic blood volume in congestive heart failure. Circulation 1958;18(4 Part 1):581–7.

61. Fallick C, Sobotka PA, Dunlap ME. Sympathetically mediated changes in capacitance: redistribution of the venous reservoir as a cause of decompensation. Circ Heart Fail 2011;4(5): 669–75.

62. Greenway CV, Oshiro G. Comparison of the effects of hepatic nerve stimulation on arterial flow, distribution of arterial and portal flows and blood content in the livers of anaesthetized cats and dogs. J Physiol 1972;227(2):487–501.

63. Rzouq F, Alahdab F, Olyaee M. New insight into volume overload and hepatorenal syndrome in cirrhosis, "the hepatorenal reflex hypothesis". Am J Med Sci 2014;348(3):244–8.

64. Kostreva DR, Castaner A, Kampine JP. Reflex effects of hepatic baroreceptors on renal and cardiac sympathetic nerve activity. Am J Physiol 1980;238(5):R390–4.

65. Koyama S, Nishida K, Terada N, et al. Reflex renal vasoconstriction on portal vein distension. Jpn J Physiol 1986;36(3):441–50.

66. Ming Z, Smyth DD, Lautt WW. Decreases in portal flow trigger a hepatorenal reflex to inhibit renal

sodium and water excretion in rats: role of adenosine. Hepatology 2002;35(1):167–75.

67. Vallon V, Muhlbauer B, Osswald H. Adenosine and kidney function. Physiol Rev 2006;86(3):901–40.

68. Hamza SM, Kaufman S. Splenorenal reflex modulates renal blood flow in the rat. J Physiol 2004; 558(Pt 1):277–82.

69. Hamza SM, Kaufman S. Role of spleen in integrated control of splanchnic vascular tone: physiology and pathophysiology. Can J Physiol Pharmacol 2009;87(1):1–7.

70. de Bold AJ, Borenstein HB, Veress AT, et al. A rapid and potent natriuretic response to intravenous injection of atrial myocardial extract in rats. Reprinted from Life Sci. 28:89-94, 1981. J Am Soc Nephrol 2001;12(2):403–9 [discussion: 403–8, 408–9].

71. Sultanian R, Deng Y, Kaufman S. Atrial natriuretic factor increases splenic microvascular pressure and fluid extravasation in the rat. J Physiol 2001; 533(Pt 1):273–80.

72. Takala J. Determinants of splanchnic blood flow. Br J Anaesth 1996;77(1):50–8.

73. Sandek A, Rauchhaus M, Anker SD, et al. The emerging role of the gut in chronic heart failure. Curr Opin Clin Nutr Metab Care 2008;11(5):632–9.

74. Sandek A, Bauditz J, Swidsinski A, et al. Altered intestinal function in patients with chronic heart failure. J Am Coll Cardiol 2007;50(16):1561–9.

75. Ding J, Magnotti LJ, Huang Q, et al. Hypoxia combined with Escherichia coli produces irreversible gut mucosal injury characterized by increased intestinal cytokine production and DNA degradation. Shock 2001;16(3):189–95.

76. Lekawanvijit S. Role of gut-derived protein-bound uremic toxins in cardiorenal syndrome and potential treatment modalities. Circ J 2015;79(10): 2088–97.

77. Evenepoel P, Meijers BK, Bammens BR, et al. Uremic toxins originating from colonic microbial metabolism. Kidney Int Suppl 2009;(114):S12–9.

78. Vanholder R, De Smet R, Glorieux G, et al. Review on uremic toxins: classification, concentration, and interindividual variability. Kidney Int 2003;63(5): 1934–43.

79. Hietbrink F, Besselink MG, Renooij W, et al. Systemic inflammation increases intestinal permeability during experimental human endotoxemia. Shock 2009;32(4):374–8.

80. Niebauer J, Volk HD, Kemp M, et al. Endotoxin and immune activation in chronic heart failure: a prospective cohort study. Lancet 1999;353(9167): 1838–42.

81. Mullens W, Abrahams Z, Skouri HN, et al. Elevated intra-abdominal pressure in acute decompensated heart failure: a potential contributor to worsening renal function? J Am Coll Cardiol 2008;51(3):300–6.

82. Mohmand H, Goldfarb S. Renal dysfunction associated with intra-abdominal hypertension and the abdominal compartment syndrome. J Am Soc Nephrol 2011;22(4):615–21.

83. De Waele JJ, De Laet I, Kirkpatrick AW, et al. Intra-abdominal hypertension and abdominal compartment syndrome. Am J Kidney Dis 2011;57(1): 159–69.

84. Mullens W, Abrahams Z, Francis GS, et al. Prompt reduction in intra-abdominal pressure following large-volume mechanical fluid removal improves renal insufficiency in refractory decompensated heart failure. J Card Fail 2008;14(6):508–14.

85. Levine B, Kalman J, Mayer L, et al. Elevated circulating levels of tumor necrosis factor in severe chronic heart failure. N Engl J Med 1990;323(4): 236–41.

86. Mann DL. Innate immunity and the failing heart: the cytokine hypothesis revisited. Circ Res 2015; 116(7):1254–68.

87. Carlstedt F, Lind L, Lindahl B. Proinflammatory cytokines, measured in a mixed population on arrival in the emergency department, are related to mortality and severity of disease. J Intern Med 1997; 242(5):361–5.

88. Ferrari R, Bachetti T, Confortini R, et al. Tumor necrosis factor soluble receptors in patients with various degrees of congestive heart failure. Circulation 1995;92(6):1479–86.

89. Testa M, Yeh M, Lee P, et al. Circulating levels of cytokines and their endogenous modulators in patients with mild to severe congestive heart failure due to coronary artery disease or hypertension. J Am Coll Cardiol 1996;28(4):964–71.

90. Colombo PC, Ganda A, Lin J, et al. Inflammatory activation: cardiac, renal, and cardio-renal interactions in patients with the cardiorenal syndrome. Heart Fail Rev 2012;17(2):177–90.

91. Hedayat M, Mahmoudi MJ, Rose NR, et al. Proinflammatory cytokines in heart failure: double-edged swords. Heart Fail Rev 2010;15(6): 543–62.

92. Dhingra S, Sharma AK, Arora RC, et al. IL-10 attenuates TNF-alpha-induced NF kappaB pathway activation and cardiomyocyte apoptosis. Cardiovasc Res 2009;82(1):59–66.

93. Engel D, Peshock R, Armstong RC, et al. Cardiac myocyte apoptosis provokes adverse cardiac remodeling in transgenic mice with targeted TNF overexpression. Am J Physiol Heart Circ Physiol 2004;287(3):H1303–11.

94. Haudek SB, Taffet GE, Schneider MD, et al. TNF provokes cardiomyocyte apoptosis and cardiac remodeling through activation of multiple cell death pathways. J Clin Invest 2007;117(9):2692–701.

95. Kaur K, Sharma AK, Dhingra S, et al. Interplay of TNF-alpha and IL-10 in regulating oxidative stress

in isolated adult cardiac myocytes. J Mol Cell Cardiol 2006;41(6):1023–30.

96. Radeke HH, Meier B, Topley N, et al. Interleukin 1-alpha and tumor necrosis factor-alpha induce oxygen radical production in mesangial cells. Kidney Int 1990;37(2):767–75.

97. Kim YS, Morgan MJ, Choksi S, et al. TNF-induced activation of the Nox1 NADPH oxidase and its role in the induction of necrotic cell death. Mol Cell 2007;26(5):675–87.

98. Kalra D, Sivasubramanian N, Mann DL. Angiotensin II induces tumor necrosis factor biosynthesis in the adult mammalian heart through a protein kinase C-dependent pathway. Circulation 2002; 105(18):2198–205.

99. Ruiz-Ortega M, Ruperez M, Lorenzo O, et al. Angiotensin II regulates the synthesis of proinflammatory cytokines and chemokines in the kidney. Kidney Int Suppl 2002;(82):S12–22.

100. Moriyama T, Fujibayashi M, Fujiwara Y, et al. Angiotensin II stimulates interleukin-6 release from cultured mouse mesangial cells. J Am Soc Nephrol 1995;6(1):95–101.

101. Tsutamoto T, Wada A, Maeda K, et al. Angiotensin II type 1 receptor antagonist decreases plasma levels of tumor necrosis factor alpha, interleukin-6 and soluble adhesion molecules in patients with chronic heart failure. J Am Coll Cardiol 2000; 35(3):714–21.

102. Prabhu SD, Chandrasekar B, Murray DR, et al. beta-adrenergic blockade in developing heart failure: effects on myocardial inflammatory cytokines, nitric oxide, and remodeling. Circulation 2000; 101(17):2103–9.

103. Anker SD, Egerer KR, Volk HD, et al. Elevated soluble CD14 receptors and altered cytokines in chronic heart failure. Am J Cardiol 1997;79(10): 1426–30.

104. Charalambous BM, Stephens RC, Feavers IM, et al. Role of bacterial endotoxin in chronic heart failure: the gut of the matter. Shock 2007;28(1):15–23.

105. Rossol M, Heine H, Meusch U, et al. LPS-induced cytokine production in human monocytes and macrophages. Crit Rev Immunol 2011;31(5):379–446.

106. Peschel T, Schonauer M, Thiele H, et al. Invasive assessment of bacterial endotoxin and inflammatory cytokines in patients with acute heart failure. Eur J Heart Fail 2003;5(5):609–14.

107. Colombo PC, Onat D, Sabbah HN. Acute heart failure as "acute endotheliitis"–Interaction of fluid overload and endothelial dysfunction. Eur J Heart Fail 2008;10(2):170–5.

108. Cheng JJ, Wung BS, Chao YJ, et al. Cyclic strain enhances adhesion of monocytes to endothelial cells by increasing intercellular adhesion molecule-1 expression. Hypertension 1996;28(3): 386–91.

109. Kawai M, Naruse K, Komatsu S, et al. Mechanical stress-dependent secretion of interleukin 6 by endothelial cells after portal vein embolization: clinical and experimental studies. J Hepatol 2002; 37(2):240–6.

110. Wang BW, Chang H, Lin S, et al. Induction of matrix metalloproteinases-14 and -2 by cyclical mechanical stretch is mediated by tumor necrosis factor-alpha in cultured human umbilical vein endothelial cells. Cardiovasc Res 2003;59(2):460–9.

111. Colombo PC, Rastogi S, Onat D, et al. Activation of endothelial cells in conduit veins of dogs with heart failure and veins of normal dogs after vascular stretch by acute volume loading. J Card Fail 2009;15(5):457–63.

112. Colombo PC, Onat D, Harxhi A, et al. Peripheral venous congestion causes inflammation, neurohormonal, and endothelial cell activation. Eur Heart J 2014;35(7):448–54.

113. Konstam MA, Kiernan MS, Bernstein D, et al. Evaluation and management of right-sided heart failure: a scientific statement from the American Heart Association. Circulation 2018;137(20): e578–622.

114. Dini FL, Demmer RT, Simioniuc A, et al. Right ventricular dysfunction is associated with chronic kidney disease and predicts survival in patients with chronic systolic heart failure. Eur J Heart Fail 2012;14(3):287–94.

115. Husain-Syed F, McCullough PA, Birk HW, et al. Cardio-pulmonary-renal interactions: a multidisciplinary approach. J Am Coll Cardiol 2015;65(22): 2433–48.

116. Rangaswami J, Bhalla V, Blair JEA, et al. Cardiorenal syndrome: classification, pathophysiology, diagnosis, and treatment strategies: a scientific statement from the American Heart Association. Circulation 2019;139(16):e840–78.

117. Brisco MA, Testani JM. Novel renal biomarkers to assess cardiorenal syndrome. Curr Heart Fail Rep 2014;11(4):485–99.

118. McCullough PA, Duc P, Omland T, et al. B-type natriuretic peptide and renal function in the diagnosis of heart failure: an analysis from the breathing not properly multinational study. Am J Kidney Dis 2003;41(3):571–9.

119. Jiang K, Shah K, Daniels L, et al. Review on natriuretic peptides: where we are, where we are going. Expert Opin Med Diagn 2008;2(10):1137–53.

120. Palazzuoli A, Ruocco G, Pellegrini M, et al. Patients with cardiorenal syndrome revealed increased neurohormonal activity, tubular and myocardial damage compared to heart failure patients with preserved renal function. Cardiorenal Med 2014; 4(3–4):257–68.

121. Colbert G, Jain N, de Lemos JA, et al. Utility of traditional circulating and imaging-based cardiac

biomarkers in patients with predialysis CKD. Clin J Am Soc Nephrol 2015;10(3):515–29.

122. Tang WH, Shrestha K, Shao Z, et al. Usefulness of plasma galectin-3 levels in systolic heart failure to predict renal insufficiency and survival. Am J Cardiol 2011;108(3):385–90.

123. Waring WS, Moonie A. Earlier recognition of nephrotoxicity using novel biomarkers of acute kidney injury. Clin Toxicol (Phila) 2011;49(8):720–8.

124. Haase M, Bellomo R, Devarajan P, et al. Accuracy of neutrophil gelatinase-associated lipocalin (NGAL) in diagnosis and prognosis in acute kidney injury: a systematic review and meta-analysis. Am J Kidney Dis 2009;54(6):1012–24.

125. Mortara A, Bonadies M, Mazzetti S, et al. Neutrophil gelatinase-associated lipocalin predicts worsening of renal function in acute heart failure: methodological and clinical issues. J Cardiovasc Med (Hagerstown) 2013;14(9):629–34.

126. Knight EL, Verhave JC, Spiegelman D, et al. Factors influencing serum cystatin C levels other than renal function and the impact on renal function measurement. Kidney Int 2004;65(4):1416–21.

127. Shlipak MG, Matsushita K, Arnlov J, et al. Cystatin C versus creatinine in determining risk based on kidney function. N Engl J Med 2013;369(10):932–43.

128. Manzano-Fernandez S, Boronat-Garcia M, Albaladejo-Oton MD, et al. Complementary prognostic value of cystatin C, N-terminal pro-B-type natriuretic Peptide and cardiac troponin T in patients with acute heart failure. Am J Cardiol 2009;103(12):1753–9.

129. Masson S, Latini R, Milani V, et al. Prevalence and prognostic value of elevated urinary albumin excretion in patients with chronic heart failure: data from the GISSI-Heart Failure trial. Circ Heart Fail 2010;3(1):65–72.

130. van de Wal RM, Asselbergs FW, Plokker HW, et al. High prevalence of microalbuminuria in chronic heart failure patients. J Card Fail 2005;11(8):602–6.

131. Jackson CE, Solomon SD, Gerstein HC, et al. Albuminuria in chronic heart failure: prevalence and prognostic importance. Lancet 2009;374(9689):543–50.

132. Tang WH, Kitai T. Intrarenal venous flow: a Window into the congestive kidney failure phenotype of heart failure? JACC Heart Fail 2016;4(8):683–6.

133. Bateman GA, Cuganesan R. Renal vein Doppler sonography of obstructive uropathy. AJR Am J Roentgenol 2002;178(4):921–5.

134. Oktar SO, Yucel C, Ozdemir H, et al. Doppler sonography of renal obstruction: value of venous impedance index measurements. J Ultrasound Med 2004;23(7):929–36.

135. Jeong SH, Jung DC, Kim SH. Renal venous Doppler ultrasonography in normal subjects and patients with diabetic nephropathy: value of venous impedance index measurements. J Clin Ultrasound 2011;39(9):512–8.

136. Iida N, Seo Y, Sai S, et al. Clinical implications of intrarenal hemodynamic evaluation by Doppler ultrasonography in heart failure. JACC Heart Fail 2016;4(8):674–82.

137. Beaubien-Souligny W, Benkreira A, Robillard P, et al. Alterations in portal vein flow and intrarenal venous flow are associated with acute kidney injury after cardiac surgery: a prospective observational cohort study. J Am Heart Assoc 2018;7(19):e009961.

138. Chitturi C, Novak JE. Diuretics in the management of cardiorenal syndrome. Adv Chronic Kidney Dis 2018;25(5):425–33.

139. Faris RF, Flather M, Purcell H, et al. Diuretics for heart failure. Cochrane Database Syst Rev 2012;2:CD003838.

140. Valente MA, Voors AA, Damman K, et al. Diuretic response in acute heart failure: clinical characteristics and prognostic significance. Eur Heart J 2014;35(19):1284–93.

141. Oh SW, Han SY. Loop diuretics in clinical practice. Electrolyte Blood Press 2015;13(1):17–21.

142. Vargo DL, Kramer WG, Black PK, et al. Bioavailability, pharmacokinetics, and pharmacodynamics of torsemide and furosemide in patients with congestive heart failure. Clin Pharmacol Ther 1995;57(6):601–9.

143. Sica DA. Pharmacotherapy in congestive heart failure: drug absorption in the management of congestive heart failure: loop diuretics. Congest Heart Fail 2003;9(5):287–92.

144. McCrindle JL, Li Kam Wa TC, Barron W, et al. Effect of food on the absorption of frusemide and bumetanide in man. Br J Clin Pharmacol 1996;42(6):743–6.

145. Gilotra NA, Princewill O, Marino B, et al. Efficacy of intravenous furosemide versus a novel, pH-neutral furosemide formulation administered subcutaneously in outpatients with worsening heart failure. JACC Heart Fail 2018;6(1):65–70.

146. Rangaswami J, McCullough PA. Efficacy of subcutaneous versus intravenous administration of furosemide in patients with worsening heart failure: the devil is in the details. JACC Heart Fail 2018;6(3):266–7.

147. Cosin J, Diez J. Torasemide in chronic heart failure: results of the TORIC study. Eur J Heart Fail 2002;4(4):507–13.

148. DiNicolantonio JJ. Should torsemide be the loop diuretic of choice in systolic heart failure? Future Cardiol 2012;8(5):707–28.

149. Wargo KA, Banta WM. A comprehensive review of the loop diuretics: should furosemide be first line? Ann Pharmacother 2009;43(11):1836–47.

150. Brater DC. Diuretic therapy. N Engl J Med 1998; 339(6):387–95.

151. Michael Felker G. Diuretic management in heart failure. Congest Heart Fail 2010;16(Suppl 1):S68–72.

152. Francis GS, Siegel RM, Goldsmith SR, et al. Acute vasoconstrictor response to intravenous furosemide in patients with chronic congestive heart failure. Activation of the neurohumoral axis. Ann Intern Med 1985;103(1):1–6.

153. Felker GM, Lee KL, Bull DA, et al. Diuretic strategies in patients with acute decompensated heart failure. N Engl J Med 2011;364(9):797–805.

154. Palazzuoli A, Pellegrini M, Ruocco G, et al. Continuous versus bolus intermittent loop diuretic infusion in acutely decompensated heart failure: a prospective randomized trial. Crit Care 2014;18(3):R134.

155. Verbrugge FH, Mullens W, Tang WH. Management of cardio-renal syndrome and diuretic resistance. Curr Treat Options Cardiovasc Med 2016;18(2):11.

156. Bart BA, Goldsmith SR, Lee KL, et al. Ultrafiltration in decompensated heart failure with cardiorenal syndrome. N Engl J Med 2012;367(24): 2296–304.

157. Chen HH, Anstrom KJ, Givertz MM, et al. Low-dose dopamine or low-dose nesiritide in acute heart failure with renal dysfunction: the ROSE acute heart failure randomized trial. JAMA 2013;310(23): 2533–43.

158. Grodin JL, Stevens SR, de Las Fuentes L, et al. Intensification of medication therapy for cardiorenal syndrome in acute decompensated heart failure. J Card Fail 2016;22(1):26–32.

159. Kramer BK, Schweda F, Riegger GA. Diuretic treatment and diuretic resistance in heart failure. Am J Med 1999;106(1):90–6.

160. Testani JM, Brisco MA, Turner JM, et al. Loop diuretic efficiency: a metric of diuretic responsiveness with prognostic importance in acute decompensated heart failure. Circ Heart Fail 2014;7(2): 261–70.

161. Singh D, Shrestha K, Testani JM, et al. Insufficient natriuretic response to continuous intravenous furosemide is associated with poor long-term outcomes in acute decompensated heart failure. J Card Fail 2014;20(6):392–9.

162. Aronson D, Burger AJ. Diuretic response: clinical and hemodynamic predictors and relation to clinical outcome. J Card Fail 2016;22(3):193–200.

163. ter Maaten JM, Dunning AM, Valente MA, et al. Diuretic response in acute heart failure-an analysis from ASCEND-HF. Am Heart J 2015;170(2):313–21.

164. Verbrugge FH, Dupont M, Bertrand PB, et al. Determinants and impact of the natriuretic response to diuretic therapy in heart failure with reduced ejection fraction and volume overload. Acta Cardiol 2015;70(3):265–73.

165. Kumar D, Bagarhatta R. Fractional excretion of sodium and its association with prognosis of decompensated heart failure patients. J Clin Diagn Res 2015;9(4):OC01–3.

166. Ellison DH. The physiologic basis of diuretic synergism: its role in treating diuretic resistance. Ann Intern Med 1991;114(10):886–94.

167. Komlosi P, Fintha A, Bell PD. Current mechanisms of macula densa cell signalling. Acta Physiol Scand 2004;181(4):463–9.

168. Kaissling B, Bachmann S, Kriz W. Structural adaptation of the distal convoluted tubule to prolonged furosemide treatment. Am J Physiol 1985;248(3 Pt 2):F374–81.

169. Ellison DH, Velazquez H, Wright FS. Adaptation of the distal convoluted tubule of the rat. Structural and functional effects of dietary salt intake and chronic diuretic infusion. J Clin Invest 1989;83(1): 113–26.

170. Rao VS, Planavsky N, Hanberg JS, et al. Compensatory distal reabsorption drives diuretic resistance in human heart failure. J Am Soc Nephrol 2017; 28(11):3414–24.

171. Knauf H, Mutschler E. Functional state of the nephron and diuretic dose-response–rationale for low-dose combination therapy. Cardiology 1994; 84(Suppl 2):18–26.

172. Rudy DW, Gehr TW, Matzke GR, et al. The pharmacodynamics of intravenous and oral torsemide in patients with chronic renal insufficiency. Clin Pharmacol Ther 1994;56(1):39–47.

173. Gehr TW, Rudy DW, Matzke GR, et al. The pharmacokinetics of intravenous and oral torsemide in patients with chronic renal insufficiency. Clin Pharmacol Ther 1994;56(1):31–8.

The Role of Multimodality Imaging in Right Ventricular Failure

Tom Kai Ming Wang, MBCHB, MD(res), Christine Jellis, MD, PhD*

KEYWORDS

- Right ventricle • Echocardiography • Magnetic resonance imaging • Computed tomography

KEY POINTS

- Sound understanding of the complex right heart anatomy and function is critical for interpretation of right ventricle imaging and pathology.
- Echocardiography remains the first-line imaging modality for right ventricular assessment, where imaging for all standard views and accurate quantitative measurements are important.
- Cardiac MRI is the gold standard for right ventricle dimensions and function, with the ability to evaluate flow, shuts, tissue characterization, and extracardiac structures.
- Complete multimodality imaging evaluation includes the tricuspid valve, right atrium, systemic veins, pulmonary circulation and disorders, left heart systolic and diastolic function, and congenital heart defects.

INTRODUCTION

Left ventricular physiology and pathology has long been the focus of cardiovascular medicine, whereas the right ventricle (RV) has traditionally been neglected and viewed as less important.[1,2] However, in more recent times, there has been greater appreciation of the clinical significance of RV pathologies, with abnormalities in size and function having strong prognostic implications across a wide range of cardiovascular diseases.[2,3] This broad spectrum of etiologies, which can manifest as RV failure include intrinsic primary RV myocardial failure due to ischemia, infiltrative processes, and toxins; secondary RV failure due to increased afterload from pulmonary hypertension or pulmonic valve stenosis; RV failure due to increased volume load from valvular regurgitation or intracardiac shunts, other complex congenital heart abnormalities, pericardial disease, and chest wall abnormalities.[3] Multimodality imaging evaluation has therefore become essential to provide adequate assessment of RV structure and function for reliable diagnostic, management, and prognostic purposes. This review provides a comprehensive overview of how to use multimodality imaging to evaluate for RV failure. Clinical cases will be used to showcase the various noninvasive techniques.

RIGHT VENTRICLE ANATOMY

The RV is a complex and often underappreciated structure. It is typically the most anterior cardiac chamber, located just behind the sternum, which increases its susceptibility to chest wall trauma. The RV does not follow a simple geometric shape, but rather wraps around the more cylindrical left ventricle (LV) and appears as triangular in the vertical planes and crescentic in transverse

Department of Cardiovascular Medicine, Heart and Vascular Institute, Cleveland Clinic, Desk J1-5, 9500 Euclid Avenue, Cleveland, OH 44195, USA
* Corresponding author.
E-mail address: jellisc@ccf.org

Cardiol Clin 38 (2020) 203–217
https://doi.org/10.1016/j.ccl.2020.01.006
0733-8651/20/© 2020 Elsevier Inc. All rights reserved.

planes. The normal adult RV has slightly larger volume, but approximately one-sixth the mass of the LV, reflecting the lower stroke work it performs.[4] Morphologically, the RV can be further distinguished from the LV in several ways identifiable with noninvasive cardiac imaging. First, it is more trabeculated and has multiple prominent muscular ridges, such as the moderator, septomarginal, and parietal bands.[5,6] Second, there is no fibrous continuity between the inlet tricuspid and outflow pulmonary valves, the former as part of the fibrous skeleton along with the aortic and mitral valves, whereas the latter from the infundibular myocardium. Furthermore, the septal tricuspid valve leaflet is apically displaced relative to the anterior mitral valve leaflet and the RV usually has 3 or more papillary muscles compared with 2 in the LV.

The RV can be divided into the trabeculated inlet portion, containing the tricuspid inflow valve and subvalvular apparatus, along with the trabeculated central chamber and smooth outflow infundibulum, which are separated by an embryologic ridge called the crista supraventricularis.[2] Alternative nomenclature for this outflow portion of the RV also includes the conus arteriosus, supracristal, or subvalvular segment. The RV free wall can be divided into basal, mid, and apical segments,

or the inferior, anterior, and infundibulum depending on convention.[5] Although the RV shares the interventricular septum with the LV, the concave nature of the septum toward the LV, with a relatively thin trabeculated RV portion, results in a proportionally smaller impact of septal motion on RV function.

The right coronary supplies most of the RV myocardium in right-dominant circulations (80% of population), with marginal branches typically supplying the anterior and lateral walls, the conal artery supplying the outflow infundibulum, and the posterior descending artery supplying the inferior wall (**Fig. 1**).[7] Interruption to this regional blood supply will result in segmental RV dysfunction and regional perfusion abnormalities seen with multimodality RV imaging. The RV inflow is demarcated from the right atrium by the tricuspid atrio-ventricular valve, while transition from the RV to the pulmonary artery is separated by the outflow pulmonic valve. Dysfunction in either of these right-sided valves can result in volume or pressure loading of the RV, which can ultimately lead to RV failure.

RIGHT VENTRICULAR FUNCTION

At the microscopic level, the RV free wall contains circumferentially oriented muscle fiber layers,

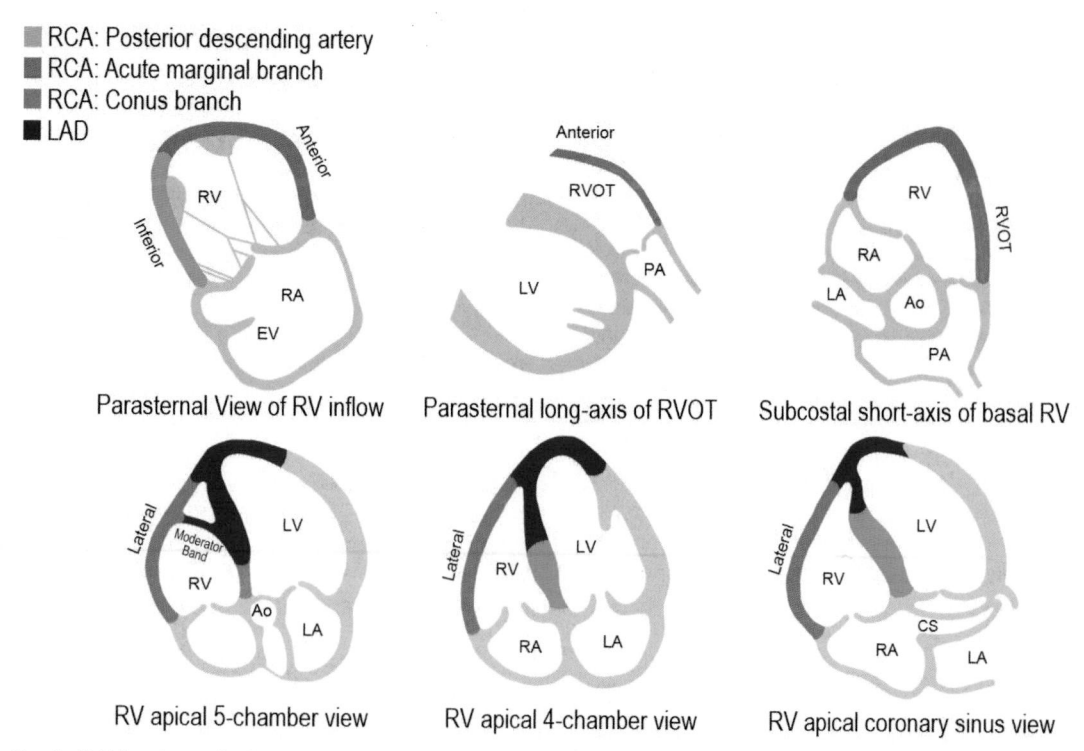

Fig. 1. RV blood supply. Ao, aorta; CS, coronary sinus; EV, Eustachian valve; LA, left atrium; LAD, left anterior descending artery; LV, left ventricle; PA, pulmonary artery; RA, right atrium; RCA, right coronary artery; RV, right ventricle; RVOT, right ventricular outflow tract.

which parallel the anterior atrioventricular groove and turn obliquely near the RV apex, before continuing in a double-helix pattern into the LV .[5] The continuity of these muscle fibers allows for RV free wall traction when the LV contracts, and contributes to ventricular interdependence. RV deep muscle fiber layers are oriented longitudinally from base to apex. These combine to enable sequential contraction of the RV starting with the inlet and the trabeculated myocardium followed by the infundibulum.[7] RV contraction is predominantly in the longitudinal direction, followed by radial. Unlike the LV, the RV has minimal contraction from rotational and twisting motion.[8]

ECHOCARDIOGRAPHY
Views of the Right Ventricle

Echocardiography remains the first-line imaging modality for assessment of the RV. On transthoracic echocardiogram there are 6 standard views for imaging the RV : (1) standard parasternal long axis view, (2) parasternal RV /tricuspid inflow view, (3) parasternal short axis view, (4) apical 4 chamber view optimized to the RV (apex at center of scanning sector with maximal RV basal diameter), (5) reverse apical 3-chamber tilt-over view, and (6) subcostal long axis view (**Fig. 2**).[9,10] Among these, (2) and (3) usually have limited windows and

reproducibility, so are less often used to for assessment. There are several challenging factors when imaging the RV by echocardiography, including its complex geometry, immediate retrosternal location, and obscured endocardial definition due to its thin free wall with relatively prominent myocardial trabeculations.[2] On transesophageal echocardiogram, further supplementary views include the mid-esophageal 4-chamber view, mid-esophageal RV inflow/outflow view, and the transgastric short axis views from base to apex.[11] However, transesophageal echocardiogram is not routinely performed for assessing the RV in the absence of other indications, given its suboptimal location in image far-field on this orientation. Optimizing echo windows is critical for RV assessment, and abnormalities in size and function should generally be confirmed on at least 2 views before making a qualitative conclusion.

Right Ventricular Dimensions

Whenever possible, quantitative assessment of the RV is preferred for assessing RV size and function. The American Society of Echocardiography and European Association of Cardiovascular Imaging guidelines for cardiac chamber quantification remain the preferred reference.[12] The main

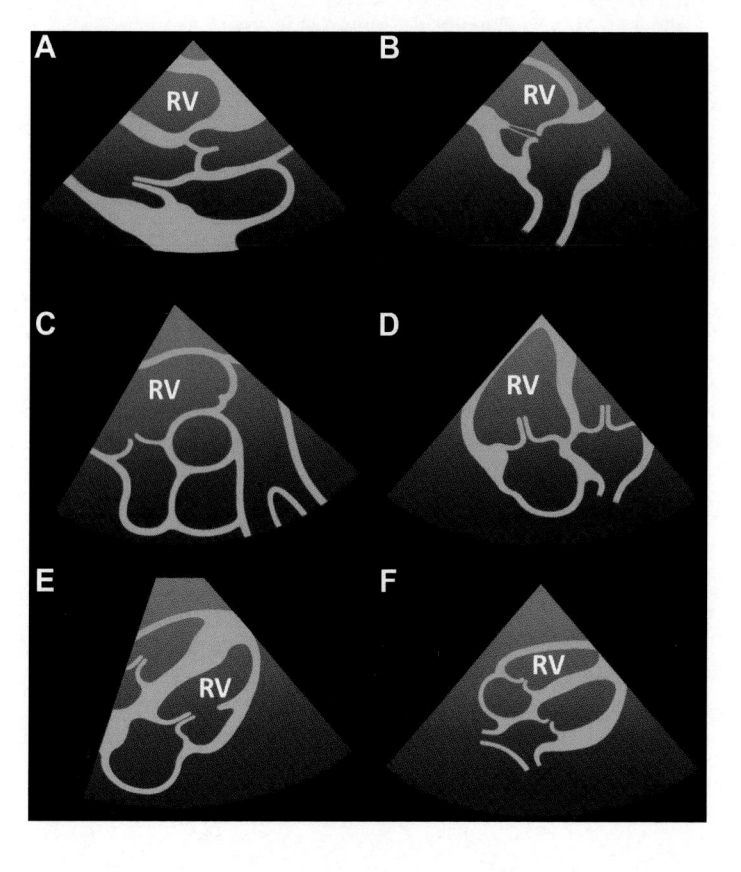

Fig. 2. Schematic representation of the transthoracic echocardiographic views for assessing the RV. (*A*) Parasternal long axis. (*B*) RV inflow. (*C*) Parasternal short axis. (*D*) RV-focused apical 4-chamber. (*E*) Reverse 3-chamber. (*F*) Subcostal long axis.

measurement parameters and normal ranges are listed in **Table 1**. Linear measurements include the RV basal, mid, and longitudinal diameters on the apical 4-chamber RV-focused view, as well as the RV outflow tract diameter on parasternal long axis, parasternal short axis proximal, and parasternal short axis distal views. It must be remembered that off-axis imaging of RV diameter will affect accuracy of RV size estimates (**Fig. 3**). RV wall thickness should be measured at end-diastole using M-mode or 2-dimensional imaging and is conventionally performed on the subcostal view at the level of the tricuspid valve chordae tendineae for reproducibility. Increased RV wall

Table 1
Normal ranges of right ventricular size and function measures on echocardiography

Echocardiographic Parameter	Normal Range
Right heart size	
Right ventricular diameter	Basal 25–41 mm Mid 19–35 mm Longitudinal 59–83 mm
Right ventricular outflow tract diameter	Parasternal long axis 20–30 mm Proximal 21–35 mm Distal 17–27 mm
Right ventricular end-diastolic area	Men 10–24 cm^2 Indexed to body surface area 5–12.5 cm^2/m^2 Women 8–20 cm^2 Indexed to body surface area 4.5–11.5 cm^2/m^2
Right ventricular end-systolic area	Men 3–15 cm^2 Indexed to body surface area 2.0–7.4 cm^2/m^2 Women 3–11 cm^2 Indexed to body surface area 1.6–6.4 cm^2/m^2
Right ventricular end-diastolic volume indexed to body surface area	Men 35–87 mL/m^2 Women 32–74 mL/m^2
Right ventricular end-systolic volume indexed to body surface area	Men 10–44 mL/m^2 Women 8–36 mL/m^2
Right ventricular wall thickness	1–5 mm
Right atrial volume	Men <39 mL/m^2 Women <33 mL/m^2
Right ventricular systolic function	
Tricuspid annular plane systolic excursion	$\geq$17 mm
Right ventricular S′ wave (pulsed Doppler)	$\geq$9.5 cm/s
Right ventricular S′ wave (color Doppler)	$\geq$6.0 cm/s
Right ventricular free wall strain	$\geq -20\%$
Fractional area change	$\geq$35%
Ejection fraction (three-dimension)	$\geq$45%
Right ventricular myocardial performance index (pulsed Doppler)	$\leq$0.43
Right ventricular myocardial performance index (tissue Doppler)	$\leq$0.54
Right ventricular diastolic function	
Tricuspid inflow E/A ratio	0.8–2.0 (can be pseudonormal)
Tricuspid inflow E wave deceleration time	119–242 ms (can be pseudonormal)
Tricuspid E/e′ ratio	$\leq$6.0
Tricuspid annular e′	$\geq$7.8 cm/s

Adapted from Lang RM, Badano LP, Mor-Avi V, Afilalo J, Armstrong A, Ernande L, et al. Recommendations for cardiac chamber quantification by echocardiography in adults: an update from the American Society of Echocardiography and the European Association of Cardiovascular Imaging. Journal of the American Society of Echocardiography: official publication of the American Society of Echocardiography. 2015 Jan;28(1):1-39.e14; with permission.

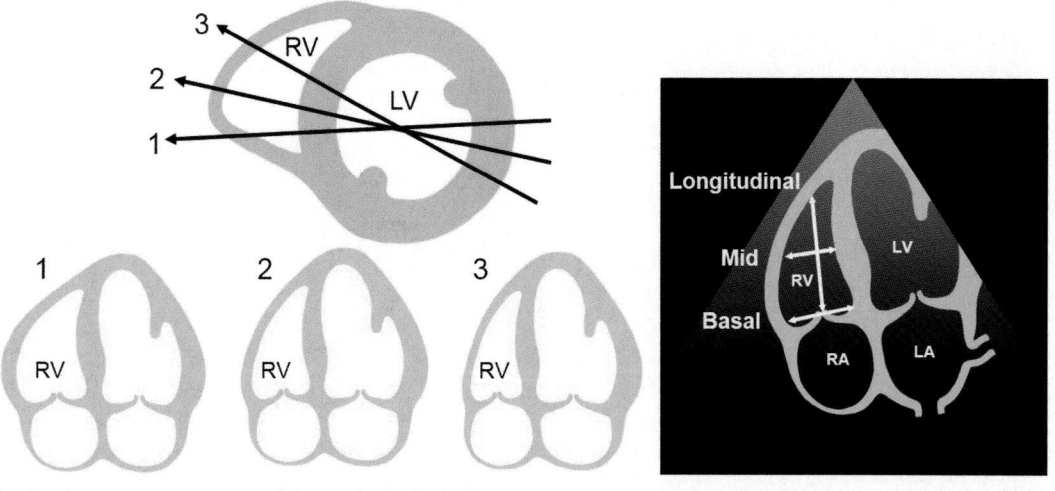

Fig. 3. Linear measurements of the RV include the basal, mid, and longitudinal diameters on the apical 4-chamber RV-focused view (view 1). Care should be taken to optimize this view to avoid underestimation of RV dimensions (views 2 and 3).

thickness suggests the presence of either RV pressure overload or infiltrative disease.

RV area can be traced on the endocardial border on either the focused RV apical 4-chamber view or the RV outflow tract.[12] Normative values differ by sex, end-diastolic or end-systolic phase (both should be measured), and whether they are indexed to body surface area. Both linear and area measurements are relatively easy and fast to obtain, but can be limited by poor endocardial definition and malaligned imaging plane, and may not accurately reflect global RV size with varying geometries. RV areas have been used to estimate volume by area-length or Simpson's methods in the past, but are no longer recommended.

Volumetric measurements are increasingly encouraged for assessing RV size, which captures the inflow, outflow, and apical regions regardless of geometry. This involves 3-dimensional multi-beat acquisition with the view containing the entire RV cavity, with adequate temporal resolution at least 20 to 25 volumes/s, with end-diastole and end-systole frames clearly established and RV trabeculae and moderator band included in the cavity calculation.[12] Limitations include the need for 3-dimensional probe, software, adequate training, and particularly adequate image quality, and larger population studies for validation of existing reference ranges. Echocardiographic RV volumes tend to underestimate compared with MRI, often because of poor visualization of the RV walls and difficulty to incorporate the entire the infundibulum, which may be up to 30% of RV volume.[13,14]

Right Ventricular Systolic Function

After assessing RV dimensions, RV systolic function is the next important step. Qualitative evaluation of the RV from all the aforementioned views should always be performed; however, integration of quantitative measures is preferred. The presence and pattern of RV segmental hypokinesis may point toward the underlying etiology of RV dysfunction as characteristic features may assist with differentiation between specific pathologies. The McConnell sign has been described in acute pulmonary embolism, where there is preserved basal and apical RV free wall contractility with severe hypokinesis of the mid-segment.[15] The rationale for this is incompletely understood, but may reflect LV tethering, regional RV free wall ischemia, or change in shape of the RV in the setting of acutely increased afterload. Regional RV hypokinesis also can be seen in the setting of myocardial infarction, with apical hypokinesis typically seen with left anterior descending artery infarction and more global RV dysfunction seen when proximal right coronary artery occlusion is the culprit.[16] Abnormal interventricular septal motion can be seen with prior cardiac surgery, and conduction abnormalities including pacing and interventricular dependence with constrictive or tamponade physiology. Septal flattening during systole is usually reflective of increased RV pressure, whereas septal flattening during diastole is seen in the setting of RV volume overload due to valvular regurgitation or a left-to-right interatrial shunt. Arrhythmogenic RV cardiomyopathy is hallmarked by fibrofatty replacement of the RV, with less frequent LV involvement. Over time, this results in aneurysmal deformation of the RV free wall and associated regional wall motion abnormalities, particularly at the apex and mid-wall segment.[17] At the extreme end of the spectrum, congenital absence of RV myocardium, known as the Uhl anomaly, is a rare condition resulting in pathognomonic severe dilation and dysfunction of the RV[18] (**Fig. 4**).

Quantitative measures of longitudinal and global RV systolic function are summarized in **Table 2**.[12] Longitudinal measures reflect the pistonlike action of the RV free wall and are often simpler and therefore more commonly performed. These include tricuspid annular plane systolic excursion (TAPSE) and myocardial tissue Doppler imaging at the tricuspid annulus during systole (RVS′). However, these parameters neglect to account for RV radial function and can be affected by loading conditions and overestimated due to RV translational motion without true contraction when LV function remains preserved.[19] TAPSE is performed using M-mode at the lateral tricuspid annulus to measure the displacement between end-diastole and peak-systole on apical views[20] (**Fig. 5**). RVS′ is taken on the same view and location using pulsed wave or color tissue Doppler imaging, to obtain the peak systolic velocity of the lateral tricuspid annulus as it moves toward the RV apex (**Fig. 6**).

To gain better appreciation of true RV function, more global measures of RV systolic function, including fractional area change (FAC), RV ejection fraction (RVEF), and RV index of myocardial performance (RIMP), should also be considered.[12] FAC is the fractional decrease in the right ventricular area from end-diastole to end-systole traced on the RV-focused apical 4-chamber view. It reflects both longitudinal and radial RV function,

although is limited by its inability to account for the RV outflow tract (**Fig. 7**). For this same reason, calculation of RVEF fraction using 2-dimensional (2D) echo cannot be performed. Three-dimensional echo capturing all borders of the RV without geometric assumptions has been validated against MRI as an accurate measure of RV function; however, it is rarely included in clinical practice, as it requires optimal simultaneous visualization of all RV walls, which is often technically difficult, even in the hands of an experienced sonographer (**Fig. 8**).[12,21] As the RV is typically larger than the LV, RVEF is normally slightly lower than LV ejection fraction. The RV myocardial performance index, also known as the RIMP or Tei index, provides global estimate of RV systolic and diastolic function.[22] It can be measured by using either pulsed wave or tissue Doppler at the lateral annulus of the tricuspid valve, with the formula (tricuspid closure to opening time − ejection time)/ejection time or (isovolumetric relaxation time + isovolumetric contraction time)/ejection time. RIMP measures are less affected by heart rate and geometric assumptions, but can be falsely abnormal in elevated right atrial pressure (**Fig. 9**).

Most recently, global longitudinal strain (GLS) of the RV has provided frame-by-frame speckle tracking of RV deformation, taking the average of percentage systolic shortening of the RV walls basal, mid, and apical segments on the RV-focused apical 4-chamber view, whereas the strain rate is the rate of the percentage shortening.[19] The RV septum may or may not be included in the RV GLS calculation, because although it adds to the complete picture of RV systolic function, it is also influenced by LV systolic function or other disease or postoperative states

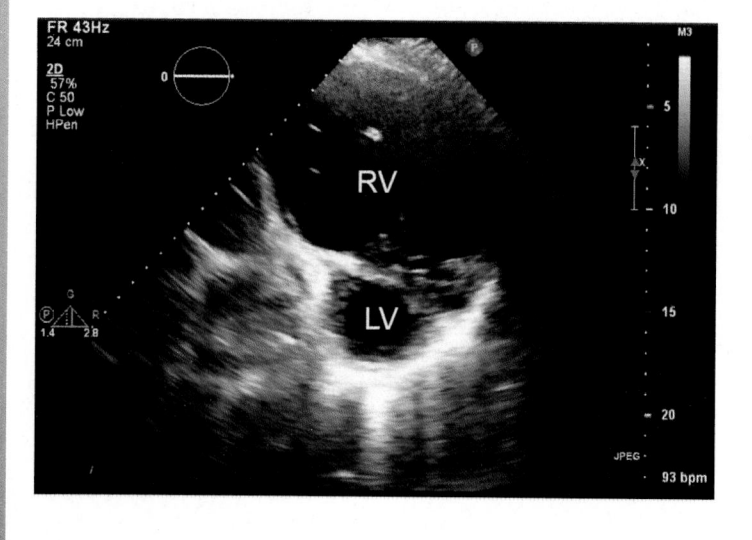

Fig. 4. Seen on this short axis parasternal view is extremely severe RV enlargement in the Uhl anomaly, a rare condition characterized by congenital absence of RV myocardium.

Table 2
Strengths and limitations of imaging modalities for right ventricular failure assessment

Modality	Advantages	Disadvantages
Transthoracic echocardiography	• First-line assessment tool • Availability • Low cost • Portable including bedside • Hemodynamic assessment (though modest accuracy) • No radiation or contrast	• Low spatial resolution • Technically difficult windows frequently encountered, right ventricle incompletely assessed • Operator dependent • Limited tissue characterization • Limited extracardiac assessment
Cardiac MRI	• Gold standard tool for chamber size and function quantification • High spatial resolution • Flow and shunt assessment • Tissue characterization • Extracardiac assessment (thoracic organs/vasculature)	• Low availability • High cost • Contrast use • Nonportable, stable patients • Long scan time, breath-hold • Contraindications: incompatible devices, claustrophobia
Computed tomography	• Adjunct or backup modality • High spatial resolution • Short scan time • Extracardiac assessment (best for lung parenchyma, also other organs/vasculature) • Coronary and calcification assessment • Procedural planning	• Radiation • Contrast use • Nonportable, stable patients • Breath-hold • Limited tissue characterization • Limited hemodynamics

that lead to abnormal septal motion (**Fig. 10**). RV strain can be influenced by image quality, artifacts, and correct positioning of reference points.[12] Strain measures are less subject to the impact of variation in loading conditions than some of the other RV functional parameters; however, it can be challenging to perform because of the thin nature of the RV free wall and suboptimal views in certain patients with poor acoustic windows, which can make tissue tracking throughout the cardiac cycle difficult. Patients with hyperinflated lungs due to chronic obstructive airways disease are often the most challenging for echo imaging, which can be especially problematic due to the need for accurate assessment of RV function and pulmonary pressures in this cohort. There are multiple vendor proprietary software options for calculation of GLS, some of which have RV strain-specific options. Range values for normal free wall RV strain can vary depending on

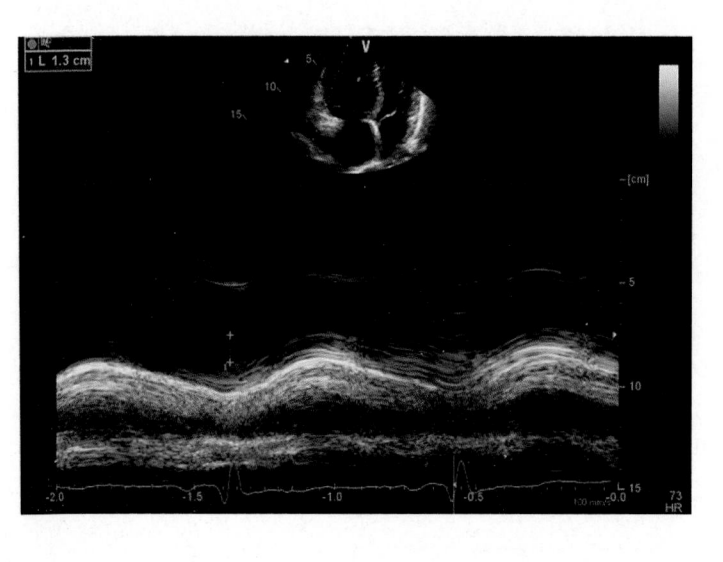

Fig. 5. TAPSE is performed using M-mode at the lateral tricuspid annulus to measure the longitudinal displacement of the RV free wall between end-diastole and peak-systole as a measure of RV function. Normal should be greater than 1.7 cm.

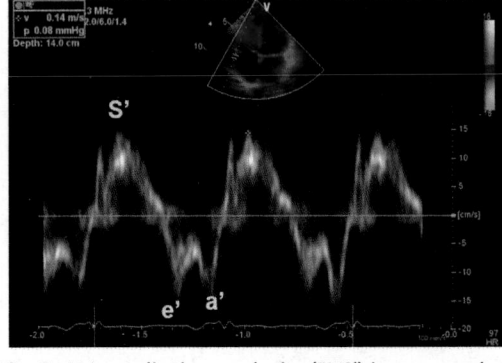

Fig. 6. RV systolic tissue velocity (RVS') is measured on an apical 4-chamber view using pulsed wave or color tissue Doppler imaging, to obtain the peak systolic velocity of the lateral tricuspid annulus as it moves toward the RV apex as a measure of longitudinal RV function. Normal should be greater than 10 cm/s.

the vendor software used, and reported at −26% ± 4% in one meta-analysis, and at less than −20% (more negative) in current guidelines.[12,23]

Other Considerations of Right Ventricular Assessment

Diastology measurements of the RV can be measured using a number of parameters analogous to LV diastology parameters. The tricuspid inflow pulsed wave Doppler provides a starting point for diastolic assessment, whereby the peak early diastolic (E wave) and late diastolic (A wave) flow velocities, along with the inflow deceleration and isovolumetric relaxation times, can be calculated.[10] This can be combined with measurement of myocardial tissue Doppler imaging

at the tricuspid annulus during diastole (RVE'), which in combination with the E wave can be used as a noninvasive estimate of RV filling pressures (RV E/E').[24] Suggested diastolic function grading from guidelines include tricuspid ratio E/A ratio less than 0.8 as impaired relaxation (grade 1, mild), E/A ratio 0.8 to 2.1 with E/E' ratio greater than 6 or hepatic vein diastolic flow predominance as pseudonormal (grade 2, moderate), and E/A ratio greater than 2.1 with deceleration time less than 120 ms as restrictive (grade 3 severe).[10] Right atrial size and filling pressure, RV wall thickness and RV systolic parameters can provide additional insights into RV diastolic function. However, the presence of atrial fibrillation and/or significant tricuspid regurgitation reduces the reliability of noninvasive measurements.

Right-sided intracardiac pressures can be estimated using the size of the inferior vena cava (IVC) on subcostal views, with larger diameters and reduced collapsibility on inspiration suggesting elevated right atrial pressure.[2,10] Current guidelines estimate normal right atrial pressure (RAP) at mean 3 mm Hg, intermediate RAP at mean 8 mm Hg (if IVC ≤2.1 cm and IVC collapsibility <50% or IVC >2.1 cm and IVC collapsibility >50%) and elevated RAP at 15 mm Hg (IVC >2.1 cm and IVC collapsibility <50%).[25] Hemodynamic information needs to be further sought when evaluating the RV, which can be in part assessed on echocardiography noninvasively. Estimates of RV stroke volume (which when multiplied by heart rate gives cardiac output) can be performed with echocardiography. This is performed using pulse wave Doppler within the RV outflow tract (RVOT) to estimate the velocity time integral (VTI), along with the area of the RVOT

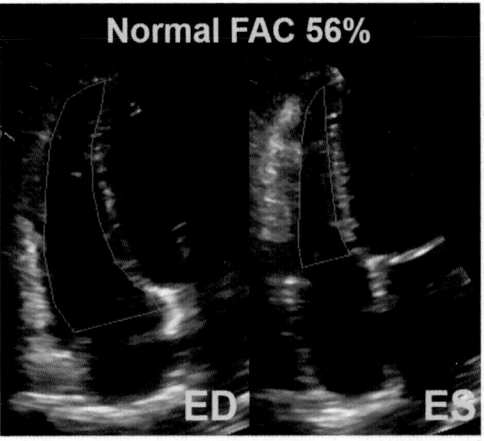
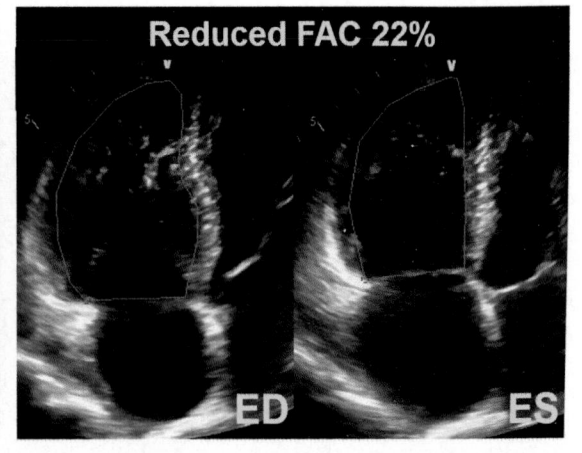

Fig. 7. FAC is the fractional decrease in the RV area from end-diastole (ED) to end-systole (ES) traced on the RV-focused apical 4-chamber view. It reflects both longitudinal and radial RV function, although is limited by its inability to account for the RVOT. Normal should be greater than 35%.

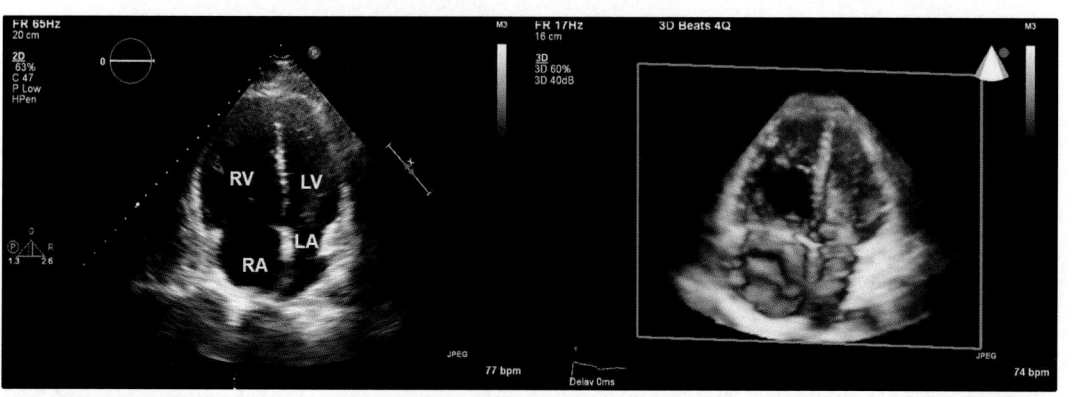

Fig. 8. Full-volume acquisition of the RV (*right*) allows semiautomated tracing of the RV endocardium during systolic and diastole to calculate RV volumes and RVEF.

(**Fig. 11**). This correlates well with invasive determinants of RV cardiac output in the absence of significant pulmonic valve regurgitation.[26]

The most common noninvasive RV hemodynamic parameter calculated by echo is RV systolic pressure (RVSP). This is performed by applying the simplified Bernoulli equation, where peak pressure is equal to $4 \times$ peak velocity[2] (**Fig. 12**).[27] In the case of the RV, the peak velocity of the tricuspid regurgitant jet gives the difference between the RVSP and RAP, which in absence of RVOT or pulmonary stenosis, is a surrogate for pulmonary arterial systolic pressure.[10] Application of the same equation to the end-diastolic pulmonary regurgitant jet velocity estimates the pulmonary artery diastolic pressure. The mean pulmonary artery pressure can then be determined. Several other methods using the pulmonary artery acceleration time, early pulmonary regurgitation velocity, and tricuspid regurgitation VTI have been devised to estimate right heart pressures. These include formulae for the noninvasive estimate of pulmonary vascular resistance, such as those described by Abbas and colleagues[26] and more recently Dahiya and colleagues.[28] LV diastolic function by echo provides a surrogate marker of left atrial pressure. When combined with pulmonary arterial pressure estimates, this can also build an overall impression of pulmonary vascular resistance.[29] For all these calculations, it must always be remembered that inaccuracies can occur due to adequate image quality, regurgitation jets, valvular pathologies, and loading conditions. The gold standard test for estimation of right heart pressures and pulmonary capillary wedge pressure remains an invasive catheter right heart hemodynamic study.

In addition to estimation of RVSP, assessment of tricuspid regurgitation (TR) mechanism and severity is integral to the understanding of RV pathophysiology.[30] In certain cases, specific etiologies of tricuspid valve dysfunction and resultant TR are evident on 2D echo imaging, such as carcinoid disease, infective endocarditis, or Ebstein anomaly (**Fig. 13**). However, notably, secondary functional causes remain the most common mechanism for TR. Whatever the mechanism of

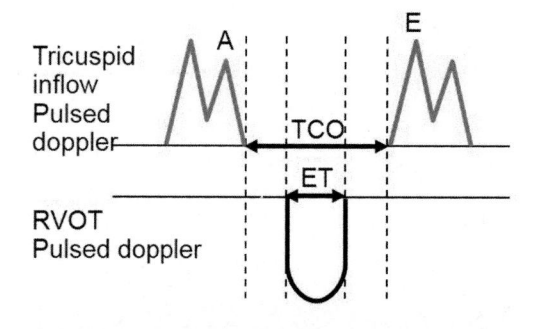

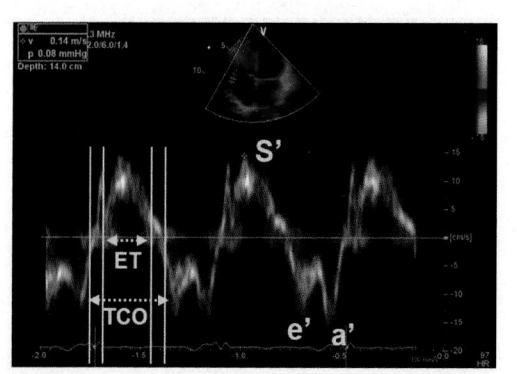

Fig. 9. RV myocardial performance index, also known as the RIMP or Tei index, provides global estimate of RV systolic and diastolic function. It can be measured by using either pulsed wave (PW) or tissue Doppler (TDI) at the lateral annulus of the tricuspid valve using the formula: tricuspid closure to opening time [TCO] – ejection time [ET])/ejection time [ET]. Normal should be <0.40 (PW); less than 0.55 (TDI).

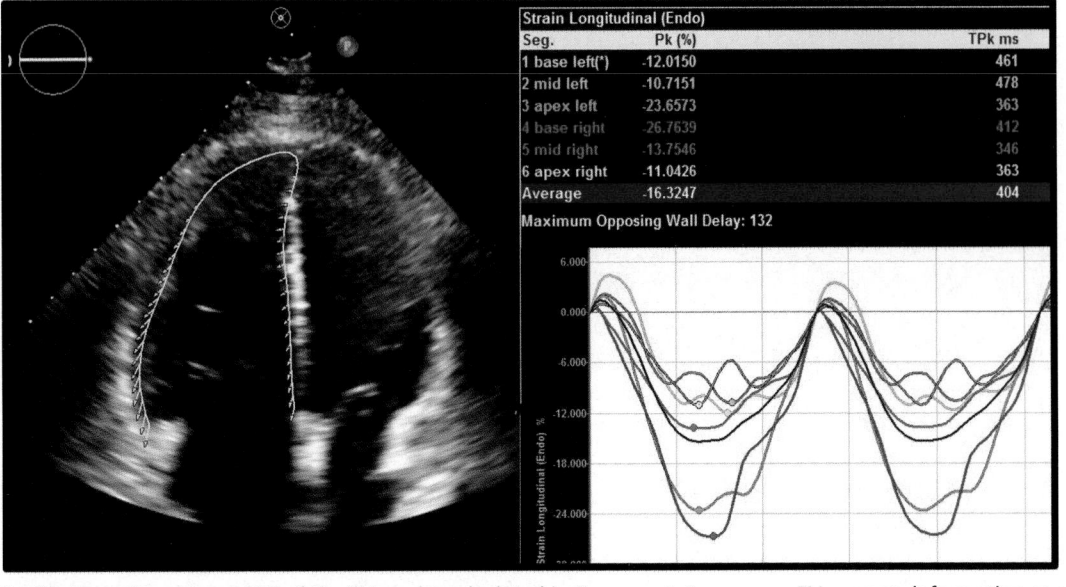

Fig. 10. Two-dimensional GLS of the RV can be calculated in 6 segments to measure RV percent deformation as a measure of systolic function. Pk, peak strain (%); Seg, segment; TPk, time to peak (milliseconds).

TR, progressive TR begets RV dilation, which over time contributes to annular dilation and further worsening of TR severity. This chicken and egg scenario is usually compensated for initially, but as TR progresses into the severe range, decompensated right-sided heart failure can develop with resultant fluid retention, hepatic congestion, and associated symptoms will require pharmacotherapy and consideration of valvular intervention. Importantly in the setting of significant tricuspid regurgitation, the lower boundary for normal RVEF should be raised to account for the increased forward flow.[31] Typically, those presenting with severe TR and RV failure will have increased perioperative risk during cardiac surgery.[32] This is due to reduced LV preload from RV dysfunction, along with underlying liver dysfunction, which can result in coagulopathy, especially if there is underlying unrecognized cirrhosis. Percutaneous tricuspid valve interventions, including replacement and clip repairs, may provide a viable alternative for these higher surgical risk candidates in the future. In all patients with RV pathology, it is always important to provide a complete echocardiographic assessment of left heart structure and function, left-sided valvular pathologies, pericardial diseases, and congenital heart lesions to provide insight into the underlying mechanism of secondary right heart dysfunction.[12,30]

CARDIAC MRI

Cardiac magnetic resonance imaging (CMR) is the gold standard for the assessment of right-sided cardiac chamber size and function.[12] The relative advantages and disadvantages of various imaging modalities are listed in **Table 2**. MRI has high spatial resolution, superior to transthoracic echocardiography, with adequate temporal resolution. RV volumes can be quantitated from a short-axis or 4-chamber cine stack. This is most typically

$$RVOT\ SV = \prod * \frac{RVOT^2}{2} * RVOT\ VTI$$

Fig. 11. RV stroke volume can be estimated using pulse wave Doppler within the RVOT to estimate the VTI, which is then multiplied by the area of the RVOT.

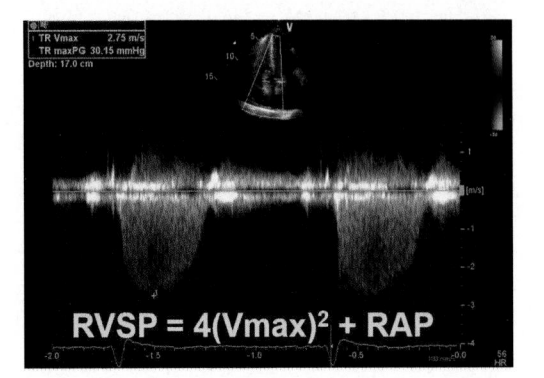

Fig. 12. The peak velocity (Vmax) of the tricuspid regurgitant jet on continuous wave Doppler plus RAP can be used to estimate the RVSP via the modified Bernoulli equation.

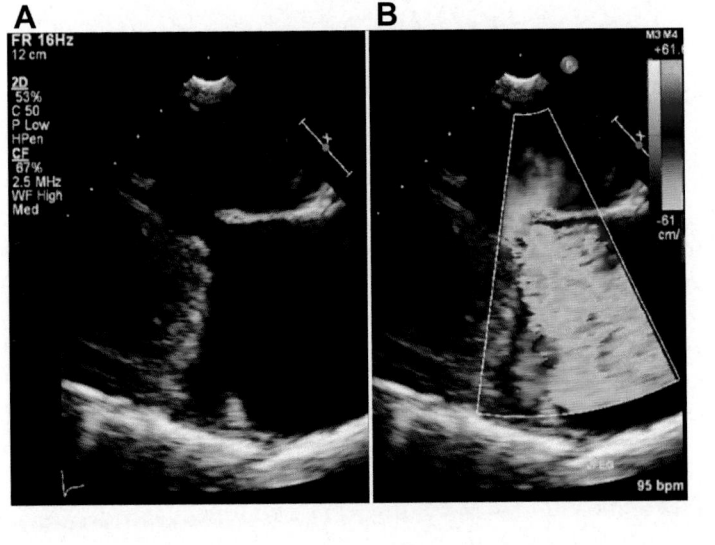

Fig. 13. Significant tricuspid valve leaflet thickening and restriction in carcinoid disease on this RV inflow view, results in failure of leaflet coaptation (*A*) and severe TR (*B*).

performed using a steady-state free precession sequence. The RV endocardium is traced on each image at both end-diastole and end-systole to give RV end-diastolic and end-systolic volumes. The difference between these volumes is used to calculate the RVEF[33] (**Fig. 14**) Additional data regarding RV function can be generated with the use of tissue tracking and MRI strain techniques, which are now beginning to be used for clinical practice.[34] Phase velocity encoding sequences can be used to quantitate flow rates. When placed at the level of the main pulmonary artery, this can be used to determine RV stroke volume and cardiac output, pulmonic regurgitant fraction, and flow velocities through the pulmonic valve. Tricuspid regurgitant fraction can also be calculated from the difference between the RV stroke volume on volumetric analysis and pulmonic valve forward flow.[2,33] Evaluation for an intracardiac shunt can also be performed by the ratio of the RV to LV stroke volumes on volumetric analysis or the pulmonic and aortic forward flow on quantitative flow (Qp:Qs). A Qp:Qs of greater than 1.2 suggests a clinically meaningful left-to-right intracardiac shunt.

Cine imaging in CMR is useful to identify RV regional dysfunction, in a similar way to that described previously using echo. However, additional information can be gleaned about the etiology of RV dysfunction with the use of tissue characterization. Edema weighted imaging with sequences such as T2 short tau inversion recovery can provide information regarding RV myocardial inflammation; however, sensitivity is suboptimal. Delayed gadolinium enhancement (DGE) provides more reliable tissue characterization, with contrast accumulating within regions of chronic fibrosis or active inflammation. The pattern, distribution, and extent of DGE can be exploited to detect and diagnose the underlying cause of LV dysfunction in conditions such as RV infarction and arrhythmogenic RV cardiomyopathy, and infiltrative processes such as cardiac sarcoidosis (**Figs. 15** and **16**). Assessment of RV diffuse fibrosis and extracellular volume can be performed using a T1 mapping technique. T1 values have been shown to correlate with RV dysfunction, provided that care is taken to ensure the region of interest is maintained on the thin RV free wall.[35] Like with echo, evaluation of the left heart, valves, pericardium, and congenital lesions (such as septal defect and anomalous pulmonary veins or coronary arteries) remains important as potential contributors to RV dysfunction.[12,30] Limitations of MRI can include cost, availability, prolonged scanning time, need for gadolinium-based contrast administration and breath-hold requirements. Although most new-generation cardiac pacing and implantable defibrillator devices are now CMR compatible, artifact from the generator or RV lead may limit diagnostic imaging quality. CMR remains contraindicated in some older, noncompatible devices. The use of CMR for assessment of the right heart is increasing, especially for those with suboptimal echo acoustic windows or when accurate assessment of RVEF is desired.

CARDIAC COMPUTED TOMOGRAPHY

Additional imaging of the right heart can be performed using cardiac computed tomography

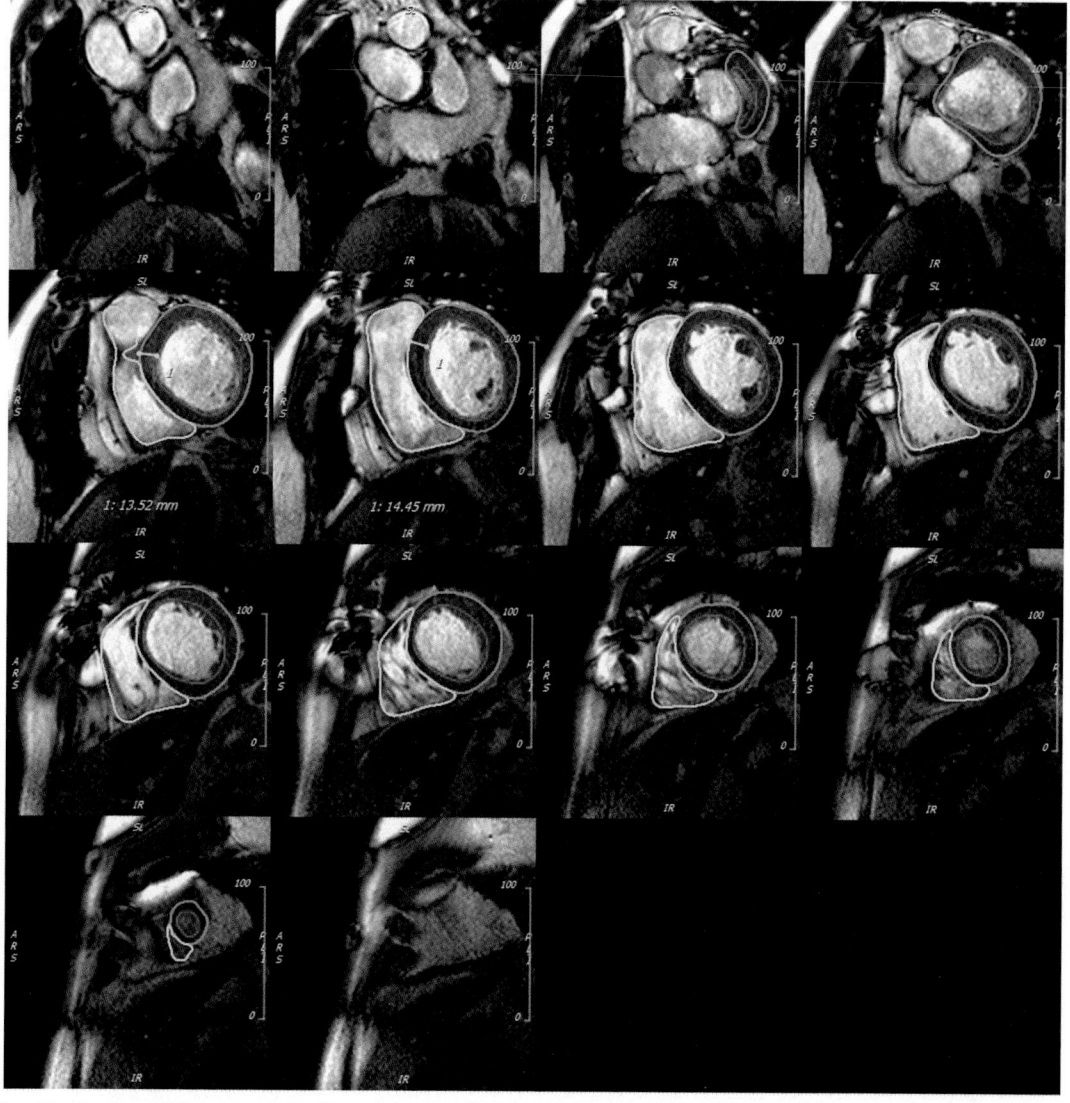

Fig. 14. Cardiac MRI short axis stack, steady-state free precession sequence, with the RV endocardium (*yellow*), LV endocardium (*red*), and LV epicardium (*green*) contoured at end-diastole. Endocardial contours are also performed at end-systole to establish ventricular volumes, which are then used to calculate biventricular ejection fractions.

(CT). Single phase-contrast imaging provides structural information about the heart and extracardiac structures, along with some myocardial tissue characterization using density measures. For subjects in whom CMR is contraindicated, image acquisition throughout the cardiac cycle can be performed using spiral retrospective imaging with electrocardiographic gating. This can then be played as a cine image or contoured for RV volumes in similar way to CMR, thereby allowing qualitative evaluation of RV function and calculation of RVEF with good spatial resolution comparable to MRI and superior to transthoracic

echocardiography.[36,37] The main limitation of this retrospective technique is increased radiation dose, so appropriate patient selection and dose minimization techniques are important considerations.

CT is now the main noninvasive imaging modality for evaluation of coronary artery disease.[38] Another advantage of CT over CMR is the ability to assess extracardiac structures for abnormalities such as pulmonary arterial thromboembolism or lung parenchymal disease.[39] CT also may be valuable to define thoracic anatomy before cardiac surgery or to assess vascular access before

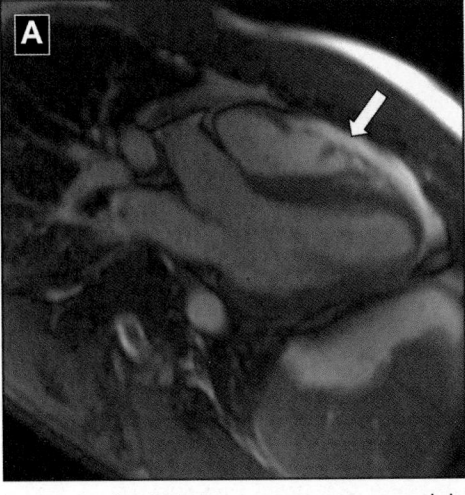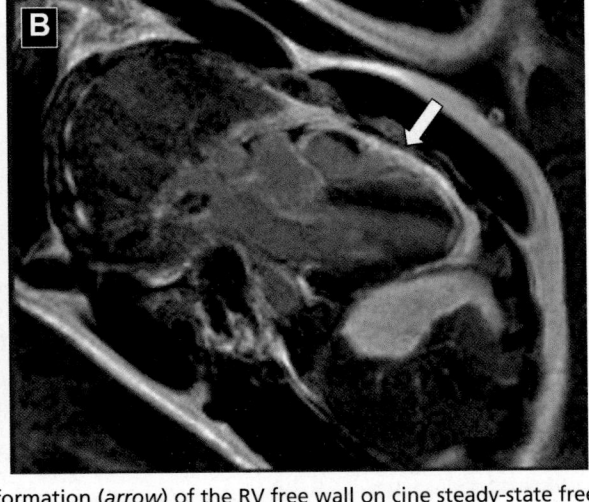

Fig. 15. Cardiac MRI demonstrates aneurysmal deformation (*arrow*) of the RV free wall on cine steady-state free precession imaging (*A*), along with fibro-fatty infiltration on delayed enhancement imaging (*arrow*) in arrhythmogenic RV cardiomyopathy (*B*).

percutaneous structural interventions.[40] The short scan time of CT is also an advantage over CMR for critically ill patients. Disadvantages include the use of ionizing radiation, need for nephrotoxic contrast, and more limited ability to assess cardiac hemodynamics. Further recent advances in CT include faster gantry rotation time and double gantry design of some scanners enabling improved temporal resolution and coverage, availability of dual-energy scanners at 2 different energy levels associated with less radiation, artifact and contrast use, and new software incorporating plaque and tissue characterization and machine

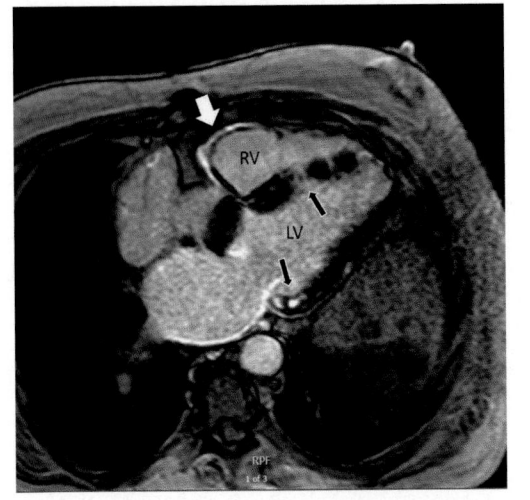

Fig. 16. Involvement of the RV in cardiac sarcoidosis, seen by DGE within the RVOT (*white arrow*) and LV (*black arrows*).

learning.[41] Like CMR, cardiac CT is sensitive to abnormal heart rhythms and inability for breath-hold. Currently for the purpose of RV assessment, CT is generally used only when MRI is unavailable or contraindicated.

NUCLEAR MEDICINE

There is a limited utility for nuclear medicine in the specific evaluation of RV function. Nuclear stress imaging can provide some qualitative data regarding RV function and size with stress compared with rest. RV involvement can sometimes be evident with cardiac PET in the setting of cardiac sarcoidosis, where focal inflammation in the free wall is evidenced by increased fluorodeoxyglucose uptake.[42]

SUMMARY

Accurate evaluation of the right heart and associated structures is critical in the setting of RV failure. Although echocardiography remains the mainstay in this arena, multimodality imaging can be useful to get a more comprehensive and quantitative assessment of RV dysfunction and associated cardiac and extracardiac conditions. Typically this additional imaging is best provided with CMR imaging techniques, although CT and nuclear imaging can be useful for specific indications. Hopefully, improved accuracy in the noninvasive assessment of RV failure with multimodality imaging will ultimately translate to better management to improve outcomes for patients with RV involvement in a variety of cardiovascular diseases.

ACKNOWLEDGMENTS

Dr Wang is supported by the National Heart Foundation of New Zealand Overseas Clinical and Research Fellowship, grant number 1775.

DISCLOSURE

The authors have nothing to disclose.

REFERENCES

1. Sheehan F, Redington A. The right ventricle: anatomy, physiology and clinical imaging. Heart 2008; 94(11):1510–5.
2. Haddad F, Hunt SA, Rosenthal DN, et al. Right ventricular function in cardiovascular disease, part I: anatomy, physiology, aging, and functional assessment of the right ventricle. Circulation 2008; 117(11):1436–48.
3. Haddad F, Doyle R, Murphy DJ, et al. Right ventricular function in cardiovascular disease, part II: pathophysiology, clinical importance, and management of right ventricular failure. Circulation 2008;117(13): 1717–31.
4. Lorenz CH, Walker ES, Morgan VL, et al. Normal human right and left ventricular mass, systolic function, and gender differences by cine magnetic resonance imaging. J Cardiovasc Magn Reson 1999;1(1):7–21.
5. Ho SY, Nihoyannopoulos P. Anatomy, echocardiography, and normal right ventricular dimensions. Heart 2006;92(Suppl 1):i2–13.
6. Farb A, Burke AP, Virmani R. Anatomy and pathology of the right ventricle (including acquired tricuspid and pulmonic valve disease). Cardiol Clin 1992;10(1):1–21.
7. Dell'Italia LJ. The right ventricle: anatomy, physiology, and clinical importance. Curr Probl Cardiol 1991;16(10):653–720.
8. Petitjean C, Rougon N, Cluzel P. Assessment of myocardial function: a review of quantification methods and results using tagged MRI. J Cardiovasc Magn Reson 2005;7(2):501–16.
9. Mitchell C, Rahko PS, Blauwet LA, et al. Guidelines for performing a comprehensive transthoracic echocardiographic examination in adults: recommendations from the American Society of Echocardiography. J Am Soc Echocardiogr 2019; 32(1):1–64.
10. Rudski LG, Lai WW, Afilalo J, et al. Guidelines for the echocardiographic assessment of the right heart in adults: a report from the American Society of Echocardiography endorsed by the European Association of Echocardiography, a registered branch of the European Society of Cardiology, and the Canadian Society of Echocardiography. J Am Soc Echocardiogr 2010;23(7):685–713 [quiz: 86–8].
11. Hahn RT, Abraham T, Adams MS, et al. Guidelines for performing a comprehensive transesophageal echocardiographic examination: recommendations from the American Society of Echocardiography and the Society of Cardiovascular Anesthesiologists. J Am Soc Echocardiogr 2013; 26(9):921–64.
12. Lang RM, Badano LP, Mor-Avi V, et al. Recommendations for cardiac chamber quantification by echocardiography in adults: an update from the American Society of Echocardiography and the European Association of Cardiovascular Imaging. J Am Soc Echocardiogr 2015;28(1):1–39.e14.
13. Kjaergaard J, Petersen CL, Kjaer A, et al. Evaluation of right ventricular volume and function by 2D and 3D echocardiography compared to MRI. Eur J Echocardiogr 2006;7(6):430–8.
14. Nesser HJ, Tkalec W, Patel AR, et al. Quantitation of right ventricular volumes and ejection fraction by three-dimensional echocardiography in patients: comparison with magnetic resonance imaging and radionuclide ventriculography. Echocardiography 2006;23(8):666–80.
15. McConnell MV, Solomon SD, Rayan ME, et al. Regional right ventricular dysfunction detected by echocardiography in acute pulmonary embolism. Am J Cardiol 1996;78(4):469–73.
16. Casazza F, Bongarzoni A, Capozi A, et al. Regional right ventricular dysfunction in acute pulmonary embolism and right ventricular infarction. Eur J Echocardiogr 2005;6(1):11–4.
17. Yoerger DM, Marcus F, Sherrill D, et al. Echocardiographic findings in patients meeting task force criteria for arrhythmogenic right ventricular dysplasia: new insights from the multidisciplinary study of right ventricular dysplasia. J Am Coll Cardiol 2005;45(6):860–5.
18. Uhl HS. A previously undescribed congenital malformation of the heart: almost total absence of the myocardium of the right ventricle. Bull Johns Hopkins Hosp 1952;91(3):197–209.
19. Giusca S, Dambrauskaite V, Scheurwegs C, et al. Deformation imaging describes right ventricular function better than longitudinal displacement of the tricuspid ring. Heart 2010;96(4):281–8.
20. Hammarstrom E, Wranne B, Pinto FJ, et al. Tricuspid annular motion. J Am Soc Echocardiogr 1991;4(2): 131–9.
21. Shimada YJ, Shiota M, Siegel RJ, et al. Accuracy of right ventricular volumes and function determined by three-dimensional echocardiography in comparison with magnetic resonance imaging: a meta-analysis study. J Am Soc Echocardiogr 2010;23(9):943–53.
22. Tei C, Dujardin KS, Hodge DO, et al. Doppler echocardiographic index for assessment of global right ventricular function. J Am Soc Echocardiogr 1996; 9(6):838–47.

23. Fine NM, Chen L, Bastiansen PM, et al. Reference values for right ventricular strain in patients without cardiopulmonary disease: a prospective evaluation and meta-analysis. Echocardiography 2015;32(5):787–96.

24. Sade LE, Gulmez O, Eroglu S, et al. Noninvasive estimation of right ventricular filling pressure by ratio of early tricuspid inflow to annular diastolic velocity in patients with and without recent cardiac surgery. J Am Soc Echocardiogr 2007;20(8):982–8.

25. Porter TR, Shillcutt SK, Adams MS, et al. Guidelines for the use of echocardiography as a monitor for therapeutic intervention in adults: a report from the American Society of Echocardiography. J Am Soc Echocardiogr 2015;28(1):40–56.

26. Abbas AE, Fortuin FD, Schiller NB, et al. A simple method for noninvasive estimation of pulmonary vascular resistance. J Am Coll Cardiol 2003;41(6):1021–7.

27. Yock PG, Popp RL. Noninvasive estimation of right ventricular systolic pressure by Doppler ultrasound in patients with tricuspid regurgitation. Circulation 1984;70(4):657–62.

28. Dahiya A, Vollbon W, Jellis C, et al. Echocardiographic assessment of raised pulmonary vascular resistance: application to diagnosis and follow-up of pulmonary hypertension. Heart 2010;96(24):2005–9.

29. Nagueh SF, Smiseth OA, Appleton CP, et al. Recommendations for the evaluation of left ventricular diastolic function by echocardiography: an update from the American Society of Echocardiography and the European Association of Cardiovascular Imaging. J Am Soc Echocardiogr 2016;29(4):277–314.

30. Zoghbi WA, Adams D, Bonow RO, et al. Recommendations for noninvasive evaluation of native valvular regurgitation: a report from the American Society of Echocardiography developed in collaboration with the society for cardiovascular magnetic resonance. J Am Soc Echocardiogr 2017;30(4):303–71.

31. Nishimura RA, Otto CM, Bonow RO, et al. 2014 AHA/ACC guideline for the management of patients with valvular heart disease: executive summary: a report of the American College of Cardiology/American Heart Association Task Force on Practice Guidelines. J Am Coll Cardiol 2014;63(22):2438–88.

32. Peyrou J, Chauvel C, Pathak A, et al. Preoperative right ventricular dysfunction is a strong predictor of 3 years survival after cardiac surgery. Clin Res Cardiol 2017;106(9):734–42.

33. Abouzeid CM, Shah T, Johri A, et al. Multimodality imaging of the right ventricle. Curr Treat Options Cardiovasc Med 2017;19(11):82.

34. Liu B, Dardeer AM, Moody WE, et al. Normal values for myocardial deformation within the right heart measured by feature-tracking cardiovascular magnetic resonance imaging. Int J Cardiol 2018;252:220–3.

35. Jellis CL, Yingchoncharoen T, Gai N, et al. Correlation between right ventricular T1 mapping and right ventricular dysfunction in non-ischemic cardiomyopathy. Int J Cardiovasc Imaging 2018;34(1):55–65.

36. Sugeng L, Mor-Avi V, Weinert L, et al. Multimodality comparison of quantitative volumetric analysis of the right ventricle. JACC Cardiovasc Imaging 2010;3(1):10–8.

37. Maffei E, Messalli G, Martini C, et al. Left and right ventricle assessment with cardiac CT: validation study vs. cardiac MR. Eur Radiol 2012;22(5):1041–9.

38. Abbara S, Blanke P, Maroules CD, et al. SCCT guidelines for the performance and acquisition of coronary computed tomographic angiography: a report of the society of cardiovascular computed tomography guidelines committee: endorsed by the North American Society for Cardiovascular Imaging (NASCI). J Cardiovasc Comput Tomogr 2016;10(6):435–49.

39. Galie N, Humbert M, Vachiery JL, et al. 2015 ESC/ERS guidelines for the diagnosis and treatment of pulmonary hypertension: the joint task force for the diagnosis and treatment of pulmonary hypertension of the European Society of Cardiology (ESC) and the European Respiratory Society (ERS): endorsed by: Association for European Paediatric and Congenital Cardiology (AEPC), International Society for Heart and Lung Transplantation (ISHLT). Eur Heart J 2016;37(1):67–119.

40. van Rosendael PJ, Kamperidis V, Kong WK, et al. Computed tomography for planning transcatheter tricuspid valve therapy. Eur Heart J 2017;38(9):665–74.

41. Commandeur F, Goeller M, Dey D. Cardiac CT: technological advances in hardware, software, and machine learning applications. Curr Cardiovasc Imaging Rep 2018. https://doi.org/10.1007/s12410-018-9459-z.

42. Manabe O, Yoshinaga K, Ohira H, et al. Right ventricular (18)F-FDG uptake is an important indicator for cardiac involvement in patients with suspected cardiac sarcoidosis. Ann Nucl Med 2014;28(7):656–63.

Right Ventricular Failure After Left Ventricular Assist Device

Rebecca Cogswell, MD[a],*, Ranjit John, MD[b], Andrew Shaffer, MD[b]

KEYWORDS

• Ventricular assist devices • Right ventricular function • Heart failure

KEY POINTS

• Right ventricular failure after left ventricular assist device (LVAD) implantation remains common in the contemporary, continuous-flow era.
• Clinically meaningful, reproducible, and consensus definitions of both early and late right ventricular failure after LVAD implantation are needed for progress in advanced heart failure.
• Right ventricular failure after LVAD implantation and post-LVAD vasoplegia share similar risk factors and physiology.
• The relative right ventricular failure that accompanies post-LVAD vasoplegia can be treated with temporary right ventricular assist device support.

INTRODUCTION

Right ventricular (RV) failure remains common after left ventricular assist device (LVAD) placement even in the contemporary continuous-flow era,[1] and remains a leading cause of morbidity and mortality after LVAD placement.[2,3] This article covers current definitions of RV failure after LVAD placement, with a focus on early RV failure. The pathophysiology, prevalence, and significance of this complication are reviewed. It also introduces the concept of RV assist device (RVAD) placement for treatment of post-LVAD vasoplegia. Risk factors for post-LVAD RV failure, treatment strategies, and future directions within the field are also covered.

DEFINITIONS

Several definitions of early RV failure after LVAD placement exist. All include unplanned RVAD placement after LVAD implantation; however, definitions vary by length and use of pulmonary vasodilators or intravenous inotropes. One of the classic definitions of early RV failure used by Kormos and colleagues[4] and others was RVAD placement after LVAD or failure to wean from inotropes within 14 days. The definition used in the MOMENTUM (Multi-Center Study of MagLev Technology in Patients Undergoing MCS Therapy With HeartMate 3™) clinical trial was RVAD implantation or inhaled nitric oxide or inotropic therapy for a duration of more than 1 week; however, this could be at any time after LVAD implantation.[1] A recent EUROMACS RV score publication used a definition of RVAD placement, pulmonary vasodilator use greater than or equal to 48 hours, or inotrope use for greater than or equal to 14 days.[5] The INTERMACS (Interagency Registry for Mechanically Assisted Circulatory Support) definition is more complicated and has acute, severe, moderate, and mild severity categories, with clinical venous congestion required for some categories.[6] Each definition has limitations. For example, an inotrope wean at 13 days versus 15 days may not be clinically meaningful, and definitions that

a Department of Medicine, Division of Cardiology, University of Minnesota, Variety Club Research Center (VCRC), 401 E. River Parkway, Minneapolis, MN 55455, USA; b Department of Surgery, Division of Cardiothoracic Surgery, University of Minnesota, 425 E River Parkway, 347, Minneapolis, MN 55455, USA
* Corresponding author.
E-mail address: cogsw014@umn.edu

Cardiol Clin 38 (2020) 219–225
https://doi.org/10.1016/j.ccl.2020.01.007

use physical examination findings have shown limitations.[7] Until a standard definition is agreed on that is clinically meaningful, easily assigned, and has a high reproducibility, progress will be hindered.

The definition of RV failure that occurs after the immediate postoperative period, termed late RV failure, is even less well defined. Part of the difficulty of studying late RV failure is the lack of serial hemodynamic data from large datasets such as INTERMACS that would be required to phenotype patients with recurrent heart failure on LVAD support.

PREVALENCE

Depending on the definition used, the prevalence of RV failure after LVAD ranges from 9% to 40%.[3,4,8,9] In the 2-year larger MOMENTUM cohort, the prevalence of RV failure was 34% in HeartMate 3 recipients; however, RVAD use was 4.1%.[1] Although this is down from the pulsatile pump era,[10] it remains high, especially given that INTERMACS 1 category patients comprised only 2% of HeartMate 3 recipients and those with expected RVAD placement were excluded from the study.[1] Collectively, these data suggest that, in real-world practice, RV failure rates are higher than observed in MOMENTUM, and that RV failure remains common in the contemporary continuous-flow era.

SIGNIFICANCE

Placement of a temporary RVAD after LVAD placement is associated with a 21% to 42% 30-day mortality.[11,12] The significance of a prolonged inotrope wean is less clear, but this was associated with 56% survival at 1 year in the HeartMate II bridge-to-transplant trial.[4] A mixed destination therapy and bridge-to-transplant population study of 114 patients found a 40% mortality at 90 days for patients who had RVAD use, prolonged inotrope or pulmonary vasodilator wean, or hypotension requiring vasopressors without sepsis.[3] Another possible outcome for patients with unplanned RVAD placement is a prolonged intensive care unit (ICU) stay and delayed overall recovery.[3] However, the concern for patients who survive the initial implant is late RV failure. However diagnosed, late right heart failure has been associated with higher complication rates and increased mortality.[13,14]

PATHOPHYSIOLOGY

In theory, single-ventricle physiology can be successful. In Fontan circulation, venous blood returns directly to the pulmonary circulation. As long as the left-sided filling pressures are low enough, the right-sided filling pressures are high enough, and as long as the pulmonary vascular resistance is low, this configuration works.[15] The existence of RV failure after LVAD implantation means that this circulatory configuration is more complicated than single-ventricle physiology.

PREOPERATIVE FACTORS

Patients who have left ventricular (LV) failure severe enough for an LVAD to be required for survival most often have concomitant RV failure. Whether the cardiac dysfunction was caused by a coronary artery disease, a genetic mutation, a virus, or toxin exposure such as chemotherapy or alcohol, the right ventricle is not spared. The chronicity of RV failure may also be important, as shown by the recent link between hemosiderosis above the knee and RV failure after LVAD placement (publication pending), because patients with these skin changes have likely had long-standing right heart failure. Longer-standing and more severe heart failure is also associated with sarcopenia and renal dysfunction, which have also been associated with poor outcomes after LVAD placement.[16,17] Pulmonary vascular resistance may also be a marker of chronicity, because long-standing increases in LV pressure lead to pulmonary vascular remodeling and ultimately a higher load for the right ventricle. Although pulmonary vascular resistance measurements change with patient optimization, this variable has been associated with the development of RV failure after LVAD placement in several separate analyses.[18,19] It may be that the RV failure that occurs after LVAD placement is a function of a right ventricle that is chronically failed, with little reserve in the setting of higher-than-normal pulmonary vascular resistance, which differs from Fontan physiology.

INTRAOPERATIVE FACTORS

Cardiopulmonary bypass, RV ischemia from hypotension, inotropes increasing myocardial demand, septal shift toward the left ventricle after turning on the LVAD, positioning the outflow graft over the right ventricle, and then closing the chest after administering intravenous fluid and blood products during surgery all likely contribute to immediate RV dysfunction after LVAD placement. Coronary artery or bypass graft injury can also occur during surgery affecting right coronary artery flow either directly or through collaterals. These factors may be mitigated with lateral thoracotomy,[20] shorter bypass times, excellent surgical technique, and delayed chest closure in complex cases.

LEFT VENTRICULAR ASSIST DEVICE/RIGHT VENTRICULAR INTERACTION

Clinicians are continuing to make progress in understanding the way the right ventricle responds to CF LVAD support. Three-dimensional echocardiography and serial hemodynamic studies have helped in this effort. The changes that occur in response to continuous-flow LVAD placement, including changing septal architecture and alterations in RV shape, can all negatively affect RV function.[21] Under normal physiologic conditions, 80% of RV function is through longitudinal shortening via the intraventricular septum.[22] After cardiothoracic surgery and opening the pericardium, there is a shift to transverse shortening.[23] Recent work by Houston and colleagues[24] using serial hemodynamic data after LVAD showed that although LVAD support decreases RV load, RV afterload sensitivity increases after LVAD implantation. It may be that this reliance on transverse motion contributes to deterioration in RV function if LVAD speeds are not high enough or if pulmonary vascular resistance remains high. Recent serial hemodynamic studies suggest that centrifugal pumps are different than axial pumps, indicating that some of the work to advanced the understanding of the right ventricle/left ventricle relationship may warrant repeating. For example, the HeartWare pump position seems to be important in achieving adequate LV unloading,[25] and this may be true for the HeartMate 3 as well.

PREDICTION OF RIGHT VENTRICULAR FAILURE

Up-front identification of patients who will develop severe right heart failure after LVAD implantation is important. Planned placement of biventricular support results in superior outcomes compared with patients receiving LVAD support with delayed institution of RVAD support.[26] For bridge-to-transplant patients, a direct-to-transplant strategy can make the difference between life and death. For destination therapy patients, unplanned RVAD placement after LVAD placement can lead to a painful and difficult ICU course with a high likelihood of death. There have been several previous studies designed to help predict those patients at high likelihood of developing RV failure following LVAD implantation. Some of the individual factors that have been identified include female gender, nonischemic heart failure cause, temporary support, and severity of tricuspid regurgitation.[12,19,27] Others have identified abnormal biochemical parameters such as increased blood urea nitrogen, bilirubin, creatinine, and aspartate aminotransferase levels, suggestive of preexisting severe multiorgan dysfunction.[28,29] Several hemodynamic variables, such as increased right atrial pressure, decreased RV stroke work index, increased pulmonary vascular resistance, increased diastolic pulmonary gradient, decrease pulmonary arterial pressure index, and tricuspid annular plane systolic excursion measured on echocardiography, have also been associated.[18,19,30,31] Several prediction models that incorporate several of these individual risk factors have been developed to capture risk of RV failure after LVAD placement. Most prediction models have not performed well outside of the derivation dataset.[3,32] This failure may be related to the fact that these models incorporate variables that are rapidly changing, such as biochemical markers (renal function, bilirubin) and central venous pressure, and echocardiographic variables can all change with LV unloading, diuresis, and inotropes. In addition, if the definition of RV failure has variables that are arbitrary (such as exact day of inotrope wean), then even variables that are clinically important in prediction of RVAD use, for example, may not perform well.

Some of the preoperative characteristics that have consistently been associated with RV failure include variables that quantify the size or pressure of the right ventricle relative to the left ventricle (central venous pressure/pulmonary capillary wedge pressure ratio, right ventricle/left ventricle size ratio) and variables that reflect how sick the patient is entering into surgery, such as those on continuous renal replacement therapy or temporary support.[3,4] Investigators are still searching for a reliable way to predict meaningful RV dysfunction after LVAD implantation. In the United States, with the bridge-to-transplant option open to patients with cardiogenic shock and with bridge-to-transplant LVADs persistently being passed by status 2 and 3 patients, the new LVAD implants will have a high percentage of destination therapy patients and bridge patients who are too critically ill to wait for transplant. With this overall sicker population receiving LVADs, higher RV failure rates may be observed than were previously seen in the continuous-flow era.

PREVENTION

Appropriate timing of advanced therapies is important because the natural history of INTERMACS 3 patients is deterioration into INTERMACS 2 and 1 categories or sudden death. In addition,

INTERMACS 4 patients have a 28% survival at 2 years without LVAD support, suggesting that a watchful waiting strategy may not be safe.[33,34] Although guidelines state to optimize patients before going to the operating room,[35] a balance exists between waiting for further optimization and proceeding, because more ICU complications and/or and further deterioration can lead to higher risk surgery or noncandidacy.

SURGICAL STRATEGIES

LVAD implant with standard median sternotomy has proved to be safe and efficient with experience over time and has shown excellent outcomes.[36,37] This approach allows performance of other interventions if needed, such as closure of patent foramen ovale or repair of aortic insufficiency. For patients at high risk for postoperative RV failure, the median sternotomy approach allows for simultaneous placement of central RV support. Central RV support is placed in the following way at our institution: the right atrium is cannulated with a 34-Fr malleable right-angle cannula for drainage and the main pulmonary artery with an 18-Fr to 22-Fr elongated 1-piece arterial (EOPA) cannula for return. This configuration can be constructed using the CentriMag pump with the addition of an oxygenator if necessary. Alternatively, a CardioHelp circuit, or similar, can be used.

The upper hemisternotomy and limited left thoracotomy (the Hanover approach) is an alternative approach to LVAD implantation and has been associated with lower rates of postoperative RV failure. The LATERAL trial of HeartWare implantation in the bridge-to-transplant population reported only 0.7% (1 out of 144) postoperative RVAD use.[20] This technique is performed by making a small upper hemisternotomy with a J into the fourth or fifth intercostal space. Aortic cannulation can be performed centrally through the upper hemisternotomy incision. The authors routinely use an 18-Fr to 22-Fr EOPA cannula for arterial access. Venous drainage is typically performed by femoral venous access. Most cases achieve excellent flow rates with a 25-Fr Bio-Medicus femoral venous drainage cannula. In select cases the right atrial appendage can be cannulated centrally for venous drainage. The authors use a 28-Fr 3-stage venous cannula in these cases. After assessment for adequate central access, a fifth or sixth left anterolateral thoracotomy is created. Intercostal nerve block with Exparel, Cryo, or Marcaine can provide improved postoperative pain control. The ventricular apical cuff is secured. Cardiopulmonary bypass is initiated for the ventricular coring, pump placement, and outflow graft anastomosis. Benefits of this technique include lower postoperative pain scores, less bleeding (which can be especially helpful in redo cases), less dissection of the intrapericardial structures, less kinking of the right coronary artery, and less violation of the pericardium.

RECOGNITION AND MANAGEMENT OF RIGHT VENTRICULAR FAILURE

Identification of RV failure after LVAD placement can be challenging. RV failure can mimic tamponade hemodynamically, and echocardiography may not be very revealing in the early postoperative period. It is common for patients with end-stage heart failure to have low blood pressure coming out of the operating room, often labeled vasoplegia. This low blood pressure is combated with vasopressors and some inotropic support until drips are weaned down, with the goal of vasopressor wean to maintain mean arterial pressure around 70 mm Hg, cardiac index more than 2.0 L/min/min², and central venous pressure between 8 and 12 mm Hg, with gradually increasing LVAD speeds to ensure adequate LV unloading. Any intraoperative lactate production should trend down, creatinine level often increases but then trends down, with urine output being maintained and aspartate transaminase/alanine transaminase ratio remaining normal.[9] Total bilirubin level often increases immediately postoperatively but then trends down.[9] If inotrope/pressor requirements are not decreasing, lactate level starts to increase, urine output is decreasing, and/or mean arterial pressure is decreasing, the diagnosis may be tamponade or RV failure. Both may have low LVAD pulsatility, high right atrial pressure, and low cardiac output. Early recognition and treatment can make the difference between survival or not. Echocardiography often shows marginal RV function (often present previously) and any postoperative hematoma may be hard to visualize. Because these diagnoses can be difficult to differentiate, some programs return to the operating room to reopen the patient. This reoperation allows any postoperative pericardial fluid or collection to be cleared and provides the right ventricle more room to fill. If the patient is not improving with opening the chest (eg, with a high ongoing pressor requirement or borderline mean arterial pressures) a temporary RVAD can be placed in the operating room, as previously described.

Early mild RV failure can be managed with inotropes, pulmonary vasodilators, decreasing the pump speed if pulmonary capillary wedge pressure is low, and with further diuresis. End-organ function and lactate should be trended often to ensure these maneuvers are successful. Escalation of vasopressors/inotropes, increasing lactate level, or decreasing urine output are signs of inadequate perfusion and signal that mechanical RV support is needed. In our practice, if the chest is already closed, a Proteck Duo temporary RVAD is placed in the cardiac catheterization laboratory. This approach shows a trend in improved survival compared with surgical RVAD.[38]

EMERGING RIGHT VENTRICULAR FAILURE PHENOTYPE

One of the emerging RV failure phenotypes is the relative RV failure in the setting of vasoplegia. If the patient's systemic vascular resistance is less than 800 dyn/s/cm^{-5} on high-dose vasopressors and the patient's blood pressure is borderline, the cardiac index between the LVAD and the chemical RVAD (inotropes) may be greater than 2 L/min/m^2; however, with this degree of vasoplegia, the cardiac index may need to be double that or more. In these cases, the classic RV failure phenotype of high central venous pressure, low pulmonary capillary wedge pressure, and low cardiac index may not be present; however, lactate level will start to increase and end-organ function will start to deteriorate if more vasopressors/inotropes are added alone. Although the LVAD speed can be increased, the right ventricle that has longstanding dysfunction and is facing abnormal pulmonary vascular resistance may not be able to compensate. In these cases, our team practice is to place a percutaneous RVAD with significant escalation of bilateral pump speeds to increase cardiac output. This practice allows vasopressors to be weaned slowly until vasoplegia resolves and then the RVAD can be weaned. The threshold for placing a percutaneous RVAD in this setting may be different from program to program; however, the natural history of vasoplegia after LVAD placement treated with vasopressors alone carries a very high mortality, suggesting an alternative strategy may be warranted.[39] In addition, there are overlapping risk factors for RV failure and vasoplegia after LVAD, and preoperative inflammatory state is associated with the development of RV failure after LVAD, suggesting an overlapping mechanism.[40] Further work in this area is warranted to understand how these physiologies are linked so that prevention and treatment strategies can be standardized.

FUTURE DIRECTIONS

Clinicians are beginning to understand more about the impact of LVAD support on RV function over time. This understanding will help define preoperative factors that matter and may help develop treatment strategies tailored to patients. A step in the right direction would be to develop a clinically meaningful, universal definition of RV failure after LVAD placement with a high repeatability. Investigators have also not identified optimal LVAD timing, because ROADMAP (Risk Assessment and Comparative Effectiveness of Left Ventricular Assist Device and Medical Management in Ambulatory Heart Failure Patients) was not a randomized clinical trial. Getting the timing right is important because the lower the INTERMACS profile, the worse the outcomes after LVAD and the higher the risk for RV failure,[41] especially for patients who are on destination therapy. For high-risk patients who are candidates for transplant, alternative strategies to transplant is what the new United Network for Organ Sharing system is designed for in the United States. Until there is a device that does the job of both ventricles with an efficacy acceptable for destination therapy, RV failure will continue to be a significant problem that limits the success of LVADs and prevents wider-scale adoption. As surgical techniques improve, shorter bypass times and lateral thoracotomy hold promise, although further data will be needed to determine the impact.

REFERENCES

1. Mehra MR, Uriel N, Naka Y, et al. A fully magnetically levitated left ventricular assist device - final report. N Engl J Med 2019;380:1618–27.
2. Dang NC, Topkara VK, Mercando M, et al. Right heart failure after left ventricular assist device implantation in patients with chronic congestive heart failure. J Heart Lung Transplant 2006;25:1–6.
3. Kalogeropoulos AP, Kelkar A, Weinberger JF, et al. Validation of clinical scores for right ventricular failure prediction after implantation of continuous-flow left ventricular assist devices. J Heart Lung Transplant 2015;34:1595–603.
4. Kormos RL, Teuteberg JJ, Pagani FD, et al. Right ventricular failure in patients with the HeartMate II continuous-flow left ventricular assist device: incidence, risk factors, and effect on outcomes. J Thorac Cardiovasc Surg 2010;139:1316–24.
5. Soliman OII, Akin S, Muslem R, et al. Derivation and validation of a novel right-sided heart failure model after implantation of continuous flow left ventricular assist devices: the EUROMACS (European Registry for Patients with Mechanical Circulatory Support) right-sided heart failure risk score. Circulation 2018;137:891–906.
6. Alabama TUo: The STS Intermacs Database. 2019, Nov 1.

7. Joly JM, El-Dabh A, Marshell R, et al. Performance of noninvasive assessment in the diagnosis of right heart failure after left ventricular assist device. ASAIO J 2019;65:449–55.

8. Potapov EV, Schweiger M, Stepanenko A, et al. Tricuspid valve repair in patients supported with left ventricular assist devices. ASAIO J 2011;57: 363–7.

9. Patel ND, Weiss ES, Schaffer J, et al. Right heart dysfunction after left ventricular assist device implantation: a comparison of the pulsatile HeartMate I and axial-flow HeartMate II devices. Ann Thorac Surg 2008;86:832–40 [discussion: 832–40].

10. Rose EA, Gelijns AC, Moskowitz AJ, et al. Long-term use of a left ventricular assist device for end-stage heart failure. N Engl J Med 2001;345:1435–43.

11. Slaughter MS, Rogers JG, Milano CA, et al. Advanced heart failure treated with continuous-flow left ventricular assist device. N Engl J Med 2009; 361:2241–51.

12. Ochiai Y, McCarthy PM, Smedira NG, et al. Predictors of severe right ventricular failure after implantable left ventricular assist device insertion: analysis of 245 patients. Circulation 2002;106: 1198–202.

13. Takeda K, Takayama H, Colombo PC, et al. Incidence and clinical significance of late right heart failure during continuous-flow left ventricular assist device support. J Heart Lung Transplant 2015;34: 1024–32.

14. Kapelios CJ, Charitos C, Kaldara E, et al. Late-onset right ventricular dysfunction after mechanical support by a continuous-flow left ventricular assist device. J Heart Lung Transplant 2015;34:1604–10.

15. Ridderbos FS, Ebels T, Berger RMF. The pulmonary vasculature: achilles heel of the Fontan circulation. Heart 2019;105:1922–3.

16. Teigen LM, John R, Kuchnia AJ, et al. Preoperative pectoralis muscle quantity and attenuation by computed tomography are novel and powerful predictors of mortality after left ventricular assist device implantation. Circ Heart Fail 2017;10 [pii:e004069].

17. Givens RC, Topkara VK. Renal risk stratification in left ventricular assist device therapy. Expert Rev Med Devices 2018;15:27–33.

18. Alnsasra H, Asleh R, Schettle SD, et al. Diastolic pulmonary gradient as a predictor of right ventricular failure after left ventricular assist device implantation. J Am Heart Assoc 2019;8:e012073.

19. Drakos SG, Janicki L, Horne BD, et al. Risk factors predictive of right ventricular failure after left ventricular assist device implantation. Am J Cardiol 2010; 105:1030–5.

20. McGee E Jr, Danter M, Strueber M, et al. Evaluation of a lateral thoracotomy implant approach for a centrifugal-flow left ventricular assist device: the LATERAL clinical trial. J Heart Lung Transplant 2019;38:344–51.

21. Sack KL, Dabiri Y, Franz T, et al. Investigating the role of interventricular interdependence in development of right heart dysfunction during LVAD support: a patient-specific methods-based approach. Front Physiol 2018;9:520.

22. Dandel M, Potapov E, Krabatsch T, et al. Load dependency of right ventricular performance is a major factor to be considered in decision making before ventricular assist device implantation. Circulation 2013;128:S14–23.

23. Raina A, Vaidya A, Gertz ZM, et al. Marked changes in right ventricular contractile pattern after cardiothoracic surgery: implications for post-surgical assessment of right ventricular function. J Heart Lung Transplant 2013;32:777–83.

24. Houston BA, Kalathiya RJ, Hsu S, et al. Right ventricular afterload sensitivity dramatically increases after left ventricular assist device implantation: a multicenter hemodynamic analysis. J Heart Lung Transplant 2016;35:868–76.

25. Imamura T, Adatya S, Chung B, et al. Cannula and pump positions are associated with left ventricular unloading and clinical outcome in patients with heartware left ventricular assist device. J Card Fail 2018;24:159–66.

26. Fitzpatrick JR 3rd, Frederick JR, Hiesinger W, et al. Early planned institution of biventricular mechanical circulatory support results in improved outcomes compared with delayed conversion of a left ventricular assist device to a biventricular assist device. J Thorac Cardiovasc Surg 2009;137:971–7.

27. Potapov EV, Stepanenko A, Dandel M, et al. Tricuspid incompetence and geometry of the right ventricle as predictors of right ventricular function after implantation of a left ventricular assist device. J Heart Lung Transplant 2008;27:1275–81.

28. Matthews JC, Koelling TM, Pagani FD, et al. The right ventricular failure risk score a pre-operative tool for assessing the risk of right ventricular failure in left ventricular assist device candidates. J Am Coll Cardiol 2008;51:2163–72.

29. Yost GL, Coyle L, Bhat G, et al. Model for end-stage liver disease predicts right ventricular failure in patients with left ventricular assist devices. J Artif Organs 2016;19:21–8.

30. Puwanant S, Hamilton KK, Klodell CT, et al. Tricuspid annular motion as a predictor of severe right ventricular failure after left ventricular assist device implantation. J Heart Lung Transplant 2008;27: 1102–7.

31. Morine KJ, Kiernan MS, Pham DT, et al. Pulmonary artery pulsatility index is associated with right ventricular failure after left ventricular assist device surgery. J Card Fail 2016;22:110–6.

32. Pettinari M, Jacobs S, Rega F, et al. Are right ventricular risk scores useful? Eur J Cardiothorac Surg 2012;42:621–6.

33. Stewart GC, Ambardekar AV, Kittleson MM. Defining ambulatory advanced heart failure: MedaMACS and beyond. Curr Heart Fail Rep 2017;14:498–506.

34. Shah KB, Starling RC, Rogers JG, et al. Left ventricular assist devices versus medical management in ambulatory heart failure patients: an analysis of INTERMACS Profiles 4 and 5 to 7 from the ROADMAP study. J Heart Lung Transplant 2018;37:706–14.

35. Feldman D, Pamboukian SV, Teuteberg JJ, et al. The 2013 International Society for Heart and Lung Transplantation guidelines for mechanical circulatory support: executive summary. J Heart Lung Transplant 2013;32:157–87.

36. Krabatsch T, Drews T, Potapov E, et al. Different surgical strategies for implantation of continuous-flow VADs-Experience from Deutsches Herzzentrum Berlin. Ann Cardiothorac Surg 2014;3:472–4.

37. Estep JD, Starling RC, Horstmanshof DA, et al. Risk assessment and comparative effectiveness of left ventricular assist device and medical management in ambulatory heart failure patients: results from the ROADMAP Study. J Am Coll Cardiol 2015;66:1747–61.

38. Coromilas EJ, Takeda K, Ando M, et al. Comparison of percutaneous and surgical right ventricular assist device support after durable left ventricular assist device insertion. J Card Fail 2019;25:105–13.

39. de Waal EEC, van Zaane B, van der Schoot MM, et al. Vasoplegia after implantation of a continuous flow left ventricular assist device: incidence, outcomes and predictors. BMC Anesthesiol 2018;18:185.

40. Tang PC, Haft JW, Romano MA, et al. Right ventricular failure following left ventricular assist device implantation is associated with a preoperative proinflammatory response. J Cardiothorac Surg 2019;14:80.

41. Kiernan MS, Grandin EW, Brinkley M Jr, et al. Early right ventricular assist device use in patients undergoing continuous-flow left ventricular assist device implantation: incidence and risk factors from the Interagency Registry for Mechanically Assisted Circulatory Support. Circ Heart Fail 2017;10 [pii: e003863].

Right Heart Failure After Left Ventricular Assist Device Placement

Medical and Surgical Management Considerations

Francis D. Pagani, MD, PhD

KEYWORDS

- Right heart failure • Mechanical circulatory assistance • Left ventricular assist device
- Right ventricular assist device • Total artificial heart • Heart transplantation • Heart failure

KEY POINTS

- Right heart failure after durable left ventricular assist device implantation occurs in approximately 20% to 40% of patients and is associated with significant morbidity and mortality.
- The medical treatment of right heart failure focuses on improving right ventricular contractility and optimizing right ventricular preload and afterload and cardiac rhythm.
- Mechanical circulatory support options for the right heart include extracorporeal membrane oxygenation and surgically implanted device options and percutaneous extracorporeal devices.
- The total artificial heart and heart transplantation remain definitive therapies for unrecoverable right heart failure refractory to optimal medical management or temporary device strategies.

INTRODUCTION

Durable left ventricular assist device (LVAD) therapy is an increasingly accepted surgical therapy for management of advanced heart failure (HF) refractory to guideline-directed medical therapy.[1] Right HF (RHF) is a known and frequent complication after durable LVAD implantation and remains an important clinical challenge preventing broader dissemination of the therapy.[2] A significant proportion of patients being evaluated for LVAD therapy have underlying biventricular dysfunction that poses a risk for RHF after durable LVAD implantation.[2] After durable LVAD implantation, RHF occurs in approximately 20% to 50% of patients.[2–8] RHF restricts LVAD output and contributes to systemic hypoperfusion and the onset of multiorgan dysfunction, increases postoperative morbidity and mortality, prolongs length of stay for the index hospitalization, and has an adverse impact on

successful bridging to heart transplantation as well as post-transplant survival.[2–8] RHF is defined by The Society of Thoracic Surgeons Interagency Registry for Mechanically Assisted Circulatory Support (Intermacs) as increases in the central venous pressure (CVP) accompanied by clinical manifestations including edema, ascites, or worsening hepatic or renal dysfunction[9,10] (**Box 1**). Severe RHF is described by Intermacs as the need for prolonged (ie, >2 weeks) postimplant inotropes, inhaled nitric oxide or intravenous pulmonary vasodilators, or the requirement for right ventricular (RV) mechanical support[9,10] (see **Box 1**). The risk of developing RHF after durable LVAD implantation is multifactorial and depends on the RV contractile state and RV preload and afterload, as well as clinical factors such as the presence of pulmonary, hepatic, and renal dysfunction. Numerous prognostic models have

Department of Cardiac Surgery, Center for Circulatory Support, Frankel Cardiovascular Center, University of Michigan, 5161 Cardiovascular Center, SPC 5864, 1500 East Medical Center Drive, Ann Arbor, MI 48109, USA
E-mail address: fpagani@umich.edu

Cardiol Clin 38 (2020) 227–238
https://doi.org/10.1016/j.ccl.2020.01.005
0733-8651/20/© 2020 Elsevier Inc. All rights reserved.

Box 1
The Society of Thoracic Surgeons Intermacs definition of RHF after durable LVAD implantation

RHF

Definition: Symptoms or findings of persistent right ventricular failure characterized by both of the following:

- Documentation of elevated CVP by:

  o Direct measurement (eg, right heart catheterization) with evidence of a CVP or right atrial pressure of greater than16 mm Hg,

    Or

  o Findings of significantly dilated inferior vena cava with absence of inspiratory variation by echocardiography,

    Or

  o Clinical findings of elevated jugular venous distension at least half way up the neck in an upright patient.

- Manifestations of elevated CVP characterized by:

  o Clinical findings of peripheral edema ($\geq$2+ either new or unresolved),

    Or

  o Presence of ascites or palpable hepatomegaly on physical examination (unmistakable abdominal contour) or by diagnostic imaging,

    Or

  o Laboratory evidence of worsening hepatic (total bilirubin >2.0 mg/dL) or renal dysfunction (creatinine >2.0 mg/dL).

If the patient meets the definition for RHF, the severity of the RHF will be graded according to the following scale.

(Note: For RHF to meet severe or severe acute severity, direct measurement of CVP or right atrial pressure must be one of the criteria.)

RHF severity grade

Mild RHF

  VAD implant admission

    Patient meets *both* criteria for RHF plus

    - Postimplant inotropes, inhaled nitric oxide or intravenous vasodilators not continued beyond postoperative day 7 after VAD implantation

      AND

    - No inotropes continued beyond postoperative day 7 after VAD implantation

  Surveillance periods (3 months, 6 months, 12 months, and every 6 months thereafter) after VAD implant

    Patient meets both criteria for RHF plus

    - No readmissions for RHF since last surveillance period

      AND

    - No inotropes since last surveillance period.

Moderate RHF

  VAD implant admission

    Patient meets both criteria for RHF plus:

    - Postimplant inotropes, inhaled nitric oxide or intravenous vasodilators continued beyond post-operative day 7 and up to postoperative day 14 after VAD implantation

Surveillance periods (3 months, 6 months, 12 months, and every 6 months hereafter) after VAD implantation

Patient meets both criteria for RHF plus:

- Limited to one[1] readmission for intravenous diuretics/vasodilators to treat RHF since last surveillance period

  AND

No inotropes since last surveillance period

Severe RHF

VAD implant admission

Patient meets both criteria for RHF plus:

- CVP or right atrial pressure of greater than 16 mm Hg

  AND

- Prolonged postimplant inotropes, inhaled nitric oxide or intravenous vasodilators continued beyond postoperative day 14 after VAD implantation

Surveillance periods (3 months, 6 months, 12 months, and every 6 months thereafter) after VAD implantation

Patient meets both criteria for RHF plus:

- Need for inotropes at any time since last surveillance period

  OR

- Two[2] or more readmissions for intravenous diuretics/vasodilators to treat RHF since last surveillance period

  OR

- Requiring RV assist device support at any time after hospital discharge

  OR

- Death at any time after discharge from the VAD implant hospitalization with RHF as the primary cause.

Severe acute RHF

VAD implant admission

Patient meets both criteria for RHF plus:

- CVP or right atrial pressure of greater than 16 mm Hg

  AND

- Need for right ventricular assist device at any time after VAD implantation

  OR

- Death during the VAD implants hospitalization with RHF as the primary cause.

been reported that examine risk factors associated with development of RHF after LVAD implantation.[4,6,7,11–20] These models generally consist of weighted clinical, hemodynamic, or echocardiographic variables. However, these models have lacked sufficient sensitivity and specificity to be relied on for preoperative clinical decision making regarding planned use of right-sided mechanical circulatory support (MCS).[4,6,7,11–20] Clinical assessment alone may be as reliable in identifying patients at risk of RHF.[21] Recent investigations using Bayesian network algorithms have improved identification of groups of risk factors and their conditional interdependency.[20]

MEDICAL STRATEGIES TO MANAGE RIGHT HEART FAILURE AFTER DURABLE LEFT VENTRICULAR ASSIST DEVICE IMPLANTATION

Medical management is the mainstay of therapy to prevent and manage RHF after LVAD implantation[2,16,22] (**Fig. 1**). Medical therapy is focused on

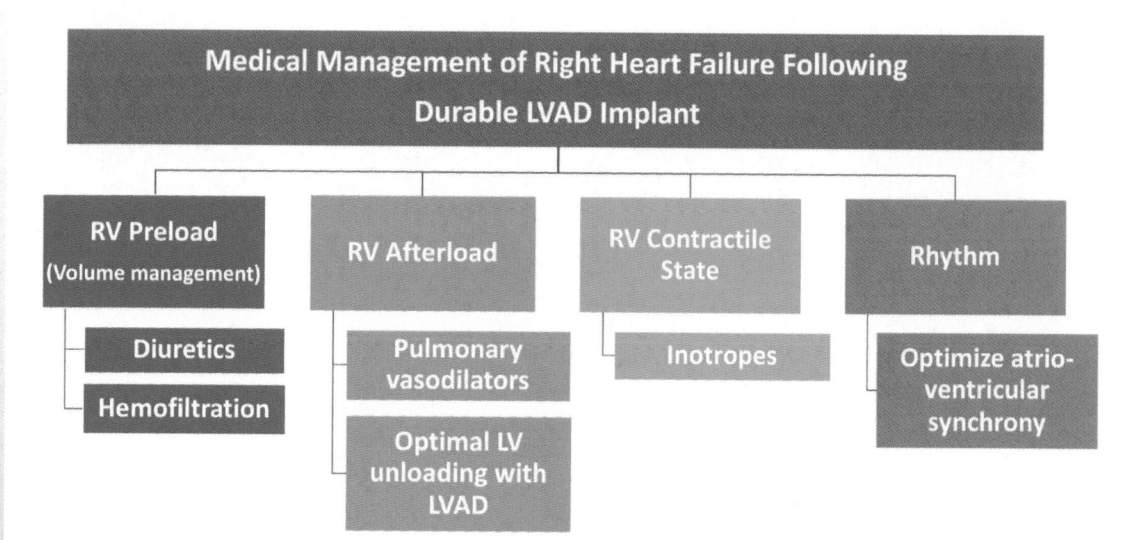

Fig. 1. Medical management of RHF after durable LVAD implant. LV, left ventricle; RV, right ventricle.

4 major areas: (1) volume management and optimization of RV preload, (2) improvement in the contractile state of the RV, (3) reduction in RV afterload, and (4) optimization of cardiac rhythm. Hemodynamic goals after LVAD implantation should optimally include a CVP goal of 8 to 12 mm Hg, with a cardiac index of 2.2 L/kg/m^2 or greater with a mean systemic perfusion pressure of 80 to 90 mm Hg.[2,22] With these hemodynamic goals, adequate systemic perfusion should be present with normalization of serum lactate levels and satisfactory cerebral, renal, and hepatic function.

Volume management is critical to prevent over-distension of the RV and prevent venous hypertension in the liver and kidneys that contribute to end-organ dysfunction. Volume overload of the RV may increase tricuspid regurgitation (TR) and result in leftward shift of the interventricular septum which can reduce left ventricular (LV) filling, worsening LVAD output and increasing venous congestion. Volume management should optimally be guided by monitoring CVP or by a pulmonary artery (PA) catheter.[23] The mainstay of volume management is appropriate diuretic use.[24] Typically, loop diuretics in combination with a thiazide diuretic are effective in achieving optimal volume status if significant renal dysfunction is not present. In cases of diuretic resistance and volume overload, use of venovenous hemofiltration should be used to optimize RV preload.[23]

Improvement in RV contractility with inotrope support is critical to the prevention and management RHF. Although several inotrope agents are available, the use of milrinone or dobutamine has several advantages over that of epinephrine or dopamine. Milrinone, and to a lesser degree dobutamine, have both inotrope and vasodilatory affects that (1) improve RV contractility and (2) elicit vasodilation of the pulmonary vasculature to decrease pulmonary vascular resistance (PVR) and reduce RV afterload.[25,26] The major disadvantage of milrinone is that its vasodilation properties are not restricted to the pulmonary vasculature and systemic hypotension may occur. Dobutamine has less vasodilator potential and thus is not as effective in decreasing the RV afterload, but has a lesser propensity to cause systemic hypotension. Additionally, dobutamine has the advantage of a much shorter half-life compared with milrinone.[26] An additional risk for the use of any inotrope is atrial or ventricular tachyarrhythmias, although milrinone is thought to be less likely to induce a tachycardia compared with dobutamine, epinephrine, or dopamine. Importantly, milrinone is partially renally cleared, and the estimated glomerular filtration rate must be considered in the determination of appropriate dosing.[25] To minimize catecholamine use and lessen the risk of exciting atrial or ventricular arrhythmias, vasopressor therapy, when needed in conjunction with inotrope therapy to counteract systemic vasodilation, can be initiated with a catecholamine-sparing regimen with vasopressin or angiotensin II in place of norepinephrine, moderate to higher doses of epinephrine or phenylephrine.[27] Maintaining a mean systemic perfusion pressure of 80 to 90 mm Hg is critical to maintaining cerebral, hepatic, and renal perfusion and providing sufficient afterload to the LVAD to prevent inappropriate LV unloading and suction events.

Optimization of RV afterload is critical to prevent or management RHF. Although LVAD therapy decreases the LV preload that has beneficial effects on RV afterload, the effects of LVAD unloading may not be observed early after LVAD implantation in the setting of chronically elevated PVR where a significant pressure gradient exists between the pulmonary diastolic pressure and the left atrial pressure. If high PVR is present in the setting of RHF, RV afterload can be reduced with pulmonary vasodilators as the primary therapy. In the acute setting, inhaled nitric oxide or inhaled or systemic administration of prostacyclins are effective in reducing PVR and decreasing RV afterload.[3,28–30] In the chronic setting of RHF, oral therapy with the endothelin receptor antagonist, bosentan, and the phosphodiesterase-5 inhibitor, sildenafil, have been shown to have important benefits in decreasing RV afterload.[31] Inhaled nitric oxide acts via the cyclic guanosine monophosphate pathway to cause pulmonary vasodilatation. Inhaled nitric oxide has been previously studied in patients with acute RHF and has been shown in combination with dobutamine to improve cardiac output and oxygenation, and to decrease PVR. Inhaled or intravenous administration of prostacyclins, that is, epoprostenol, act via the cyclic adenosine monophosphate pathway to result in potent pulmonary vasodilatation, systemic vasodilatation, and inhibition of platelet aggregation.[32] Inhaled administration of epoprostenol is thought to have a lower risk of causing significant systemic hypotension compared with the intravenous administration.

Ventilator management is critical to optimizing RV afterload. Increasing mean airway pressures significantly increase RV afterload and exacerbates RHF. Thus, excessive tidal volumes and positive end-expiratory pressure increase the PA pressure, CVP, and RV afterload. Optimal ventilator settings should be selected to obtain satisfactory systemic oxygenation; optimal ventilation reduces the risk of hypercapnia at the lowest mean airway pressures.

Optimal rhythm management in the setting of RHF is important to maximizing RV output. Maintaining sinus rhythm at optimal heart rates of 80 to 110 beats per minute maximizes RV output and contractility. Efforts should be made to restore sinus rhythm in patients with atrial arrhythmias given the contribution of atrial contraction to cardiac output in RHF. The placement of temporary pacing wires at the time of LVAD implantation permits the option of treating bradyarrhythmias with atrial or atrioventricular pacing or using liberal pharmacologic suppression of tachyarrhythmias with the option of temporary pacing, if needed.

Digoxin is of value in controlling atrial tachyarrhythmias in the setting of RHF and additionally improves RV contractility.[33] Amiodarone is also an effective antiarrhythmic agent in controlling atrial and ventricular arrhythmias.

MANAGEMENT OF THE LEFT VENTRICULAR ASSIST DEVICE SPEED CONTROL IN THE SETTING OF RIGHT HEART FAILURE

Although LVAD unloading of the LV may decrease RV afterload and improve RV contractility, LVAD support has important hemodynamic effects that may adversely impact RV function and exacerbate RHF. LVAD unloading of the LV results in the loss of the intraventricular septal contribution to RV function and contributes to a decrease in RV contractility.[34,35] Further, leftward septal shift, caused by inappropriate LV unloading from high LVAD speeds, may result in RV distension and TR.[34,35] Further, augmented output by the LVAD device may result in increased preload to the RV, further exacerbating RV distension and TR. Management of the LVAD device is thus important in the prevention and management of RHF. Early device management should focus on maintaining device speeds sufficient to obtain satisfactory hemodynamic goals without inappropriate LV unloading.[22,36] Early in the postoperative setting, LVAD speed control should focus on maintaining a rightward or neutral position of the interventricular septum and limiting cardiac output. As RV function improves, LVAD speeds can be increased to accommodate the increase in LV preload.[22,36]

Maintaining appropriate systemic perfusion pressure in the setting of LVAD support is another important aspect to facilitate device management. Vasodilation or low systemic perfusion pressures result in inappropriate unloading of the LV by the LVAD that can contribute to leftward septal shift and suction events. Suction events prevent adequate LVAD output and may additionally cause ventricular arrhythmias.

INTRAOPERATIVE STRATEGIES TO MANAGE RIGHT HEART FAILURE ASSOCIATED WITH LEFT VENTRICULAR ASSIST DEVICE THERAPY

A variety of intraoperative factors may result in worsening right heart function. Surgical technique that limits the duration of cardiopulmonary bypass time and aortic cross-clamp time, if needed, is important in reducing the risk of RV injury after durable LVAD implantation. Recent evidence suggests that RV function may be less impaired by using a minimally invasive surgical approach with an anterior lateral thoracotomy and limited upper sternotomy as compared with a complete median sternotomy approach.[37] Additionally, durable LVAD implantation without the use of cardiopulmonary bypass (ie, off pump surgery) may decrease systemic inflammation and the need for blood transfusion, as well as preserving RV function.[38] Importantly, careful attention to bleeding can limit the requirement for transfusion, which may prevent inflammation and transfusion-related lung injury that adversely impacts systemic oxygenation, PVR, and, subsequently, RV afterload.[38] Proper deairing techniques during weaning from cardiopulmonary bypass could also prevent air embolism to the right coronary artery resulting in RV ischemia.[17] Delayed sternal closure is also an effective strategy to manage coagulopathy to prevent cardiac tamponade and not further impair RV function by mechanical compression. This approach has been demonstrated not to increase postoperative risk of infection, although its potential benefit has recently been brought into question.[39,40]

Significant mitral valve and tricuspid valve disease is frequently present in patients presenting for durable LVAD implantation. Moderate to severe functional TR is present in approximately 40% to 50% of patients undergoing LVAD implantation and persists in 23% to 40% of patients after durable LVAD implantation.[41–45] TR is usually secondary to annular dilation and leaflet tethering, and is generally associated with worse RV function and/or elevated PVR. Patients with significant preoperative TR have more tricuspid valve annular enlargement and lower RV stroke work and are at greater risk for postoperative RHF.[41–45] Despite the potential favorable effects of the LVAD on reducing RV afterload, the severity of TR does not always improve after LVAD implantation owing to interventricular septal shift, RV dilation and increase in RV preload from the LVAD.[45] Although the presence of postoperative significant TR has been shown to be associated with worse clinical outcomes, including a longer duration of inotrope support, a greater need for RV assist device (RVAD) support, a longer hospital stay, and a trend toward worse survival, concomitant tricuspid valve repair at the time of LVAD implantation has not been conclusively shown to improve outcomes or decrease the risk of RHF.[45–53]

Significant MR is frequently present in patients with advanced HF and is associated with a worse prognosis.[54,55] More than 50% of patients presenting for durable LVAD evaluation have at least moderate MR at the time of LVAD implantation.[54,55] In the majority of patients, significant MR resolves with LVAD support owing to the significant unloading of the LV.[56–60] Persistent secondary MR after LVAD implantation has been demonstrated to have detrimental hemodynamic and clinical effects, and is associated with persistent pulmonary hypertension, worse RV function, and worse survival.[57,59] Whether concomitant mitral valve repair or replacement to address MR improves outcomes, specifically RV function, is unknown and remains controversial.

MECHANICAL CIRCULATORY SUPPORT DEVICE THERAPIES TO MANAGE RIGHT HEART FAILURE AFTER DURABLE LEFT VENTRICULAR ASSIST DEVICE IMPLANTATION

Right-sided MCS is reserved for patients refractory to optimal medical management of RHF. The appropriate timing of intervention is critical in optimizing patient outcomes to prevent delays in instituting MCS therapy and causing unnecessary morbidity and mortality. Temporary MCS device options for RHF, in setting of durable LVAD support, can be used as a bridge to recovery of the right heart, bridge to heart transplantation along with support of the durable LVAD, or as a bridge to a durable right-sided MCS device implant if temporary MCS for right heart support was initially provided and temporary MCS cannot be withdrawn and durable biventricular support is needed to facilitate patient discharge from the hospital.[61–63] Durable MCS device strategies for management of RHF include concomitant durable RVAD implant with durable LVAD implantation or implantation of a total artificial heart. These latter 2 options assume recovery of the right heart is highly unlikely and the patient needs permanent biventricular support as a bridge to heart transplantation or as destination therapy.

In the setting of early RHF after durable LVAD implantation, recent observations suggests that approximately 42% to 75% of patients may recover sufficient right heart function to permit explantation of the right-sided MCS device.[61–63] Thus, the appropriate application of right-sided MCS is essential to maximize the possibility of myocardial recovery. Studies have shown that planned or early RVAD implantation is associated with superior outcomes compared with delayed or rescue placement.[64,65]

There are no standard hemodynamic thresholds to initiate temporary MCS support for RHF and the decision depends on a number of important clinical indicators and experience. Low cardiac output assessed hemodynamically by a cardiac index of less than 2.0 L/min/m^2 with a CVP of greater than 15 mm Hg supports a diagnosis of RHF in the setting of normal LVAD operation. If hemodynamic parameters consistent with RHF are accompanied by evidence of inadequate systemic perfusion (eg, elevated serum lactate, evidence of renal and/or hepatic dysfunction) despite optimal medical management, MCS for right heart support should be initiated. A common mistake in the management of RHF is the failure to promptly institute MCS before the occurrence of significant renal or hepatic injury. The goal of temporary right-sided MCS device placement is to support the failing RV and preserve LVAD preload and end-organ perfusion in the hopes that there will be gradual and consistent improvement in RV and/or pulmonary injury, which permits weaning of the right heart support device.

A challenge in the management of patients who present with clinical evidence of biventricular failure is discriminating between patients who have primary RV involvement necessitating true concomitant RV and LV support from those with RHF caused primarily by left-sided heart disease, where LVAD support alone may be sufficient. Importantly, not all patients who present with biventricular dysfunction require biventricular support at the time of operation. However, determining which patients can be adequately supported by isolated LV support is challenging because clinical and hemodynamic predictors have low specificity with regard to identifying patients requiring right-sided circulatory support. Patients with biventricular dysfunction who initially receive isolated LV support should be monitored closely for clinical deterioration and evidence of worsening RHF should lead to rapid deployment of right-sided support mechanical support.

Among patients with RHF secondary to left-sided failure, LVAD support may provide sufficient improvement in right heart function as a consequence of RV unloading from LV decompression. Clinical experience along with prognostic models permit estimations of the probability of recovery of the right heart to guide a decision as to whether to use a strategy of durable (ie, total artificial heart) versus temporary right-sided support devices.[4,6,7,11,12,14–19,66,67] The appropriate type of MCS device used to support the right heart is determined by whether the pathogenesis of the RHF is a primary RV insult (ie, myocardial stunning or infarction) or is the result of disease of the pulmonary vasculature or parenchyma. Typically, acute RHF from a primary pathogeneses of the RV lends itself to application with temporary implantable or percutaneous RVADs. Acute forms of RHF dominated by pathology of the pulmonary vasculature or parenchyma may be more appropriately treated with extracorporeal membrane oxygenation (ECMO) as opposed to a surgical implanted or percutaneous RVAD because

increased pulmonary blood flow from an RVAD, in the setting of pulmonary hypertension, may further increase PA pressure and increase the risk of pulmonary hemorrhage or exacerbate further pulmonary interstitial edema.[68]

Temporary MCS device options to support the right heart include newer percutaneous devices designed specifically for RV support and include the Impella RP (Abiomed, Inc., Danvers, MA; http://www.abiomed.com/impella/impella-rp) 394 and TandemHeart pVAD with the PROTEK Duo cannula (TandemLife, Inc., Pittsburgh, PA; http://www.tandemlife.com/protekduo-kit/).[69,70] The Impella RP is a microaxial temporary extracorporeal VAD that is placed percutaneously through the femoral vein and positioned with the distal tip in the PA. The microaxial pump positioned within the catheter drains blood from the right atrium and pumps it into the PA. The efficacy and safety of this device were investigated in The Use of Impella RP Support System in Patients With Right Heart Failure: A Clinical Safety and Probable Benefit Study (RECOVER RIGHT), a prospective, multicenter, single-arm outcomes trial.[69] Two groups of patients with RHF were enrolled, the first after LVAD placement and the second consisting of a mixture of patients after cardiotomy, after transplantation, and with acute myocardial infarction. The primary outcome was a combined end point of either survival at 30 days or hospital discharge or survival to next therapy (ie, transplantation or surgical RVAD). Thirty patients were enrolled with 73% survival to discharge. The major complication was postoperative bleeding, which occurred in 36.6% of patients. The PROTEK Duo cannula is a dual-lumen coaxial cannula positioned via the internal jugular vein, with its distal tip in the PA and connected to an extracorporeal centrifugal blood pump.[71] Because of its internal jugular cannulation site, this configuration permits ambulation during support. These devices provide an option for MCS because of the ease of device insertion and removal, and obviate the need for surgical sternotomy for removal.

ECMO represents a viable alternative for acute MCS support for RHF after LVAD implantation that is either caused by primary RV failure or is a consequence of primary pulmonary pathology, including the presence of systemic oxygen desaturation.[72] The benefits of ECMO are that it can be applied easily in the operating room or percutaneously at the bedside for the initiation of emergent support and it addresses pathologies of the pulmonary system that are not addressed with isolated RV mechanical support. The most common ECMO support configuration instituted in the operating room for right heart support is using right atrial (RA) cannulation for venous drainage with arterial outflow to the PA. This configuration provides RV support and maintains systemic oxygenation and preload to the LVAD. However, a drawback of this configuration is that flow to the lungs is increased and could exacerbate an underlying pulmonary injury if that was the inciting cause of the RHF. Additionally, this configuration requires redo sternotomy for decannulation in most instances. Another support configuration is using RA cannulation for venous drainage but arterial outflow is delivered with cannulation of the right superior pulmonary vein. The advantages of this configuration are that it provides RV support, maintains systemic oxygenation and preload to the LVAD, and diverts flow from the pulmonary system that prevents further potential injury to the pulmonary vasculature. Similar to the RA to PA ECMO support configuration, decannulation requires redo sternotomy. Additional ECMO support configurations can include femoral venous drainage and arterial outflow to the femoral artery. This configuration, more likely instituted in the postoperative setting, can be achieved either percutaneously or by surgical cut down on the femoral vessels. In this configuration, a major drawback is the difficulty of balancing flow through the ECMO circuit to maintain sufficient systemic oxygenation while maintaining sufficient residual pulmonary flow to fill the LV and provide adequate preload to the LVAD. If inadequate pulmonary gas exchange is present, deoxygenated blood from the lungs that returns to the LV and is ejected by the LVAD could result in systemic hypoxemia to the upper torso, and coronary and cerebral circulations. Other peripheral support configurations include internal jugular cannulation for venous drainage and arterial outflow to the axillary artery obtained with surgical cutdown. The advantages of this peripheral cannulation strategy include a lower risk of cerebral hypoxemia in the setting of pulmonary parenchymal disease and the ability to facilitate ambulation.[72] The complications of ECMO have been well-chronicled in the literature.[72,73]

Surgical options for right heart support remain important for patients experiencing intraoperative acute RHF after implantation of a durable LVAD.[4,63] Surgical implantation of an RVAD involves cannulation of the RA or RV for venous drainage and cannulation of the PA for arterial outflow. The cannulas are connected to an extracorporeal centrifugal flow pump such as the CentriMag (Abbott Labs, Chicago, IL) or Revolution (LivaNova, London, UK).[63,74] Numerous reports have detailed the use of a surgically implanted temporary RVAD after LVAD and have

demonstrated that this strategy is effective in supporting the patient through acute RHF during the postoperative period. Importantly, surgically implanted systems, such as the CentriMag, have greater flow capacity compared with percutaneous systems (ie, Impella or PROTEK Duo catheter). Although effective, a surgically placed RVAD typically requires a repeat sternotomy if not placed at the same time as the LVAD, and a second surgery is usually required to remove the device at the time of RV recovery. However, recent surgical techniques have been described that permit RVAD decannulation without the need for redo sternotomy.[75,76]

Long-term, durable MCS device options for irrecoverable forms of RHF after LVAD implantation are limited and data on durable device therapy for the RV largely comes from single center reports and is not well-studied.[77–79] For patients with advanced refractory RHF after LVAD implantation, whether on temporary RV support or not, few long-term MCS options are available. Two potential options exist in this circumstance: (1) reoperation with placement of a durable ventricular assist device used for RV support or (2) LVAD explant, cardiectomy, and placement of a total artificial heart system. Whether MCS support with newer, durable, implantable continuous flow VADs could be of benefit in patients with refractory RHF with a contraindication to transplantation is unknown. The off-label use of durable MCS devices in the setting of RHF caused by chronic significant pulmonary hypertension is controversial, and rigorous data on its efficacy in this setting are lacking. Typically, durable devices used for long-term or permanent RV support have been designed for LV support, and their use for RV support represents an off-label or unapproved indication. The most frequently used durable VAD for chronic RV support has been the HVAD (Medtronic, Inc, Minneapolis, MN), which is a small, continuous flow centrifugal device with magnetic and hydrodynamic levitation of the internal impellor.[80] Small, single-center observational series have demonstrated successful application of this device for long-term RV support. The inflow cannula of the device has been positioned within the diaphragmatic surface of the RV, anterior surface of the RV, or RA, with the outflow connected to the PA. However, the use of durable continuous flow rotary pumps for RV support raises many issues of feasibility, including the increased risk of thrombus generated in the venous system embolizing to the pump.

In a multicenter analysis of data from Intermacs, 19 participating centers implanted durable VAD devices for long-term RV support in 38 patients; 11 patients died with the device in place, 9 patients received a heart transplant, and 18 remained alive on support with the durable RVAD in place.[78] Overall survival outcomes were 68% at 6 months and 62% at 12 months. The LVAD was placed in the left ventricle apex in 91% of cases, and in 9% the location was not specified. The RVAD was placed in the RV in 50%, RA in 37%, and not specified in 13%. In a subgroup analysis of inlet cannula site position, RA cannulation was associated with a trend toward higher survival compared with RV cannulation. Adverse event burdens in this cohort were high and included infection (50%), bleeding (44%), respiratory failure (31.6%), and malfunction (26.3%); neurologic dysfunction (26.3%); renal dysfunction (18.4%); and arrhythmia (18.4%). These data suggested that the use of durable, intracorporeal, continuous flow centrifugal pumps for management of advanced biventricular HF is associated with high morbidity and mortality.

The total artificial heart (TAH) represents an alternative therapy for biventricular support for the failing RV and LV. The most used TAH is the Syncardia TAH-t (Syncardia Systems, LLC, Tucson, AZ).[81,82] The Syncardia TAH-t is a pneumatically driven pulsatile device currently approved for bridge to transplantation in the United States. The device is available in 50- and 70-cm sizes and is being investigated as a destination therapy indication. The use of the TAH may be advantageous over biventricular assist device support options in clinical situations, such as arrhythmogenic RV cardiomyopathy, restrictive cardiomyopathies, biventricular failure with significant intraventricular thrombus burden, very large body size, and failed transplantation.

In an recent analysis from Intermacs, 450 patients (87% men; mean age, 50 years) receiving the Syncardia TAH-t between June 2006 and April 2017 were evaluated for long-term outcomes.[83] The 2 most common diagnoses were dilated cardiomyopathy (50%) and ischemic cardiomyopathy (20%). Risk factors for RHF were present in 82% of patients. Most patients were Intermacs Profile 1 (43%) or 2 (37%) at implantation. There were 266 patients who eventually underwent transplantation, and 162 died. Overall 3-, 6-, and 12-month actuarial survival rates were 73%, 62%, and 53%, respectively. Risk factors for death included older age ($P<.001$), need for preimplantation dialysis ($P = .006$), higher creatinine ($P = .008$) and lower albumin ($P = .001$) levels, and implantation at a low-volume center ($\leq$10 TAHs; $P = .001$). Competing outcomes analysis showed 71% of patients in high-volume centers were alive on the device or had undergone transplantation at 12 months after TAH implantation versus 57% in low-volume centers ($P = .003$).

In patients with persistent RHF after LVAD implantation, cardiac transplantation represents the best treatment option for those candidates meeting eligibility criteria for transplantation. The major consideration in determining cardiac transplant candidacy is identifying the mechanism of RHF and whether this is attributed to RV failure or pulmonary vascular disease. In patients with pulmonary hypertension, elevated PVR, generally above 5 Wood units, significantly increases the early mortality risk of cardiac transplantation. Additionally, the presence of an RVAD at the time of cardiac transplantation has additional adverse prognostic impact on survival. Outcomes for isolated cardiac transplantation are generally excellent, and 1-year survival is approximately 90% in the most recent era for all patients based on registry data. However, the presence of RVAD support before heart transplantation is associated with a relative mortality hazard of 3.03 after transplantation.[84,85]

DISCLOSURE

The author has no relevant disclosures to report.

REFERENCES

1. Mehra MR, Uriel N, Naka Y, et al. A fully magnetically levitated left ventricular assist device - final report. N Engl J Med 2019;380:1618–27.
2. Argiriou M, Kolokotron SM, Sakellaridis T, et al. Right heart failure post left ventricular assist device implantation. J Thorac Dis 2014;6(suppl 1):S52–9.
3. Kukucka M, Potapov E, Stepanenko A, et al. Acute impact of left ventricular unloading by left ventricular assist device on the right ventricle geometry and function: effect of nitric oxide inhalation. J Thorac Cardiovasc Surg 2011;141:1009–14.
4. Dang NC, Topkara VK, Mercando M, et al. Right heart failure after left ventricular assist device implantation in patients with chronic congestive heart failure. J Heart Lung Transplant 2006;25:1–6.
5. Patel ND, Weiss ES, Schaffer J, et al. Right heart dysfunction after left ventricular assist device implantation: a comparison of the pulsatile HeartMate I and axial-flow HeartMate II devices. Ann Thorac Surg 2008;86:832–40.
6. Matthews JC, Koelling TM, Pagani FD, et al. The right ventricular failure risk score a pre-operative tool for assessing the risk of right ventricular failure in left ventricular assist device candidates. J Am Coll Cardiol 2008;51:2163–72.
7. Kormos RL, Teuteberg JJ, Pagani FD, et al. Right ventricular failure in patients with the HeartMate II

continuous-flow left ventricular assist device: incidence, risk factors, and effect on outcomes. J Thorac Cardiovasc Surg 2010;139:1316–24.

8. Baumwol J, Macdonald PS, Keogh AM, et al. Right heart failure and "failure to thrive" after left ventricular assist device: clinical predictors and outcomes. J Heart Lung Transplant 2011;30:888–95.

9. Kormos RL, Cowger J, Pagani FD, et al. The Society of Thoracic Surgeons Intermacs database annual report: evolving indications, outcomes, and scientific partnerships. J Heart Lung Transplant 2019;38:114–26.

10. Intermacs. Available at: https://www.uab.edu/medicine/intermacs/. Assessed November 1, 2019.

11. Atluri P, Goldstone AB, Fairman AS, et al. Predicting right ventricular failure in the modern, continuous flow left ventricular assist device era. Ann Thorac Surg 2013;96:857–63.

12. Drakos SG, Janicki L, Horne BD, et al. Risk factors predictive of right ventricular failure after left ventricular assist device implantation. Am J Cardiol 2010; 105:1030–5.

13. Wang Y, Bonde P, Uber B, et al. Cost-sensitive decision tree model for optimal identification of need for right ventricular support. Proceedings of the 10th IEEE International Conference on Information Technology and Applications in Biomedicine; 2010. p. 1–4.

14. Wang Y, Simon M, Bonde P, et al. Prognosis of right ventricular failure in patients with left ventricular assist device based on decision tree with SMOTE. IEEE Trans Inf Technol Biomed 2012;16:383–90.

15. Wang Y, Simon MA, Bonde P, et al. Decision tree for adjuvant right ventricular support in patients receiving a left ventricular assist device. J Heart Lung Transplant 2012;31:140–9.

16. Meineri M, Van Rensburg AE, Vegas A. Right ventricular failure after LVAD implantation: prevention and treatment. Best Pract Res Clin Anaesthesiol 2012;26:217–29.

17. Fitzpatrick JR III, Frederick JR, Hsu VM, et al. Risk score derived from pre–operative data analysis predicts the need for biventricular mechanical circulatory support. J Heart Lung Transplant 2008;27: 1286–92.

18. Kukucka M, Stepanenko A, Potapov E, et al. Right-to-left ventricular end-diastolic diameter ratio and prediction of right ventricular failure with continuous-flow left ventricular assist devices. J Heart Lung Transplant 2011;30:64–9.

19. Grant AD, Smedira NG, Starling RC, et al. Independent and incremental role of quantitative right ventricular evaluation for the prediction of right ventricular failure after left ventricular assist device implantation. J Am Coll Cardiol 2012;60:521–8.

20. Loghmanpour NA, Kormos RL, Kanwar MK, et al. A Bayesian model to predict right ventricular failure following left ventricular assist device therapy. JACC Heart Fail 2016;4:711–21.

21. Kormos RL, Gasior TA, Kawai A, et al. Transplant candidate's clinical status rather than right ventricular function defines need for univentricular versus biventricular support. J Thorac Cardiovasc Surg 1996; 111:773–82.

22. Slaughter MS, Pagani FD, Rogers JG, et al. Clinical management of continuous-flow left ventricular assist devices in advanced heart failure. J Heart Lung Transplant 2010;29(4 Suppl):S1–39.

23. Yancy CW, Jessup M, Bozkurt B, et al. 2013 ACCF/AHA guideline for the management of heart failure: a report of the American College of Cardiology Foundation/American Heart Association Task Force on Practice guidelines. Circulation 2013;128: e240–327.

24. Felker GM, Lee KL, Bull DA, et al, NHLBI Heart Failure Clinical Research Network. Diuretic strategies in patients with acute decompensated heart failure. N Engl J Med 2011;364:797–805.

25. Movsesian M, Stehlik J, Vandeput F, et al. Phosphodiesterase inhibition in heart failure. Heart Fail Rev 2009;14:255–63.

26. Ruffolo RR. The pharmacology of dobutamine. Am J Med Sci 1987;294:244–8.

27. Holmes CL, Patel BM, Russell JA, et al. Physiology of vasopressin relevant to management of septic shock. Chest 2001;120:989–1002.

28. Argenziano M, Choudhri AF, Moazami N, et al. Randomized, double-blind trial of inhaled nitric oxide in LVAD recipients with pulmonary hypertension. Ann Thorac Surg 1998;65:340–5.

29. Potapov E, Meyer D, Swaminathan M, et al. Inhaled nitric oxide after left ventricular assist device implantation: a prospective, randomized, double-blind, multicenter, placebo-controlled trial. J Heart Lung Transplant 2011;30:870–8.

30. Tedford RJ, Hemnes AR, Russell SD, et al. PDE5A inhibitor treatment of persistent pulmonary hypertension after mechanical circulatory support. Circ Heart Fail 2008;1:213–9.

31. Baker WL, Radojevic J, Gluck JA. Systematic review of phosphodiesterase-5 inhibitor use in right ventricular failure following left ventricular assist device implantation. Artif Organs 2016;40:123–8.

32. Inglessis I, Shin JT, Lepore JJ, et al. Hemodynamic effects of inhaled nitric oxide in right ventricular myocardial infarction and cardiogenic shock. J Am Coll Cardiol 2004;44:793–8.

33. Rich S, Seidlitz M, Dodin E, et al. The short-term effects of digoxin in patients with right ventricular dysfunction from pulmonary hypertension. Chest 1998;114:787–92.

34. Salamonsen RF, Mason DG, Ayre PJ. Response of rotary blood pumps to changes in preload and afterload at a fixed speed setting are unphysiological when compared with the natural heart. Artif Organs 2011;35:E47–53.

35. Santamore WP, Dell'Italia LJ. Ventricular interdependence: significant left ventricular contributions to right ventricular systolic function. Prog Cardiovasc Dis 1998;40:289–308.

36. Feldman D, Pamboukian SV, Teuteberg JJ, et al. The 2013 International Society for Heart and Lung Transplantation guidelines for mechanical circulatory support: executive summary. J Heart Lung Transplant 2013;32:157–87.

37. Pasrija C, Sawan MA, Sorensen E, et al. Less invasive left ventricular assist device implantation may reduce right ventricular failure. Interact Cardiovasc Thorac Surg 2019;29:592–8.

38. Makdisi G, Wang IW. Minimally invasive is the future of left ventricular assist device implantation. J Thorac Dis 2015;7:E283–8.

39. Stulak JM, Romans T, Cowger J, et al. Delayed sternal closure does not increase late infection risk in patients undergoing left ventricular assist device implantation. J Heart Lung Transplant 2012;31:1115–9.

40. Yanagida R, Rajagopalan N, Davenport DL, et al. Delayed sternal closure does not reduce complications associated with coagulopathy and right ventricular failure after left ventricular assist device implantation. J Artif Organs 2018;21:46–51.

41. Piacentino VR, Ganapathi AM, Stafford-Smith M, et al. Utility of concomitant tricuspid valve procedures for patients undergoing implantation of a continuous-flow left ventricular device. J Thorac Cardiovasc Surg 2012;144:1217–21.

42. Nakanishi K, Homma S, Han J, et al. Usefulness of tricuspid annular diameter to predict late right sided heart failure in patients with left ventricular assist device. Am J Cardiol 2018;122:115–20.

43. Potapov EV, Stepanenko A, Dandel M, et al. Tricuspid incompetence and geometry of the right ventricle as predictors of right ventricular function after implantation of a left ventricular assist device. J Heart Lung Transplant 2008;27:1275–81.

44. Atluri P, Fairman AS, MacArthur JW, et al. Continuous flow left ventricular assist device implant significantly improves pulmonary hypertension, right ventricular contractility, and tricuspid valve competence. J Card Surg 2013;28:770–5.

45. Song HK, Gelow JM, Mudd J, et al. Limited utility of tricuspid valve repair at the time of left ventricular assist device implantation. Ann Thorac Surg 2016;101:2168–74.

46. Kukucka M, Stepanenko A, Potapov E, et al. Impact of tricuspid valve annulus dilation on mid-term survival after implantation of a left ventricular assist device. J Heart Lung Transplant 2012;31:967–71.

47. Piacentino VR, Williams ML, Depp T, et al. Impact of tricuspid valve regurgitation in patients treated with implantable left ventricular assist devices. Ann Thorac Surg 2011;91:1342–6.

48. Zhigalov K, Szczechowicz M, Mashhour A, et al. Left ventricular assist device implantation with concomitant tricuspid valve repair: is there really a benefit? J Thorac Dis 2019;11:S902–12.

49. Maltais S, Topilsky Y, Tchantchaleishvili V, et al. Surgical treatment of tricuspid valve insufficiency promotes early reverse remodeling in patients with axial-flow left ventricular assist devices. J Thorac Cardiovasc Surg 2012;143:1370–6.

50. Saeed D, Kidambi T, Shalli S, et al. Tricuspid valve repair with left ventricular assist device implantation: is it warranted? J Heart Lung Transplant 2011;30:530–5.

51. Robertson JO, Grau-Sepulveda MV, Okada S, et al. Concomitant tricuspid valve surgery during implantation of continuous-flow left ventricular assist devices: a Society of Thoracic Surgeons database analysis. J Heart Lung Transplant 2014;33:609–17.

52. Dunlay SM, Deo SV, Park SJ. Impact of tricuspid valve surgery at the time of left ventricular assist device insertion on postoperative outcomes. ASAIO J 2015;61:15–20.

53. Han J, Takeda K, Takayama H, et al. Durability and clinical impact of tricuspid valve procedures in patients receiving a continuous-flow left ventricular assist device. J Thorac Cardiovasc Surg 2016;151:520–7.e1.

54. Asgar AW, Mack MJ, Stone GW. Secondary mitral regurgitation in heart failure: pathophysiology, prognosis, and therapeutic considerations. J Am Coll Cardiol 2015;65:1231–48.

55. Patel JB, Borgeson DD, Barnes ME, et al. Mitral regurgitation in patients with advanced systolic heart failure. J Card Fail 2004;10:285–91.

56. Robertson JO, Naftel DC, Myers SL, et al. Concomitant mitral valve procedures in patients undergoing implantation of continuous-flow left ventricular assist devices: an INTERMACS database analysis. J Heart Lung Transplant 2018;37:79–88.

57. Kassis H, Cherukuri K, Agarwal R, et al. Significance of residual mitral regurgitation after continuous flow left ventricular assist device implantation. JACC Heart Fail 2017;5:81–8.

58. Morgan JA, Brewer RJ, Nemeh HW, et al. Left ventricular reverse remodeling with a continuous flow left ventricular assist device measured by left ventricular end-diastolic dimensions and severity of mitral regurgitation. ASAIO J 2012;58:574–7.

59. Ertugay S, Kemal HS, Kahraman U, et al. Impact of residual mitral regurgitation on right ventricular systolic function after left ventricular assist device implantation. Artif Organs 2017;41:622–7.

60. Choi JH, Luc JGY, Moncho Escriva E, et al. Impact of concomitant mitral valve surgery with LVAD placement: systematic review and meta-analysis. Artif Organs 2018;42:1139–47.

61. Cheung AW, White CW, Davis MK, et al. Short-term mechanical circulatory support for recovery from acute right ventricular failure: clinical outcomes. J Heart Lung Transplant 2014;33:794–9.

62. Morgan JA, John R, Lee BJ, et al. Is severe right ventricular failure in left ventricular assist device recipients a risk factor for unsuccessful bridging to transplant and post-transplant mortality. Ann Thorac Surg 2004;77:859–63.

63. John R, Long JW, Massey HT, et al. Outcomes of a multicenter trial of the Levitronix CentriMag ventricular assist system for short-term circulatory support. J Thorac Cardiovasc Surg 2011;141:932–9.

64. Salna M, Shudo Y, Teuteberg JJ, et al. Planned concomitant left and right ventricular assist device insertion to avoid long-term biventricular mechanical support: bridge to right ventricular recovery. Heart Surg Forum 2018;21:E412–4.

65. Fitzpatrick JR 3rd, Frederick JR, Hiesinger W, et al. Early planned institution of biventricular mechanical circulatory support results in improved outcomes compared with delayed conversion of a left ventricular assist device to a biventricular assist device. J Thorac Cardiovasc Surg 2009;137:971–7.

66. Morine KJ, Kiernan MS, Pham DT, et al. Pulmonary artery pulsatility index is associated with right ventricular failure after left ventricular assist device surgery. J Card Fail 2016;22:110–6.

67. Kiernan MS, Grandin EW, Brinkley M Jr. Early right ventricular assist device utilization in patients undergoing continuous-flow left ventricular assist device implantation: incidence and risk factors from INTERMACS. Circ Heart Fail 2017;10:1–10.

68. Verbelen T, Verhoeven J, Goda M, et al. Mechanical support of the pressure overloaded right ventricle: an acute feasibility study comparing low and high flow support. Am J Physiol Heart Circ Physiol 2015;309:H615–24.

69. Anderson MB, Goldstein J, Milano C, et al. Benefits of a novel percutaneous ventricular assist device for right heart failure: the prospective RECOVER RIGHT study of the Impella RP device. J Heart Lung Transplant 2015;34:1549–60.

70. Schmack B, Weymann A, Popov AF, et al. Concurrent left ventricular assist device (LVAD) implantation and percutaneous temporary RVAD support via CardiacAssist Protek-Duo TandemHeart to preempt right heart failure. Med Sci Monit Basic Res 2016;22:53–7.

71. Aggarwal V, Einhorn BN, Cohen HA. Current status of percutaneous right ventricular assist devices: first-in-man use of a novel dual lumen cannula. Catheter Cardiovasc Interv 2016;88:390–6.

72. Makdisi G, Wang IW. Extra corporeal membrane oxygenation (ECMO): review of a lifesaving technology. J Thorac Dis 2015;7:E166–76.

73. Zangrillo A, Landoni G, Biondi-Zoccai G, et al. A meta-analysis of complications and mortality of extracorporeal membrane oxygenation. Crit Care Resusc 2013;15:172–8.

74. Bhama JK, Kormos RL, Toyoda Y, et al. Clinical experience using the Levitronix CentriMag system for temporary right ventricular mechanical circulatory support. J Heart Lung Transplant 2009;28:971–6.

75. Park I, Cho YH, Chung SR, et al. Temporary right ventricular assist device insertion via left thoracotomy after left ventricular assist device implantation. J Thorac Cardiovasc Surg 2019;52:105–8.

76. Saxena P, Marasco SF. Tunneling a pulmonary artery graft: a simplified way to insert and remove a temporary right ventricular assist device. Tex Heart Inst J 2015;42:540–2.

77. Strueber M, Meyer AL, Malehsa D, et al. Successful use of the HeartWare HVAD rotary blood pump for biventricular support. J Thorac Cardiovasc Surg 2010;140:936–7.

78. Arabía FA, Milano CA, Mahr C, et al. Biventricular support with intracorporeal, continuous flow, centrifugal ventricular assist devices. Ann Thorac Surg 2018;105:548–55.

79. Krabatsch T, Stepanenko A, Schweiger M, et al. Alternative technique for implantation of biventricular support with HeartWare implantable continuous flow pump. ASAIO J 2011;57:333–5.

80. Bernhardt AM, De By TM, Reichenspurner H, et al. Isolated permanent right ventricular assist device implantation with the HeartWare continuous-flow ventricular assist device: first results from the European Registry for patients with mechanical circulatory support. Eur J Cardiothorac Surg 2015;48:158–62.

81. Cook JA, Shah KB, Quader MA, et al. The total artificial heart. J Thorac Dis 2015;7:2172–80.

82. Copeland JG, Smith RG, Arabia FA, et al, CardioWest Total Artificial Heart Investigators. Cardiac replacement with a total artificial heart as a bridge to transplantation. N Engl J Med 2004;351:859–67.

83. Arabía FA, Cantor RS, Koehl DA, et al. Interagency registry for mechanically assisted circulatory support report on the total artificial heart. J Heart Lung Transplant 2018;37:1304–12.

84. Colvin M, Smith JM, Skeans MA, et al. OPTN/SRTR 2015 annual data report: heart. Am J Transplant 2017;17(suppl 1):286–356.

85. Lund LH, Edwards LB, Kucheryavaya AY, et al. The Registry of the International Society for Heart and Lung Transplantation: thirty-second official adult lung and heart-lung transplantation report–2015; focus theme: early graft failure. J Heart Lung Transplant 2015;34:1264–77.

Right Ventricular Failure and Congenital Heart Disease

Payton Kendsersky, MD[a],*, Cary Ward, MD[b]

KEYWORDS

- Right ventricle • Congenital heart disease • Tetralogy • Transposition

KEY POINTS

- The overall mortality of ACHD patients with heart failure is significantly higher than patients with ACHD without heart failure.
- The significance of right ventricular physiology in the development of heart failure in ACHD patients is increasingly recognized.
- Congenital malformations, palliations, residual defects, and their resultant physiology impact the RV through both pressure and volume loading.

INTRODUCTION

Survivorship into adulthood of patients with congenital heart disease (CHD) lesions has been due in large part to improvement in prenatal detection, novel surgeries and procedural interventions, and the development of specialized adult CHD (ACHD) care.[1] As patients survive further into adulthood, the long-term complications of congenital and repaired physiology have been more clearly elucidated. A major source of health care use in ACHD patients is a result of the treatment for heart failure.[2] The overall mortality of patients with ACHD with heart failure stands at around 4%, which is significantly higher than patients with ACHD without heart failure, even after controlling for age and comorbidities.[2] Historically, the contribution of left ventricle (LV) dysfunction has received more attention, owing in part to a better understanding of its morphology and contribution to normal hemodynamics, resulting in the right ventricular (RV) moniker "the forgotten ventricle."[3] However, it is now well-understood that the LV and RV, which share a pericardium, septum, and myocardial fibers, cannot be considered singularly. Growing understanding of the mechanical and neurohormonal coupling that exists between the 2 ventricles has subsequently provided insight into the altered biventricular mechanics of CHD.[4] Congenital malformations, palliations, residual defects, and their resultant physiology impact the RV, and this relationship influences morbidity and mortality. LV mechanics and ventricular–ventricular interactions are adversely affected in both the pressure loaded and volume loaded RVs—isolated volume overloading being associated with decreased LV ejection fraction, and pressure overloading being associated with preserved LV ejection fraction.[5] For this discussion, we therefore categorize right-sided congenital heart defects into RV pressure and volume overloading lesions, focusing on atrial septal defects, Ebstein anomaly, tetralogy of Fallot (TOF), transposition of the great vessels, and single RV physiology.

RIGHT VENTRICULAR VOLUME OVERLOAD

There are several congenital lesions that influence cardiac function by overloading the RV with volume, including atrial septal defects, atrialization of the RV (Ebstein anomaly), and corrected TOF.

[a] Duke University Medical Center, Box 2819, Durham, NC 27710, USA; [b] Division of Cardiovascular Medicine, Duke University Medical Center, Box 2819, Durham, NC 27710, USA
* Corresponding author.
E-mail address: payton.kendsersky@duke.edu

Cardiol Clin 38 (2020) 239–242
https://doi.org/10.1016/j.ccl.2020.02.002

The RV is able to tolerate an excess of volume for a long time, mainly owing to the compliance of a thin-walled RV, a more distensible right atrium as compared with the left atrium, and a roomier tricuspid valve as compared with the left-sided mitral valve.[4] Despite this adaptation of the right heart to volume overloading, it is well-understood that long-standing volume overload of the RV leads to adverse ventricular interdependence and LV dysfunction resulting from myofibril rearrangement, decreased myofiber preload, and altered chamber geometry.[6]

Atrial Septal Defects

An atrial septal defect is a communication between the atria resulting from a deficiency of tissue in the septum and can be subdivided according to anatomic location. The 3 most common types of atrial septal defects (ASDs) include ostium secundum, ostium primum, and sinus venosus. Of these 3 defects, ostium secundum is the most common type, accounting for about 70% of all cases.[7–9] Ostium secundum defects classically involve the fossa ovalis and can be associated with anomalous pulmonary venous return to the right atrium. Defects of the septum inferior to the fossa ovalis include ostium primum defects, which occur immediately adjacent to the tricuspid and mitral valves in a portion of the atrioventricular canal. The least commonly occurring sinus venosus defects, around 6% of cases, straddle an otherwise intact septum, but represent a biatrial connection of the superior vena cava.[7] Common to all subtypes of ASD is volume overloading of the RV, right atrium, and pulmonary vasculature. In a small percentage of cases of unrepaired ASD, Eisenmenger physiology can develop, characterized by reversal of the intracardiac shunt, cyanosis, and RV hypertrophy and failure. RV failure can also develop in unrepaired ASDs later in life, even in the absence of Eisenmenger syndrome, as the left-to-right shunt magnitude increases with progressive LV stiffness associated with aging.[10] In this case, it is both volume and pressure loading that begets right heart failure. ASDs do not close spontaneously, but surgical or percutaneous closure of the ASD results in varying degrees of reversal of the increased mortality and morbidities (ie, heart failure, arrhythmia, and thromboembolic events) associated with unrepaired defects. Current guidelines recommend closure of an ASD in patients with RV enlargement, regardless of symptoms.[11] Patients who do not undergo ASD closure have worse long-term outcomes, including decreased functional capacity, greater degrees of pulmonary arterial hypertension, and more atrial arrhythmias.[12] Studies by Kodaira and colleagues[12] and Takaya and colleagues[13] have also demonstrated that in patients with moderate or severe tricuspid regurgitation in the setting of an unrepaired ASD, tricuspid regurgitation severity, and heart failure symptoms were improved for the vast majority of patients who underwent percutaneous closure.

Ebstein Anomaly

Ebstein anomaly has a wide range of clinical presentations, but is uniformly characterized by abnormalities of the RV and tricuspid valve. The anterior leaflet of the tricuspid valve is attached normally to the annulus, whereas varying portions of the posterior and septal leaflets are displaced downward attaching to the RV wall below the annulus.[6,13] In other words, there is an atrialization of the RV and varying degrees of tricuspid regurgitation. Often there is an associated atrial communication in the form of a patent foramen ovale. For patients surviving into adulthood with an Ebstein anomaly, mortality is largely due to heart failure and arrhythmias.[13] In adulthood, a combination of severe tricuspid regurgitation, severe right atrium dilation, and reduced effective RV size can result in inadequate antegrade flow and progression to RV failure. In addition to the impact of volume overload, the natural history of RV failure in Ebstein anomaly also owes to increased arrhythmia burden, as RV cardiomyocytes preserve ventricular specificity despite anatomic atrialization.[14] One study confirmed an association between myocardial fibrosis and supraventricular arrhythmias in this population and suggests that chronic RV volume overload contributes to the development of said fibrosis.[15]

Tetralogy of Fallot

Characterized by a large ventricular septal defect with overriding aorta, obstruction of pulmonary blood flow, and RV hypertrophy, TOF is among the most common cyanotic congenital cardiac defects.[6] Among the first lesions to be corrected surgically, TOF represents a model not only of the impact of abnormal physiology of the defect, but also of repair physiology. Classically, infundibular pulmonary stenosis owing to hypertrophy and deviation of the infundibular septum, as well as malformation and stenosis of the pulmonary valve result in obstruction of pulmonary blood flow.[4] Currently, severe pulmonary regurgitation (PR) is the most common residual lesion seen in adulthood after repair; significant pulmonary annular hypoplasia requires a transannular patch, which disrupts the valve architecture.[16] Although the surgical approach to the repair of TOF has shifted recently to a transatrial–transpulmonary approach, more than 60% of TOF repairs still use transannular patch enlargement according to the Society for Thoracic Surgery database.[17] Over time, the resulting severe PR precipitates RV dilation and tricuspid regurgitation, likely in combination with a component of tricuspid valve trauma. Electrical remodeling of the heart after TOF repair also impacts the synchronicity and function of the RVs and LVs.[14]

In a 1993 review of patients who had undergone repair of TOF from 1955 to 1960, 22 late deaths were discovered: 10 of these were due to sudden cardiac death and 3 of heart failure. Since then, significant advances in the care of patients with repaired TOF have revealed the connections between PR, RV dilation, longer QRS duration, and ventricular arrhythmias.[18] There is now recognition that it is important to correct significant PR before the RV dilatation and dysfunction becomes too advanced. The 2018 American College of Cardiology/American Heart Association Adult Congenital Heart Disease guidelines recommend regular surveillance of the RV by cardiac MRI to evaluate for size and RV fibrosis.[11] Pulmonary valve replacement is suggested for patients with severe PR and symptoms, as well as for patients with severe PR and mild to moderate RV dysfunction and/or severe RV dilation, even in the absence of symptoms.[11] The option of a transcatheter pulmonary valve is also available and thousands have been implanted since they became available in 2000.[19] However, the transcatheter pulmonary valves have specific anatomic requirements that limit their use in a native RV outflow tract, including a uniform diameter from the RV outflow tract to the pulmonary artery bifurcation and adequate pulmonary artery length. They are most commonly used in dysfunctional RV to pulmonary artery conduits or as a second procedure in a preexisting but dysfunctional bioprosthetic pulmonary valve.[19]

RIGHT VENTRICULAR PRESSURE OVERLOAD

Surgical palliation of several different forms of CHD, including D-transposition of the great arteries and hypoplastic left heart syndrome requires reassignment of the RV from its role in the low-resistance pulmonary circuit to supporting the systemic circulation. The same is true for the physiology of L-transposition of the great arteries or congenitally corrected transposition of the great arteries. These systemic RV systems represent instances of RV pressure overload, leading to RV dysfunction and failure.

Transposition of the Great Arteries

Discordant ventriculoarterial connection underlying D-transposition of the great arteries results in displaced aorta and pulmonary artery, so that the morphologic RV supports the systemic circulation and the morphologic LV supports the pulmonary circulation. These parallel circuits are incompatible with life and require atrial or arterial switch operations.[20] The long-term outcomes of the newer arterial switch operations remain to be elucidated, but the complications of the older atrial switch operations, the Mustard and Senning procedures, include RV dysfunction in adult survivors of the correction.[21] The RV coupled to the high-pressure systemic circulation, leading to an increased risk of RV dilatation and failure.[22] In these patients, there may also be a contribution of myocardial perfusion defects and RV fibrosis.[4]

The role of medical therapy in a patient with systemic RV dysfunction related to an atrial switch procedure is unclear. Currently, there is not sufficient evidence to recommend the use of angiotensin-converting enzyme inhibitors, beta-blockers, or aldosterone inhibitors in this population. Although patients with a systemic RV are at risk for ventricular arrhythmias, there is also not enough evidence to recommend primary prevention implantable cardioverter-defibrillators in this population.[11]

Single Right Ventricle Physiology

The most common of the functional single ventricle palliations is the Fontan procedure, which reroutes systemic venous return directly to the pulmonary artery, eliminating the need for a functional pulmonary ventricle. This palliation comes at the expense of a chronic increase in the central venous pressure. Many of the long-term problems associated with Fontan physiology are a result of chronically increased central venous pressure, including liver disease, coagulation factor abnormalities and resultant thromboembolic events, and protein-losing enteropathy. In instances of hypoplasia or total absence of the LV, the Fontan palliation also results in a morphologic RV supporting systemic circulation.[16,23] The high resistance systemic circulation pressure overloads the RV, leading to higher likelihood of RV dilation, tricuspid regurgitation, and RV failure in these patients over time as compared with patients with a systemic LV. As in Ebstein anomaly, in a cohort of late Fontan survivors, myocardial fibrosis was associated with arrhythmia and adverse ventricular mechanics.[22] The medical management of patients with a single ventricle is the same regardless of the morphology of that ventricle.[11]

DISCLOSURE

The authors have nothing to disclose.

REFERENCES

1. Konstam MA, Kiernan MS, Bernstein D, et al. Evaluation and management of right-sided heart failure: a scientific statement from the American Heart Association. Circulation 2018;137(20). https://doi.org/10.1161/CIR.0000000000000560.

2. Mazor Dray E, Marelli AJ. Adult congenital heart disease. Cardiol Clin 2015;33(4):503–12.

3. Tretter JT, Redington AN. The forgotten ventricle? Circ Cardiovasc Imaging 2018;11(3). https://doi.org/10.1161/circimaging.117.007410.

4. Davlouros PA. The right ventricle in congenital heart disease. Heart 2006;92(suppl_1):i27–38.

5. Voges I, Al-Mallah MH, Scognamiglio G, et al. Right heart-pulmonary circulation unit in congenital heart diseases. Heart Fail Clin 2018;14(3):283–95.

6. Walker RE, Moran AM, Gauvreau K, et al. Evidence of adverse ventricular interdependence in patients with atrial septal defects. Am J Cardiol 2004;93(11):1374–7.

7. Fuster V. Chapter 84: congenital heart disease in adults. Hurst's the heart, 13th edition: two volume set. New York: McGraw Hill Professional; 2011.

8. Webb G, Gatzoulis MA. Atrial septal defects in the adult. Circulation 2006;114(15):1645–53.

9. Pradat P, Francannet C, Harris JA, et al. The epidemiology of cardiovascular defects, Part I: a study based on data from three large registries of congenital malformations. Pediatr Cardiol 2003;24(3):195–221.

10. Konstam MA, Idoine J, Wynne J, et al. Right ventricular function in adults with pulmonary hypertension with and without atrial septal defect. Am J Cardiol 1983;51(7):1144–8.

11. Stout KK, Daniels CJ, Aboulhosn JA, et al. 2018 AHA/ACC guideline for the management of adults with congenital heart disease: a report of the American College of Cardiology/American Heart Association Task Force on clinical practice guidelines. J Am Coll Cardiol 2019;139(14):e698–800.

12. Kodaira M, Kawamura A, Okamoto K, et al. Comparison of clinical outcomes after transcatheter vs. Minimally invasive cardiac surgery closure for atrial septal defect. Circ J 2017;81(4):543–51.

13. Takaya Y, Akagi T, Kijima Y, et al. Functional tricuspid regurgitation after transcatheter closure of atrial septal defect in adult patients. JACC Cardiovasc Interv 2017;10(21):2211–8.

14. Attenhofer Jost CH, Connolly HM, Dearani JA, et al. Ebstein's anomaly. Circulation 2007;115(2):277–85.

15. Kumar S, Tedrow UB, Triedman JK. Arrhythmias in adult congenital heart disease. Cardiol Clin 2015;33(4):571–88.

16. Ciepłucha A, Trojnarska O, Kociemba A, et al. Clinical aspects of myocardial fibrosis in adults with Ebstein's anomaly. Heart Vessels 2018;33(9):1076–85.

17. Wald RM, Marie Valente A, Marelli A. Heart failure in adult congenital heart disease: emerging concepts with a focus on tetralogy of Fallot. Trends Cardiovasc Med 2015;25(5):422–32.

18. Hutter P. The arterial switch operation twenty years later. J Am Coll Cardiol 1998;31(2):287A.

19. Graham TP. Congenitally corrected transposition of the great arteries: ventricular function at the time of systemic atrioventricular valve replacement predicts long-term ventricular function. J Am Coll Cardiol 2012;2012:118–9.

20. Filippov AA, del Nido PJ, Vasilyev NV. Management of systemic right ventricular failure in patients with congenitally corrected transposition of the great arteries. Circulation 2016;134(17):1293–302.

21. Brida M, Diller G-P, Gatzoulis MA. Systemic right ventricle in adults with congenital heart disease. Circulation 2018;137(5):508–18.

22. Rathod RH, Prakash A, Powell AJ, et al. Myocardial fibrosis identified by cardiac magnetic resonance late gadolinium enhancement is associated with adverse ventricular mechanics and ventricular Tachycardia late after Fontan operation. J Am Coll Cardiol 2010;55(16):1721–8.

23. Gewillig M. The Fontan circulation. Heart 2005;91(6):839–46.

Right Heart Failure in Pulmonary Hypertension

Steven Cassady, MD[a], Gautam V. Ramani, MD[b],*

KEYWORDS

- Pulmonary hypertension • Pulmonary arterial hypertension • Right ventricle
- Right ventricular failure • Right heart failure

KEY POINTS

- Right heart failure is a major source of morbidity and mortality in pulmonary hypertension.
- Right ventricular failure in pulmonary hypertension is characterized by alterations in cellular metabolism, the development of right ventricular ischemia, and activation of the renin–angiotensin–aldosterone system.
- Pharmacologic treatment of right heart failure in pulmonary hypertension focuses primarily on optimizing preload, enhancing right ventricular contractility, and decreasing right ventricular afterload.
- Mechanical circulatory support, including extracorporeal membrane oxygenation is increasing used as a bridge to recovery or transplantation in right heart failure refractory to pharmacologic treatments.

INTRODUCTION AND EPIDEMIOLOGY

Pulmonary hypertension (PH), previously defined as a mean pulmonary artery pressure of greater than 25 mm Hg, has recently been redefined by the Sixth World Symposium on Pulmonary Hypertension as a mean pulmonary artery pressure of greater than 20 mm Hg along with a pulmonary vascular resistance (PVR) of 3 or more Wood units for precapillary disease.[1] Multiple etiologies for the disease, codified in the World Health Organization group classification system, underlie the shared mechanism of elevated pulmonary arterial pressure resulting in an increase in right ventricular (RV) afterload.[1] This increase in afterload results in a spectrum of mechanical and biochemical changes, both adaptive and maladaptive, that may lead to the syndrome of right heart failure (RHF).

In the context of PH, RHF can be defined as an increased afterload resulting in dysfunction of the RV that produces a syndrome with the clinical signs and symptoms of heart failure.[2] In PH, RVF can present acutely, with hemodynamic instability and cardiogenic shock, as well as a more chronically, with symptoms developing over a period of months. Chronic RVF results from longstanding increases in RV afterload that ultimately overwhelm the compensatory mechanisms of the RV. RHF produces symptoms related to impaired cardiac output as well as systemic venous congestion.[3]

RHF is the leading cause of death in pulmonary arterial hypertension (PAH), although the lack of a strict definition of RHF makes its true prevalence in PH difficult to determine. RV dysfunction seems to be a strong predictor of poor clinical outcomes in PAH, which itself has a baseline 5-year survival of only 57%. Patients with PAH with RHF who require intensive care unit admission and inotropic support have been shown to have a mortality rate exceeding 40%.[4,5] Routine surveillance of RV function is a critical aspect of PH management,

[a] Division of Pulmonary and Critical Care Medicine, Department of Medicine, University of Maryland School of Medicine, 110 South Paca Street, 2nd Floor, Baltimore, MD 21201, USA; [b] Division of Cardiovascular Medicine, Department of Medicine, University of Maryland School of Medicine, 110 South Paca Street, 7th Floor, Baltimore, MD 21201, USA
* Corresponding author.
E-mail address: gramani@som.umaryland.edu

Cardiol Clin 38 (2020) 243–255
https://doi.org/10.1016/j.ccl.2020.02.001

and improvement in RV function is associated with improved outcomes. Although the role of the RV in PAH cannot be overstated, the specific relationship between aspects of RV function and prognosis is not yet well-understood. The current armamentarium of medications for PAH act primarily on the pulmonary vasculature, with only secondary effects on the RV.

PATHOPHYSIOLOGY

The development of RHF in PH is primarily a result of the downstream effects of increased RV afterload. Although there are differences in the pathophysiologic mechanisms underlying different groups of PH, a common element is an increase in RV loading conditions. Group 3 PH is characterized by parenchymal lung disease and hypoxia, which lead to PH, and Group 2 PH is characterized by pathology downstream from the pulmonary vasculature in the left heart causing pressure elevation. PAH is characterized by progressive changes to the pulmonary vasculature, including fibromuscular intimal thickening, in situ thrombosis, and smooth cell hypertrophy. Relentless remodeling leads to a decrease in the cross-sectional area of the pulmonary vasculature, leading to an elevated PVR, which in turn increases RV pressures. These progressive changes result in fixed remodeling of the vessels and sustained increases in PVR.

Ongoing pressure increases in the pulmonary vasculature lead to a variety of mechanical changes in the RV, which have been divided into adaptive and maladaptive phenotypes. Despite the common presence of increased RV afterload as the cause behind these changes, different etiologies of PH have shown markedly different patterns of RV adaptation, with differing prognoses as a result; notably, the right ventricle in Eisenmenger syndrome does not share the same propensity for maladaptive change as in other diseases such as PAH.[6]

Differences in early compensatory changes seem to determine the risk of future RV compensation.[6] In the adaptive phenotype of RV compensation, increases in RV afterload lead to cardiomyocyte hypertrophy along with some degree of myocardial fibrosis, analogous to the remodeling seen in the left ventricle when confronted with chronically high afterload.[7,8] In the early stages of this remodeling, RV hypertrophy allows the right ventricle to remain isovolumic, with the increase in cardiomyocyte growth allowing for increased contractility to match the rise in pulmonary arterial elastance.[9] As a result of this compensation, RV systolic pressure and RV end-diastolic volume increase.

In the maladaptive phenotype of compensation, RV dilatation and systolic dysfunction are prominent features. RV dilatation leads to tricuspid annular dilatation, poor coaptation of the valvular leaflets, and functional tricuspid regurgitation.[10] With worsened systolic function, the right heart is less able to compensate for the increased pulmonary arterial elastance; indeed, the finding of increasing right atrial pressure alongside increasing PVR raises concern for right heart decompensation.[11] Pressure and volume overload of the RV lead to a septal shift toward the LV, compressing the left ventricular cavity and further decreasing cardiac output in what is termed interventricular dependence. Accompanying delays in RV contraction have also been observed in PAH, further compromising left ventricular filling.[12] It is thought that both processes—reduced RV stroke volume and interventricular interdependence—are responsible for reduced left-sided output in RHF.

The demands on the right ventricle confronted with chronically high afterload lead to outsize metabolic demands and an increase in blood flow (**Fig. 1**).[13] Underlying the mechanical changes that lead to RV failure are numerous biochemical alterations, of which the most significant is a change in cellular metabolism toward a state of decreased energy efficiency. RV cardiomyocytes have been observed to undergo a complex metabolic rewiring, shifting from oxidative phosphorylation to the much less efficient process of glycolysis, along with upregulations in glutaminolysis and fatty acid oxidation.[14–16] Increased RV long-chain fatty acids, ceramides, and triglycerides suggest an additional component of altered fatty acid metabolism and lipotoxicity.[17] A marked shift away from oxidative phosphorylation is thought to underlie maladaptive mechanical changes in the right ventricle and increase the likelihood of eventual decompensation.[18] Mitochondrial dysfunction has also been recognized to play a key role in underlying changes of PH; with the shift toward glycolysis, mitochondria in PH become hyperpolarized and apoptosis resistant, preventing mitophagy, the process through which damaged mitochondria are normally removed, and further hampering efficient cellular metabolism.[19] Many of these metabolic changes are mediated by the transcription factors hypoxia-inducible factor 1α and hypoxia-inducible factor-2α, which are implicated in the process of pulmonary arterial remodeling in PAH and stabilized by oxidative stress, hypoxia, and inflammation.[20,21]

RV ischemia is a key consideration in worsening performance in PH, and the hypertrophied RV is vulnerable to subendocardial ischemia. The right

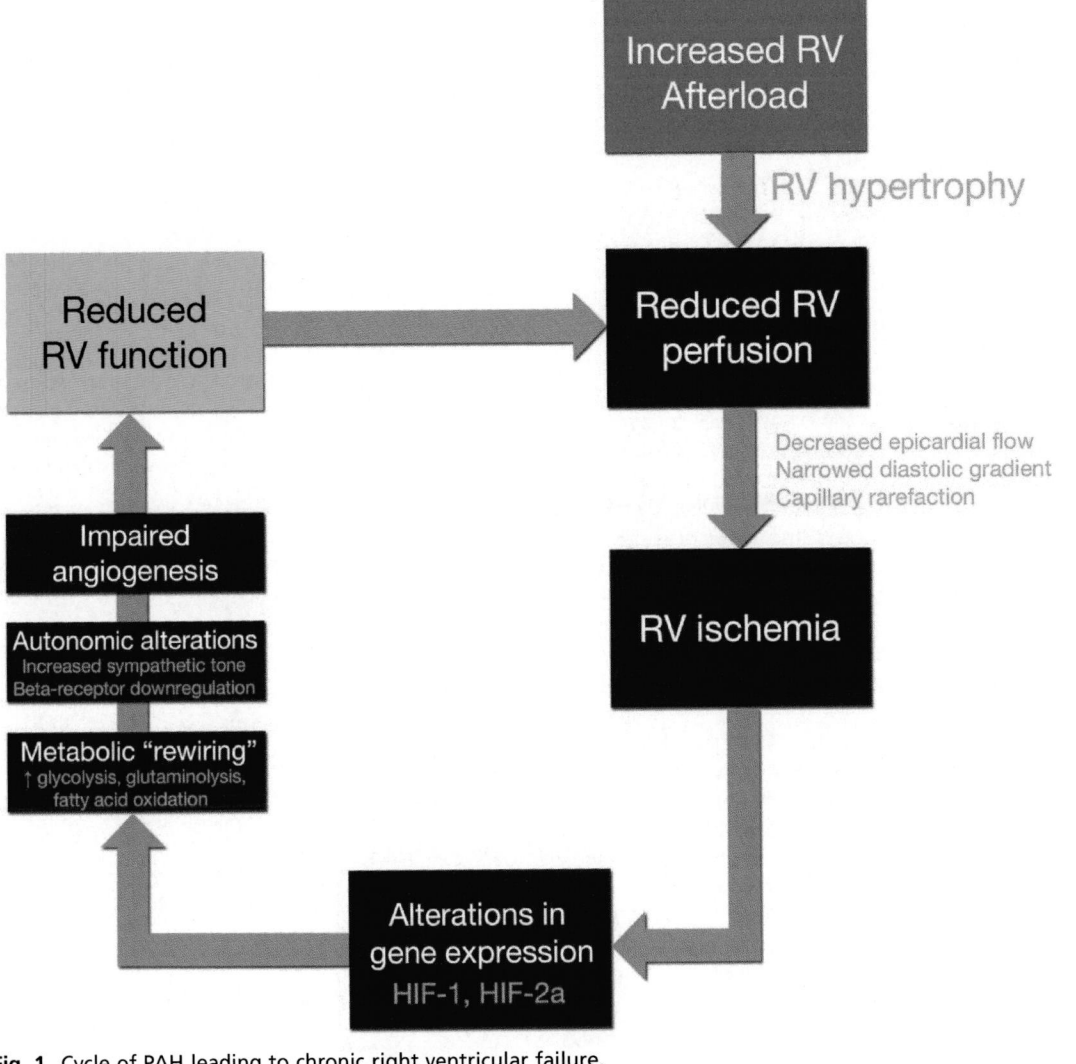

Fig. 1. Cycle of PAH leading to chronic right ventricular failure.

coronary artery perfuses the RV in both systole and diastole, and coronary artery filling in both phases is affected. Increases in pulmonary artery pressure decrease the gradient between RV systolic pressure and aortic pressure, resulting in a decreased epicardial systolic flow and rarefaction of capillaries in the ventricular wall. Furthermore, increasing RV end-diastolic pressure leads to a narrowing of the diastolic gradient between right and left sides of the heart that can worsen ischemia.[22]

Finally, the autonomic nervous system and the renin–angiotensin–aldosterone system play major roles in the pathogenesis of PAH.[23] Heightened adrenergic stimulation drives the compensatory mechanisms that preserve cardiac systolic function in the face of increased RV afterload, but leads to myocardial dysfunction if persistent over the long term.[24] In addition, chronically increased adrenergic tone leads to a downregulation of myocardial beta receptors in the right ventricle and depletion of norepinephrine stores.[24] A recent study using nuclear imaging in a small group of patients with PAH suggests there may be frank sympathetic dysfunction in PAH proportional to disease severity, significantly worse than controls and similar to what is observed in left-sided heart failure with a reduced ejection fraction.[25] The renin–angiotensin–aldosterone system activation results both by direct beta-adrenergic stimulation of renin release and by local changes in angiotensin II receptors in the right ventricle.[24] However, unlike in chronic left heart failure, treatments targeting the renin–angiotensin–aldosterone system and the beta-adrenergic system have not yet been shown to improve outcomes in PAH, which is discussed elsewhere in this article.

PRESENTATION

Acute and Chronic Right Heart Failure in Pulmonary Hypertension

As described elsewhere in this article, acute increases in RV afterload lead to RV dilation, compressing the left ventricle and decreasing left ventricular filling through the mechanism of ventricular interdependence. Precipitants of acute decompensated heart failure are listed in **Box 1**. Signs and symptoms of acute decompensated RHF reflect systemic hypoperfusion and include decreased mental status, tachycardia, cool extremities, hypotension, and diaphoresis. Physical examination reveals jugular venous distension, right-sided S3, and the holosystolic murmur suggestive of tricuspid regurgitation. Signs of hepatic congestion, including hepatomegaly, right upper abdominal pain owing to capsular distension, and peripheral edema may be present if an element of chronic failure was present previously. This finding may be reflected in laboratory values that show elevated transaminases and bilirubin. Acute kidney injury, the result of poor forward flow and systemic venous congestion, may be seen.

The clinical presentation of chronic RHF reflects the effects of venous congestion as more insidious forms of the end-organ effects seen in acute RHF. Peripheral edema is a common feature.[26] Prolonged elevation of venous systemic pressure leads to right atrial stretch, resulting in an increased frequency of atrial tachyarrhythmias.[27] Chronic venous congestion, as in left heart failure, also leads to end-organ dysfunction of the liver, kidneys, and gastrointestinal tract. Congestion, poor forward flow, and the effects of neurohormonal activation (collectively termed type 2 cardiorenal syndrome) lead to chronic kidney dysfunction, which has been strongly associated with higher mortality in patients with PAH.[28,29] Exercise intolerance owing to insufficient reserve in cardiac output is the second major clinical feature of RHF and has been shown to be a strong predictor of survival.[3,5]

Because there are no specific laboratory markers for right heart dysfunction, biomarkers should be interpreted in the context of the patient and are better proven for prognosis in specific types of PH. Serum troponin is the most commonly used biomarker of myocardial injury and elevations also been shown to independently predict mortality in patients with PH.[30] Brain natriuretic peptide and N-terminal pro b-type natriuretic peptide have been shown to be useful more for prognosis of RV dysfunction from PAH and are used as part of the REVEAL 2.0 calculator for predicting mortality at the time of PAH diagnosis.[31]

DIAGNOSTIC TOOLS AND IMAGING

Imaging in Pulmonary Hypertension Right Ventricular Failure

Although the history and physical examination are valuable, imaging studies are essential in the management of PH in RV failure. Quantifying RV function is valuable in identifying high-risk patients and guiding treatments. Furthermore, imaging studies provide insight into the severity of PH, potential underlying etiologies, and comorbid conditions, such as pericardial effusions and mitral valve disease. Routine imaging of the RV is performed using nuclear modalities, echocardiography, and cardiac MRI.

In routine clinical practice, transthoracic echocardiography is most often performed for RV function assessment and is the first step in the diagnostic algorithm in patients with suspected PH.[32] In addition to quantitative and qualitative assessment of RV function, transthoracic echocardiography allows assessment of the peak tricuspid regurgitant velocity, which is used to calculate the pulmonary artery systolic pressure. **Fig. 2.** shows an echocardiogram of a patient with PH presenting with acute RV failure.

Cardiac MRI is considered the gold standard to assess RV size and function given the complex, 3-dimensional structure of the RV.[33] Although cardiac MRI does not involve the use of ionizing radiation, the need for breath holds and the prolonged time in the scanner limit its use in critically ill patients. In addition to providing accurate end-diastolic and systolic volumes for RV ejection fraction calculation, cardiac MRI also provides valuable information on RV mass, regional wall motion, late gadolinium enhancement, and pulmonary arterial flow.

Box 1
Precipitants of decompensated RHF in PH
Pulmonary embolism
Sepsis
Pneumonia
Respiratory failure/acute respiratory distress syndrome
Hypovolemia
Cardiac tamponade
Constrictive pericarditis
Severe tricuspid insufficiency
RV ischemia or infarct

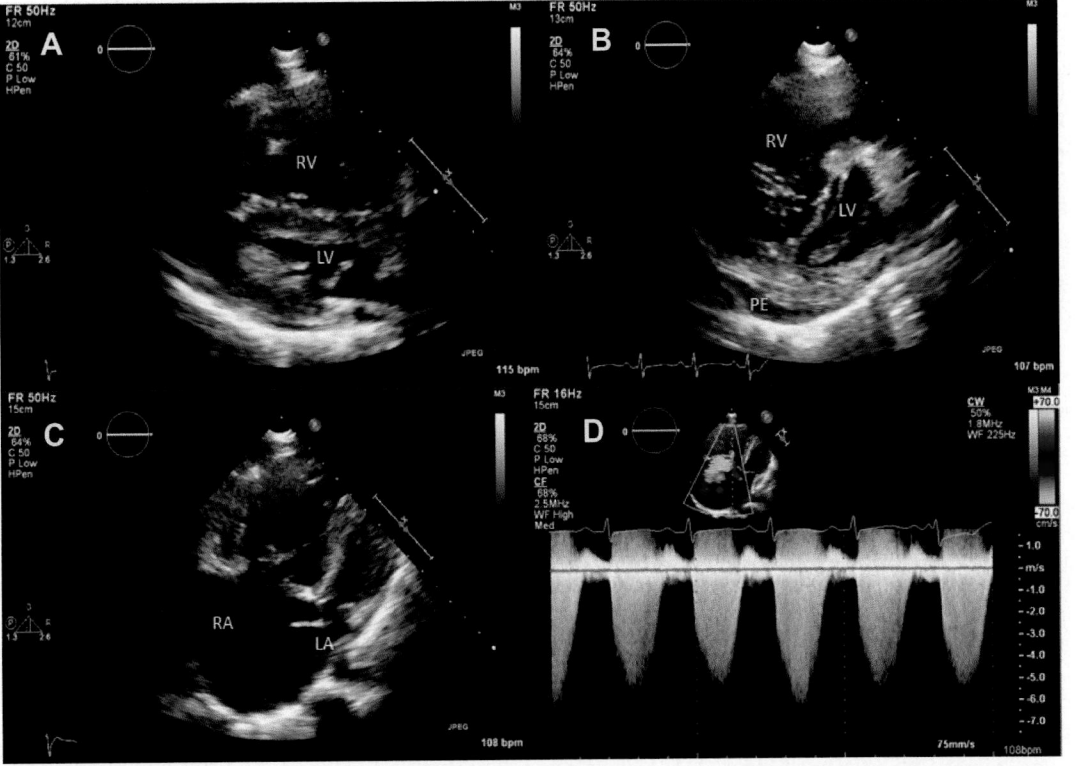

Fig. 2. Echocardiographic findings of PH in RHF. (*A*) A parasternal long axis image, revealing marked LV compression by the dilated and dysfunctional right ventricle. (*B*) A parasternal short axis image, revealing profound systolic and diastolic septal flattening, and a pericardial effusion (PE) is seen. (*C*) Apical 4-chamber view, showing the interatrial septum bowing toward the left atrium. (*D*) Continuous wave Doppler showing an elevated tricuspid regurgitant velocity compatible with PH. LA, left atrium; LV, left ventricle; RA, right atrium; RV, right ventricle.

Radionuclide techniques, including first pass radionuclide angiography and gated blood pool single photon emission computed tomography, are older techniques that provide reliable and reproducible measurements of the RV ejection fraction.[34]

Medical Management of Right Ventricular Failure in Pulmonary Hypertension

Acute management of RV failure in PH focuses on optimizing RV preload, enhancing RV contractility, and reducing RV afterload. Additional emphasis is placed on correcting atrial rhythm disorders, maintaining systemic blood pressure, and correcting problems with oxygenation and ventilation.

Congestion is almost always present when RV failure develops in PH. Classical teaching has long been that the failing right ventricle is preload dependent, and elements of critical illness such as sepsis, volume loss, and positive-pressure ventilation may decrease right-sided preload significantly. However, a careful approach to volume status is needed to ensure that excess preload does not further decompensate the RV through worsened ventricular dilation and resultant tricuspid regurgitation and ischemia from increased RV wall tension.[35] If the volume status cannot be determined clinically, placement of a central venous catheter or pulmonary artery catheter should be considered. Empirically administering intravenous fluids in a hypotensive patient with acute RHF in a whom the volume status is unknown may lead to rapid hemodynamic deterioration. When adequately dosed, diuretics can lead to rapid symptomatic and hemodynamic improvements. If urine output is inadequate despite adequate diuretic dosing, or renal failure develops, renal replacement therapy should be considered.

Decreasing RV afterload with pulmonary arterial vasodilators is a critical aspect of management in PH, although unlike in chronic PH there are few studies to guide their use in acute decompensated PH. The ideal vasodilator would be a drug with rapid onset and short half-life that preferentially reduces the PVR preferentially over the systemic vascular resistance and minimally impacts oxygenation. Because the pulmonary vasodilators commonly used in acute heart failure are nonselective, they decrease PVR and RV afterload but carry the risk of adversely affecting hemodynamics by reducing systemic blood pressure and the risk of worsening V/Q mismatch. It is also critical to realize that pulmonary arterial vasodilators have only been shown to improve long terms outcomes in patients with group 1 and group 4 PH, and that there is potential for harm when used in patients with other PH groups. In acutely ill patients with group 2 PH, where elevated pulmonary artery pressures are secondary to increased left-sided pressures, pulmonary vasodilator use increases the transpulmonary gradient and may further increase left-sided filling pressures, leading to pulmonary edema and further decompensation.[36]

Both inhaled epoprostenol and inhaled nitric oxide have been studied in diverse patient populations and have been shown to have beneficial effects on oxygenation and PVR. Theoretically, inhaled agents have fewer systemic side effects, and by virtue of their delivery to functional, ventilated alveoli may be less detrimental to V/Q matching. Nitric oxide is a potent nonspecific vasodilator, but owing to its very short half-life and inhaled method of delivery, produces relatively little systemic hypotension. Its use is associated with decreases in PVR and resultant improvements in cardiac output, and it has been shown to favorably improve systemic oxygenation through improvement in V/Q matching.[36,37]

Intravenous epoprostenol and treprostinil are rapidly titratable prostacyclin agents with potent vasodilatory effects that are well-established in the treatment of PAH. Both agents decrease PVR and enhance cardiac output, and long-term epoprostenol use has been shown to improve survival in patients with PAH.[38,39] The inhaled form of epoprostenol is frequently used in the intensive care unit and, like inhaled nitric oxide, is more selective by virtue of its delivery than intravenous prostanoids and carries less risk of systemic hypotension.[40] The role of parenteral prostacyclins in decompensated PH from nongroup 1 etiologies is uncertain, and caution should be exercised, especially in those with group 2 PH owing to decreased survival observed with their long-term use.[41] Phosphodiesterase-5 inhibitors are more commonly used in the outpatient setting, but may also have usefulness in less acutely ill patients with RHF. Sildenafil is available in both oral and intravenous formulations, and its three times daily dosing permits fairly rapid dose titration. It reduces RV afterload and appears to directly increase RV contractility in vitro in the hypertrophied RV, in which upregulation of phosphodiesterase-5

receptors has been shown.[42] Given its systemic administration, it may have a greater tendency toward systemic hypotension than inhaled vasodilators.[40]

Inotropic agents should be considered to enhance RV contractility and improve oxygen delivery once factors to ensure RV perfusion have been optimized. Both milrinone and dobutamine are widely used in clinical practice, and both have the beneficial effects of augmenting cardiac inotropy and lowering PVR. Milrinone is a selective phosphodiesterase-3 inhibitor that acts by slowing cyclic adenosine monophosphate degradation in cardiomyocytes, and may lower PVR to a greater extent than that of dobutamine.[43] Dobutamine, which acts principally on beta$_1$-adrenergic receptors, has also been shown to improve PVR and RV–pulmonary artery coupling.[44] Although both drugs have systemic vasodilatory effects, milrinone is more likely to cause systemic hypotension and may accumulate in renal failure. The lowest possible doses to achieve improved tissue perfusion should be used, because atrial and ventricular arrhythmias are more common with escalating doses.

When hypotension develops, either owing to inotropes or pulmonary arterial vasodilators, maintaining tissue perfusion and supporting the systemic blood pressure is paramount, especially because the hypertrophied and dilated RV is highly susceptible to subendocardial ischemia. Systemic pressures should be kept at least above the RV systolic pressure to ensure right-sided coronary perfusion. Vasodilators or inotropic drugs should not be abandoned or discontinued solely for hypotension. Vasopressors support the systemic blood pressure, improve coronary perfusion, and potentially decrease the degree of right-to-left interatrial shunting and hypoxia which may result from a patent foramen ovale.

The ideal vasopressor for RHF would preferentially increase the systemic vascular resistance, while having minimal effect on the PVR. Vasopressors in common use include the catecholaminergic vasopressors norepinephrine and phenylephrine, as well as the noncatecholaminergic vasopressin. Norepinephrine acts primarily on alpha-adrenergic receptors to produce vasoconstriction and is considered to be a first-line vasopressor in RV failure. It increase systemic vascular resistance, and, to a lesser extent, PVR, although significant effects on the pulmonary vasculature are not seen except at higher doses in animal models.[44] Improvements in RV myocardial oxygen delivery through increases in systemic vascular resistance have been demonstrated in a small study of patients with RV failure and septic shock, although increases in PVR were also noted.[45] Norepinephrine additionally has inotropic effects mediated by beta₁-adrenergic receptors and has shown beneficial effects on RV contractility in animal models.[46] Phenylephrine acts exclusively on alpha-adrenergic receptors to cause systemic vasoconstriction and has been shown to improve right coronary perfusion, but should be avoided in RV failure because it significantly increases mean pulmonary artery pressure and PVR, leading to worsening of RV function.[47] Vasopressin acts on the V1 receptor to induce systemic vasoconstriction and has been shown to produce pulmonary vasodilation at low doses (0.01–0.03 U/min) through nitric oxide–dependent pathways, and to decrease PVR and improve RV dilatation in animal models of PH.[48,49] However, higher doses have been shown to cause pulmonary vasoconstriction through sensitization to circulating catecholamines (**Table 1**).[50]

Sinus tachycardia is almost always present and is a reflection of the higher heart rate required to maintain cardiac output with a decreased stroke volume. However, atrial tachyarrhythmias, including atrial flutter and atrial fibrillation, are poorly tolerated, because the atrial contraction, or atrial kick, is a key contributor to the stroke volume in PH. Indeed, atrial tachyarrhythmias are associated with worsened functional status and survival in patients with PH.[27] In hemodynamically unstable patients with atrial arrhythmias, urgent cardioversion may be considered.

Hypoxia and acidosis resulting from hypercapnea have adverse effects on the pulmonary vasculature, because both conditions produce pulmonary vasoconstriction and thus increase the RV afterload. Ensuring adequate oxygenation and ventilation to keep acid–base balance and oxygen tension as close to normal values as possible is, therefore, paramount in the patient with RHF. Supplemental oxygen should be provided to keep systemic saturation above 92%. High-flow nasal cannula, although not yet comprehensively studied in the setting of acute RHF, provide supplemental oxygen with the added benefits of washout of CO_2 from anatomic dead space and a modicum of positive end-expiratory pressure.[51] Noninvasive ventilation modalities such as bilevel positive-pressure ventilation can be used to decrease respiratory work and enhance oxygenation and ventilation. Should noninvasive methods prove to be inadequate, or there is concern for the patient's ability to protect their airway, intubation may be required, and should be undertaken with great care in this patient population. The sedation required for intubation commonly causes hypotension, and minimization of sedative doses

as well as judicious use of vasopressors before sedation are advised.

Ventilation strategies in RHF using either noninvasive or mechanical ventilation carry special considerations that may differ from those typically used in the intensive care unit. Tidal volumes should be titrated so that they are not so low as to cause atelectasis or so high that they result in elevated plateau pressures, because both extremes may compromise pulmonary blood flow and worsen RV afterload.[52] During each breath in positive-pressure ventilation, the increase in alveolar pressure increases pleural pressure and thus right atrial pressure, reducing venous return and RV preload. The presence of positive end-expiratory pressure throughout the respiratory cycle further compromises venous return by increasing both pleural pressure and intra-abdominal pressure, which narrows the hepatic veins and superior vena cava.[53] In the compromised, preload-dependent right heart, this decrease in venous return can progress to hemodynamic collapse. Increased positive end-expiratory pressure also causes an increase in lung volume throughout the respiratory cycle, proportionally increasing the resistance of alveolar vessels and increasing net PVR and thus RV afterload.[54] Therefore, both tidal volume and positive end-expiratory pressure should be kept at the lowest reasonable levels to optimize the filling and function of the failing right heart.

In patients who continue to exhibit signs and symptoms of hypoperfusion, refractory congestion, or impaired oxygenation/ventilation despite maximal medical therapy, mechanical circulatory support may be indicated. For patients with RV failure owing to PH, mechanical circulatory support has been used as a bridge to recovery amid worsening PH, as a bridge to transplantation, and increasingly as a rescue option after pulmonary endarterectomy.[55,56]

Extracorporeal membrane oxygenation is being used with increasing frequency in cases of RV failure where medical therapy has failed. In centers with relevant expertise, venoarterial extracorporeal membrane oxygenation can be started to rapidly unload the right ventricle and augment its systolic function, rapidly improving tissue perfusion and end-organ oxygenation without increasing blood flow through the pulmonary circulation. In severely ill patients with underlying PH in whom it is felt that hypoxia and hypercapnea from respiratory failure are driving features of their decompensation, venovenous extracorporeal membrane oxygenation may be considered as an alternative. This form of extracorporeal membrane oxygenation augments end-organ oxygenation and carbon dioxide

Table 1
Vasoactive therapies in RV failure

Vasoactive Medication	Target Receptor	Primary Action	Considerations
Norepinephrine	α1, α2 (strong) β1 (moderate)	Peripheral vasoconstriction (major) Inotropy, chronotrophy (minor)	Tachyarrhythmia risk Potential for myocardial ischemia Considered first line for systemic hypotension in RHF
Epinephrine	β1, β2 (strong) α1, α2 (moderate)	Inotropy, chronotrophy (major) Peripheral vasoconstriction (major)	Tachyarrhythmia risk Potential for myocardial ischemia Associated with increased peripheral lactate
Vasopressin	V1	Peripheral vasoconstriction	Considered second-line Decreased risk of tachyarrhythmia, myocardial ischemia vs catecholamines[80] May decrease PVR
Phenylephrine	α1	Peripheral vasoconstriction	Less risk of cardiac ischemia or tachyarrhythmia Neutral or decreased cardiac output; may worsen RV output Increases mean pulmonary artery pressure and PVR Minimal usefulness in RHF
Dobutamine	β1 > β2	Inotropy, chronotropy (↑cardiac output) Peripheral vasodilation	Shorter half-life than milrinone Less systemic hypotension than milrinone Higher chronotropy and frequency of tachyarrhythmias
Milrinone	Phospho-diesterase-3	Inotropy, chronotropy (↑cardiac output) Peripheral vasodilation	Greater reductions in LV end-diastolic pressure/RV end-diastolic pressure and fewer tachyarrhythmias than dobutamine More risk of systemic hypotension than dobutamine Contraindicated in severe renal dysfunction

clearance, but does not augment the function of the right ventricle.

Because the cause of the RV failure in PH is related to increased afterload, RV assist devices have emerged as a method to augment RV function and increase flow into the poorly compliant vasculature. Both implantable centrifugal pump designs such as the HeartMate III (Abbott Laboratories, Chicago, IL; which is designed for left ventricular use) and percutaneously placed impeller-based designs like the Abiomed (Danvers, MA) Impella RP (specific to RV support) have been developed and may allow for longer term treatment strategies than extracorporeal membrane oxygenation. Animal studies of RV assist devices have that shown RV unloading during diastole and improvement of cardiac output in the setting of acutely increased PVR.[57] Owing to safety concerns, including the risk of pulmonary hemorrhage, their use thus far has been limited to a bridge to transplantation in end-stage disease.[58]

Chronic Management

Decongestion, achieved through diuretics or renal replacement therapy modalities, decreases interventricular dependence and improves left ventricular filling, increasing stroke volume and overall cardiac output. Loop diuretics have long been considered first-line agents for this purpose. Venous congestion resulting in cardiorenal syndrome, hypotension, and oliguric acute kidney injury may blunt the response to diuretics, requiring escalation with the addition of thiazide diuretics, escalation to renal replacement therapies, and/or inotropic agents to augment forward flow to the kidneys.

In chronic RHF, where RV dysfunction is a result of ongoing PH, afterload reduction is the backbone of chronic RHF management and prevention. Countering the increase in PVR allows for enhancement of forward flow from the right ventricle and augmentation of RV perfusion through relief of wall tension, curbing downstream effects of RV ischemia and oxidative stress. The current armamentarium of pulmonary vasodilators includes phosphodiesterase-5 inhibitors, endothelin-receptor antagonists, soluble guanylate cyclase inhibitors, and prostacyclin derivatives. Guidance for choosing specific long-term pulmonary vasodilator treatment in the patient with World Health Organization group I PAH is a complex and ever-expanding topic that is outside the scope of this review.

A number of strategies used in the management of left heart failure that target the renin–angiotensin–aldosterone system are being studied as applied to the right heart in patients with PH, including beta-blockers, angiotensin-converting enzyme inhibitors/angiotensin receptor antagonists, and aldosterone antagonists, as well as resynchronization therapy. Both increases in baseline sympathetic nervous activity and renin–angiotensin–aldosterone system activation are contributing factors to PAH and may represent therapeutic targets.[59,60] Animal studies of beta-blockers have shown mixed results, and small clinical studies have not consistently shown robust clinical improvements.[61–64] Given the potential for deterioration of RV function with beta blockers, these therapies are generally avoided in RHF.[65] Studies of angiotensin-converting enzyme inhibitors and angiotensin receptor antagonists have also not shown significant improvement in hemodynamics or exercise tolerance, and there remains concern about systemic hypotension in this patient population.[66] Aldosterone blockade continues to be a target of interest but has shown mixed results, with one trial combining use with ambrisentan showing nonstatistically significant improvements in N-terminal pro b-type natriuretic peptide and 6-minute walking distance compared with ambrisentan alone.[67] A recent single-center study found that patients with group I PAH taking aldosterone receptor antagonists had a significantly greater rate of hospitalizations than those who did not.[68] Finally, sympathetic ganglion block, pulmonary denervation, and sympathetic renal denervation are being explored with some promise in animal models.[69–71]

In selected patients with severe PH who have failed maximal medical therapies, balloon atrial septostomy may be performed as a palliative therapy for treatment of RV failure or as a bridge therapy for transplantation, although its precise role in the management of PH and RV failure remains unclear.[72] The procedure is thought to ameliorate RV failure through reduction of RV preload, enhanced filling of the left ventricle, and improvement in systemic oxygen delivery despite a reduction in arterial oxygen saturation.[73] Balloon atrial septostomy seems to significantly improve clinical symptoms, hemodynamic parameters, and at least short-term survival in advanced PAH.[74,75]

Prevention of Right Heart Failure in Pulmonary Hypertension

RV function is a key prognostic marker in PH. Consequently, preservation of RV function and prevention of deterioration are crucial tenets of PH care. In addition to the strategies used for chronic management of existing RV dysfunction, careful attention should be focused on risk factor reduction, including screening for related conditions, such as lung disease, that may contribute to PH and/or RV dysfunction and goal-directed treatment of such conditions. Obesity is a well-known risk factor for cardiomyopathy, and a correlative relationship between higher body mass index and RV dysfunction has been described in patients with PH, highlighting weight management as an issue that requires ongoing attention.[76,77] High prevalence rates of obstructive sleep apnea and nocturnal hypoxemia in patients with existing PH warrant routine screening with polysomnography.[78]

Monitoring of PH, including routine use of the 6-minute walk test, echocardiography, and use of biomarkers such as brain natriuretic peptide are valuable in identifying clinical worsening, which may occur before the development of overt clinical RV failure and signal the need for more aggressive treatment to prevent this outcome. Finally, although elective surgical procedures under anything more than local anesthesia should be avoided if at all possible in PAH, it is recommended that patients who are to undergo them should be referred to centers with expertise in PAH management.[79]

SUMMARY

RHF is the leading cause of mortality in patients with PAH and is the result of a complex series of changes prompted by chronic increases in RV afterload. Despite an increasingly broad arsenal of available PAH-specific treatments, mortality rates in this patient group remain especially high. Increasing understanding of the complex pathophysiologic changes that underlie PAH, such as metabolic dysregulation and neurohormonal effects on the right heart, will hopefully produce new or effectively repurposed treatments to further improve patient survival and quality of life.

DISCLOSURE

The authors have nothing to disclose.

REFERENCES

1. Simonneau G, Montani D, Celermajer DS, et al. Haemodynamic definitions and updated clinical classification of pulmonary hypertension. Eur Respir J 2019;53(1) [pii:1801913].
2. Mehra MR, Park MH, Landzberg MJ, et al. Right heart failure: toward a common language. J Heart Lung Transplant 2014;33(2):123–6.
3. Vonk-Noordegraaf A, Haddad F, Chin KM, et al. Right heart adaptation to pulmonary arterial hypertension: physiology and pathobiology. J Am Coll Cardiol 2013;62(25 Suppl):D22–33.
4. Campo A, Mathai SC, Le Pavec J, et al. Outcomes of hospitalisation for right heart failure in pulmonary arterial hypertension. Eur Respir J 2011;38(2):359–67.
5. Benza RL, Gomberg-Maitland M, Elliott CG, et al. Predicting survival in patients with pulmonary arterial hypertension: the REVEAL risk score calculator 2.0 and comparison with ESC/ERS-based risk assessment strategies. Chest 2019;156(2):323–37.
6. van der Bruggen CEE, Tedford RJ, Handoko ML, et al. RV pressure overload: from hypertrophy to failure. Cardiovasc Res 2017;113(12):1423–32.
7. Ryan JJ, Huston J, Kutty S, et al. Right ventricular adaptation and failure in pulmonary arterial hypertension. Can J Cardiol 2015;31(4):391–406.
8. Handoko ML, de Man FS, Allaart CP, et al. Perspectives on novel therapeutic strategies for right heart failure in pulmonary arterial hypertension: lessons from the left heart. Eur Respir Rev 2010;19(115):72–82.
9. Kuehne T, Yilmaz S, Steendijk P, et al. Magnetic resonance imaging analysis of right ventricular pressure-volume loops: in vivo validation and clinical application in patients with pulmonary hypertension. Circulation 2004;110(14):2010–6.
10. Rana B, Robinson S, Francis R, et al. Tricuspid regurgitation and the right ventricle: risk stratification and timing of intervention. Echo Res Pract 2019;6(1):R25–39.
11. Konstam MA, Kiernan MS, Bernstein D, et al. Evaluation and management of right-sided heart failure: a scientific statement from the American Heart Association. Circulation 2018;137(20):e578–622.
12. Marcus JT, Gan CT, Zwanenburg JJ, et al. Interventricular mechanical asynchrony in pulmonary arterial hypertension: left-to-right delay in peak shortening is related to right ventricular overload and left ventricular underfilling. J Am Coll Cardiol 2008;51(7):750–7.
13. van Wolferen SA, Marcus JT, Westerhof N, et al. Right coronary artery flow impairment in patients with pulmonary hypertension. Eur Heart J 2008;29(1):120–7.
14. Piao L, Fang YH, Parikh K, et al. Cardiac glutaminolysis: a maladaptive cancer metabolism pathway in the right ventricle in pulmonary hypertension. J Mol Med (Berl) 2013;91(10):1185–97.
15. Piao L, Fang YH, Cadete VJ, et al. The inhibition of pyruvate dehydrogenase kinase improves impaired cardiac function and electrical remodeling in two models of right ventricular hypertrophy: resuscitating the hibernating right ventricle. J Mol Med (Berl) 2010;88(1):47–60.
16. Archer SL, Fang YH, Ryan JJ, et al. Metabolism and bioenergetics in the right ventricle and pulmonary vasculature in pulmonary hypertension. Pulm Circ 2013;3(1):144–52.
17. Brittain EL, Talati M, Fessel JP, et al. Fatty acid metabolic defects and right ventricular lipotoxicity in human pulmonary arterial hypertension. Circulation 2016;133(20):1936–44.
18. Drake JI, Bogaard HJ, Mizuno S, et al. Molecular signature of a right heart failure program in chronic severe pulmonary hypertension. Am J Respir Cell Mol Biol 2011;45(6):1239–47.
19. Marshall JD, Bazan I, Zhang Y, et al. Mitochondrial dysfunction and pulmonary hypertension: cause, effect, or both. Am J Physiol Lung Cell Mol Physiol 2018;314(5):L782–96.
20. Culley MK, Chan SY. Mitochondrial metabolism in pulmonary hypertension: beyond mountains there are mountains. J Clin Invest 2018;128(9):3704–15.
21. Hashimoto T, Shibasaki F. Hypoxia-inducible factor as an angiogenic master switch. Front Pediatr 2015;3:33.
22. Bogaard HJ, Abe K, Vonk Noordegraaf A, et al. The right ventricle under pressure: cellular and

molecular mechanisms of right-heart failure in pulmonary hypertension. Chest 2009;135(3):794–804.

23. Vaillancourt M, Chia P, Sarji S, et al. Autonomic nervous system involvement in pulmonary arterial hypertension. Respir Res 2017;18(1):201.

24. Bristow MR, Quaife RA. The adrenergic system in pulmonary arterial hypertension: bench to bedside (2013 Grover Conference series). Pulm Circ 2015; 5(3):415–23.

25. Mercurio V, Pellegrino T, Bosso G, et al. EXPRESS: cardiac sympathetic dysfunction in pulmonary arterial hypertension: lesson from left-sided heart failure. Pulm Circ 2019 [Epub ahead of print].

26. Harjola VP, Mebazaa A, Celutkiene J, et al. Contemporary management of acute right ventricular failure: a statement from the heart failure association and the working group on pulmonary circulation and right ventricular function of the European Society of Cardiology. Eur J Heart Fail 2016;18(3): 226–41.

27. Tongers J, Schwerdtfeger B, Klein G, et al. Incidence and clinical relevance of supraventricular tachyarrhythmias in pulmonary hypertension. Am Heart J 2007;153(1):127–32.

28. Shah SJ, Thenappan T, Rich S, et al. Association of serum creatinine with abnormal hemodynamics and mortality in pulmonary arterial hypertension. Circulation 2008;117(19):2475–83.

29. Nickel NP, O'Leary JM, Brittain EL, et al. Kidney dysfunction in patients with pulmonary arterial hypertension. Pulm Circ 2017;7(1):38–54.

30. Xu SL, Yang J, Zhang CF, et al. Serum cardiac troponin elevation predicts mortality in patients with pulmonary hypertension: a meta-analysis of eight cohort studies. Clin Respir J 2019;13(2):82–91.

31. Benza RL, Gomberg-Maitland M, Miller DP, et al. The REVEAL Registry risk score calculator in patients newly diagnosed with pulmonary arterial hypertension. Chest 2012;141(2):354–62.

32. Frost A, Badesch D, Gibbs JSR, et al. Diagnosis of pulmonary hypertension. Eur Respir J 2019; 53(1).

33. Surkova E, Muraru D, Iliceto S, et al. The use of multimodality cardiovascular imaging to assess right ventricular size and function. Int J Cardiol 2016; 214:54–69.

34. Ramani GV, Gurm G, Dilsizian V, et al. Noninvasive assessment of right ventricular function: will there be resurgence in radionuclide imaging techniques? Curr Cardiol Rep 2010;12(2):162–9.

35. Vonk Noordegraaf A, Westerhof BE, Westerhof N. The relationship between the right ventricle and its load in pulmonary hypertension. J Am Coll Cardiol 2017;69(2):236–43.

36. Creagh-Brown BC, Griffiths MJ, Evans TW. Bench-to-bedside review: inhaled nitric oxide therapy in adults. Crit Care 2009;13(3):221.

37. Pepke-Zaba J, Higenbottam TW, Dinh-Xuan AT, et al. Inhaled nitric oxide as a cause of selective pulmonary vasodilatation in pulmonary hypertension. Lancet 1991;338(8776):1173–4.

38. Rubin LJ, Mendoza J, Hood M, et al. Treatment of primary pulmonary hypertension with continuous intravenous prostacyclin (epoprostenol). Results of a randomized trial. Ann Intern Med 1990;112(7): 485–91.

39. McLaughlin VV, Shillington A, Rich S. Survival in primary pulmonary hypertension: the impact of epoprostenol therapy. Circulation 2002;106(12): 1477–82.

40. Hill NS, Preston IR, Roberts KE. Inhaled therapies for pulmonary hypertension. Respir Care 2015;60(6): 794–802 [discussion: 802–5].

41. Califf RM, Adams KF, McKenna WJ, et al. A randomized controlled trial of epoprostenol therapy for severe congestive heart failure: the Flolan International Randomized Survival Trial (FIRST). Am Heart J 1997;134(1):44–54.

42. Nagendran J, Archer SL, Soliman D, et al. Phosphodiesterase type 5 is highly expressed in the hypertrophied human right ventricle, and acute inhibition of phosphodiesterase type 5 improves contractility. Circulation 2007;116(3):238–48.

43. Eskandr AM, Metwally AA, Abu Elkassem MS, et al. Dobutamine and nitroglycerin versus milrinone for perioperative management of pulmonary hypertension in mitral valve surgery. A randomized controlled study. J Cardiothorac Vasc Anesth 2018;32(6): 2540–6.

44. Kerbaul F, Rondelet B, Motte S, et al. Effects of norepinephrine and dobutamine on pressure load-induced right ventricular failure. Crit Care Med 2004;32(4):1035–40.

45. Schreuder WO, Schneider AJ, Groeneveld AB, et al. Effect of dopamine vs norepinephrine on hemodynamics in septic shock. Emphasis on right ventricular performance. Chest 1989;95(6):1282–8.

46. Hirsch LJ, Rooney MW, Wat SS, et al. Norepinephrine and phenylephrine effects on right ventricular function in experimental canine pulmonary embolism. Chest 1991;100(3):796–801.

47. Rich S, Gubin S, Hart K. The effects of phenylephrine on right ventricular performance in patients with pulmonary hypertension. Chest 1990;98(5): 1102–6.

48. Evora PR, Pearson PJ, Schaff HV. Arginine vasopressin induces endothelium-dependent vasodilatation of the pulmonary artery. V1-receptor-mediated production of nitric oxide. Chest 1993;103(4): 1241–5.

49. Sugawara Y, Mizuno Y, Oku S, et al. Effects of vasopressin during a pulmonary hypertensive crisis induced by acute hypoxia in a rat model of pulmonary hypertension. Br J Anaesth 2019;122(4):437–47.

50. Leather HA, Segers P, Berends N, et al. Effects of vasopressin on right ventricular function in an experimental model of acute pulmonary hypertension. Crit Care Med 2002;30(11):2548–52.

51. Helviz Y, Einav S. A systematic review of the high-flow nasal cannula for adult patients. Crit Care 2018;22(1):71.

52. Biondi JW, Schulman DS, Matthay RA. Effects of mechanical ventilation on right and left ventricular function. Clin Chest Med 1988;9(1):55–71.

53. Jardin F, Vieillard-Baron A. Right ventricular function and positive pressure ventilation in clinical practice: from hemodynamic subsets to respirator settings. Intensive Care Med 2003;29(9):1426–34.

54. Disselkamp M, Adkins D, Pandey S, et al. Physiologic approach to mechanical ventilation in right ventricular failure. Ann Am Thorac Soc 2018;15(3):383–9.

55. Sugiyama K, Suzuki S, Fujiyoshi T, et al. Extracorporeal membrane oxygenation after pulmonary endarterectomy for chronic thromboembolic pulmonary hypertension. J Card Surg 2019;34(6):428–34.

56. Donahoe L, Granton J, McRae K, et al. Role of extracorporeal life support after pulmonary endarterectomy: a single-centre experience. Interact Cardiovasc Thorac Surg 2016;23(1):74–8.

57. Verbelen T, Burkhoff D, Kasama K, et al. Systolic and diastolic unloading by mechanical support of the acute vs the chronic pressure overloaded right ventricle. J Heart Lung Transpl 2017;36(4):457–65.

58. Westerhof BE, Saouti N, van der Laarse WJ, et al. Treatment strategies for the right heart in pulmonary hypertension. Cardiovasc Res 2017;113(12):1465–73.

59. Ciarka A, Doan V, Velez-Roa S, et al. Prognostic significance of sympathetic nervous system activation in pulmonary arterial hypertension. Am J Respir Crit Care Med 2010;181(11):1269–75.

60. de Man FS, Tu L, Handoko ML, et al. Dysregulated renin-angiotensin-aldosterone system contributes to pulmonary arterial hypertension. Am J Respir Crit Care Med 2012;186(8):780–9.

61. Farha S, Saygin D, Park MM, et al. Pulmonary arterial hypertension treatment with carvedilol for heart failure: a randomized controlled trial. JCI Insight 2017;2(16) [pii:95240].

62. Provencher S, Herve P, Jais X, et al. Deleterious effects of beta-blockers on exercise capacity and hemodynamics in patients with portopulmonary hypertension. Gastroenterology 2006;130(1):120–6.

63. Bogaard HJ, Natarajan R, Mizuno S, et al. Adrenergic receptor blockade reverses right heart remodeling and dysfunction in pulmonary hypertensive rats. Am J Respir Crit Care Med 2010;182(5):652–60.

64. Andersen S, Schultz JG, Andersen A, et al. Effects of bisoprolol and losartan treatment in the hypertrophic and failing right heart. J Card Fail 2014;20(11):864–73.

65. Perros F, de Man FS, Bogaard HJ, et al. Use of beta-blockers in pulmonary hypertension. Circ Heart Fail 2017;10(4):e003703.

66. Leier CV, Bambach D, Nelson S, et al. Captopril in primary pulmonary hypertension. Circulation 1983;67(1):155–61.

67. Maron BA, Waxman AB, Opotowsky AR, et al. Effectiveness of spironolactone plus ambrisentan for treatment of pulmonary arterial hypertension (from the [ARIES] study 1 and 2 trials). Am J Cardiol 2013;112(5):720–5.

68. Corkish M, Devine L, Clarke M, et al. EXPRESS: rates of hospitalization associated with the use of aldosterone receptor antagonists in patients with pulmonary arterial hypertension. Pulm Circ 2019 [Epub ahead of print].

69. Na S, Kim OS, Ryoo S, et al. Cervical ganglion block attenuates the progression of pulmonary hypertension via nitric oxide and arginase pathways. Hypertension 2014;63(2):309–15.

70. Chen SL, Zhang H, Xie DJ, et al. Hemodynamic, functional, and clinical responses to pulmonary artery denervation in patients with pulmonary arterial hypertension of different causes: phase II results from the Pulmonary Artery Denervation-1 study. Circ Cardiovasc Interv 2015;8(11):e002837.

71. Liu Q, Song J, Lu D, et al. Effects of renal denervation on monocrotaline induced pulmonary remodeling. Oncotarget 2017;8(29):46846–55.

72. Sandoval J, Gomez-Arroyo J, Gaspar J, et al. Interventional and surgical therapeutic strategies for pulmonary arterial hypertension: beyond palliative treatments. J Cardiol 2015;66(4):304–14.

73. Koeken Y, Kuijpers NH, Lumens J, et al. Atrial septostomy benefits severe pulmonary hypertension patients by increase of left ventricular preload reserve. Am J Physiol Heart Circ Physiol 2012;302(12):H2654–62.

74. Sandoval J, Gaspar J, Pena H, et al. Effect of atrial septostomy on the survival of patients with severe pulmonary arterial hypertension. Eur Respir J 2011;38(6):1343–8.

75. Khan MS, Memon MM, Amin E, et al. Use of balloon atrial septostomy in patients with advanced pulmonary arterial hypertension: a systematic review and meta-analysis. Chest 2019;156(1):53–63.

76. Wong CY, O'Moore-Sullivan T, Leano R, et al. Association of subclinical right ventricular dysfunction with obesity. J Am Coll Cardiol 2006;47(3):611–6.

77. Friedman SE, Andrus BW. Obesity and pulmonary hypertension: a review of pathophysiologic mechanisms. J Obes 2012;2012:505274.

78. Jilwan FN, Escourrou P, Garcia G, et al. High occurrence of hypoxemic sleep respiratory disorders in

precapillary pulmonary hypertension and mechanisms. Chest 2013;143(1):47–55.

79. Scientific leadership council consensus statement: elective surgery. 2018, Pulmonary Hypertension Association. Available at: www.PHAssociation.org. Accessed December 12, 2019.

80. McIntyre WF, Um KJ, Alhazzani W, et al. Association of vasopressin plus catecholamine vasopressors vs catecholamines alone with atrial fibrillation in patients with distributive shock: a systematic review and meta-analysis. JAMA 2018;319(18): 1889–900.

Surgical and Percutaneous Interventions for Chronic Thromboembolic Pulmonary Hypertension

William R. Auger, MD, FCPP

KEYWORDS

- Chronic thromboembolism • Chronic thromboembolic pulmonary hypertension
- WHO group IV pulmonary hypertension • Pulmonary thromboendarterectomy
- Balloon pulmonary angioplasty

KEY POINTS

- Chronic thromboembolic pulmonary hypertension results from unresolved pulmonary thromboembolism in approximately 3% of long-term survivors of an acute pulmonary embolic event(s).
- Chronic thromboembolic pulmonary hypertension is an under-recognized disease that is potentially curable.
- Pulmonary thromboendarterectomy is a unique cardiothoracic surgical procedure shown to result in marked improvements in pulmonary hemodynamics and functional status in selected patients with chronic thromboembolic pulmonary hypertension.
- Balloon pulmonary angioplasty is a catheter-based intervention that has shown promise in improving pulmonary hemodynamics in patients with chronic thromboembolic pulmonary hypertension deemed to be unsuitable for operative intervention.

INTRODUCTION

The last several decades have witnessed considerable steps forward in our understanding of the natural history and epidemiology of chronic thromboembolic pulmonary hypertension (CTEPH). Fueled by this understanding, worldwide experience with this disease has expanded exponentially, prompting the recent observation that "CTEPH and its recognition and treatment have become global endeavors."[1] Since 2012 in particular, advancements in the management of both operable and inoperable CTEPH have been particularly noteworthy. Although pulmonary thromboendarterectomy remains the treatment option with the greatest potential for a cure, distal vessel endarterectomy, balloon pulmonary angioplasty, and pulmonary hypertension (PH) targeted medical therapy are the most recent therapeutic developments for patients with distal vessel chronic thromboembolic disease. As a result, not only is disease recognition of substantial import, but the determination of which patient with CTEPH is operable versus nonsurgical takes on greater significance because the treatment algorithm for the 2 patient groups is distinctly different, each posing unique challenges. This assessment is most appropriately made with the input of a multidisciplinary team of experienced clinicians versed in the diagnostic difficulties presented by this patient population.[2] This article focuses on the interventions available for managing the pulmonary vascular obstructive component of CTEPH: pulmonary thromboendarterectomy, pulmonary thromboembolism (PTE) (or pulmonary endarterectomy [PEA]) for the surgical removal of chronic thrombotic disease from the pulmonary

Pulmonary Hypertension and CTEPH Research Program, Temple Heart and Vascular Institute, Temple University, Lewis Katz School of Medicine, 3401 North Broad Street, Philadelphia, PA 19140, USA
E-mail address: Bill.Auger@tuhs.temple.edu

Cardiol Clin 38 (2020) 257–268
https://doi.org/10.1016/j.ccl.2020.01.003
0733-8651/20/© 2020 Elsevier Inc. All rights reserved.

arteries, and balloon pulmonary angioplasty, a catheter-based intervention to manage the vascular compromise in pulmonary vessels involved with chronic thromboembolic disease.

PATIENT ASSESSMENT

The current World Health Organization's PH classification has categorized CTEPH as group IV PH and defined it as the presence of an elevated pulmonary arterial pressure (mean pulmonary artery pressure of >25 mm Hg) in the setting of persistent perfusion defects from organized thromboembolism diagnosed by lung ventilation–perfusion scintigraphy, computed tomography, and angiography of the chest and/or magnetic resonance angiography of the pulmonary vasculature.[2] This definition presumes the absence of coexisting left heart disease, which might be substantially contributing to the PH.

CTEPH is considered to be a relatively rare complication of an acute pulmonary embolic event or recurrent events, with a number of medical factors identified as placing patients at risk for developing this disease[3] (**Box 1**). It is estimated at an annual incident rate for diagnosed and undiagnosed CTEPH in the United States and Europe at 3 to 5 cases per 100,000 population.[4] CTEPH is also felt to be underdiagnosed given the nonspecific nature of presenting symptoms, the frequently absent history of known venous thromboembolic events, and often misinterpreted diagnostic studies. As is the case with pulmonary arterial hypertension, if left untreated, the natural history of misdiagnosed and untreated CTEPH carries a poor prognosis with the development of right heart failure and death. Further underscoring the significance of establishing the diagnosis of CTEPH is that surgical endarterectomy provides an opportunity for a potential remedy for this form of PH, and as such, making the distinction between CTEPH and other pulmonary vascular diseases bears considerable consequence.

Patients having experienced an acute pulmonary embolic event(s) with persistent cardiopulmonary symptoms after a defined course of antithrombotic therapy, all patients with diagnose PH, and patients with exertional dyspnea or progressive exercise intolerance without explanation following an evaluation are individuals in whom CTEPH should be considered.[5,6] Screening patients for PH and right ventricular dysfunction with echocardiography, as well as, using lung ventilation–perfusion scintigraphy for the detection of unmatched perfusion defects represent the recommended initial studies in the assessment for chronic thromboembolic disease and

CTEPH.[2,7,8] However, diagnostic testing with computed tomography angiography of the chest, magnetic resonance angiography, and/or catheter-based pulmonary angiography are essential to definitively establish the presence of chronic thromboembolic disease.[8,9] Computed tomography angiography of the chest has the advantage of a broader interpretative experience with radiologists, as well as providing essential information about the pulmonary circulation, the mediastinum, and the lung parenchyma to address alternative diagnoses and cardiopulmonary comorbidities. However, as interpretation difficulties of computed tomography imaging do exist, especially at the level of the segmental and subsegmental vessels,[10] the performance of conventional catheter-based pulmonary angiography continues to be of considerable value. This finding is especially relevant given the availability of distal vessel endarterectomy and balloon pulmonary angioplasty, where intervention at this vascular level has documented efficacy.[11,12] Although more

---

Box 1
Risk factors for CTEPH

Related to pulmonary embolic event

  PH and right ventricular dysfunction at initial presentation

  History of recurrent pulmonary emboli

  Large thrombus burden

  Idiopathic pulmonary embolus

  Delay in diagnosis, greater than 2 weeks

Associated medical conditions

  Prothrombotic states: Antiphospholipid syndromes (lupus anticoagulant, anticardiolipin antibodies)

    Elevated factor VIII

    Elevated von Willebrand factor

    Dysfibrinogenemia

  Splenectomy

  Non-group O blood group

  Hypothyroidism/thyroid replacement therapy

  Prolonged presence of intravascular devices (? infected): venous catheters, pacemaker wires, ventriculoatrial shunts

  Pelvic vein compression from uterine masses/fibroids

  History of malignancy

  Possibly chronic inflammatory conditions: osteomyelitis, inflammatory bowel disease

advanced imaging testing include SPECT VQ scanning,[13] dual energy computed tomography,[14] and optical coherence tomography,[15] their ultimate place in the diagnostic algorithm for patients with suspected CTEPH has not been established. Additionally, they are not widely available and are most often used at experienced centers where research and advanced diagnostics are being addressed.

Once the diagnosis of CTEPH has been established, determination of operability is the next essential step. Despite advancements in diagnostics and expanding surgical experience, there remains considerable subjectivity in this assessment. Experience with interpretation of the diagnostic studies and knowledge of the capabilities the surgical team at a specialized center for PTE surgery will dictate which chronic thromboembolic lesions can be endarterectomized (**Fig. 1**). As surgical experience is gained, not only is it possible to resect main pulmonary artery and lobar level disease, but also more distal, segmental and subsegmental chronic thromboembolic lesions. As discussed elsewhere in this article, additional steps in decision making extend beyond the determination of operable versus inoperable disease. Surgical risks are an essential calculation in those patients with technically operable disease, and for those without an endarterectomy option, the presence of chronic thromboembolic lesions technically amenable to angioplasty[16] needs to be discerned, most often by clinicians with expertise in this intervention.

An essential component of defining surgical candidacy is the assessment of perioperative risks. A properly performed right heart catheterization is necessary to accurately determine the severity of PH and the degree of right heart dysfunction in patients with CTEPH undergoing surgical evaluation. Despite the decrease in perioperative risks among experienced CTEPH centers worldwide, the severity of PH and right heart dysfunction continues to impact mortality outcomes after endarterectomy. In a recent report, with the expansive experience of the San Diego group, there has been a declining overall operative mortality risk of 2.2% after thromboendarterectomy surgery in 500 patients operated between 2006 and 2010. Nonetheless, in this same group, those patients with a preoperative pulmonary vascular resistance of greater than 1000 d/s/cm^{-5} experienced a mortality rate of 4.1% compared with 1.6% in those patients with a pulmonary vascular resistance of less than 1000 d/s/cm^{-5}.[17] A subsequent report from de Perrot and colleagues[18] compared postendarterectomy outcomes in those patients with CTEPH with a preoperative total pulmonary vascular resistance of greater than (n = 26) or less than (n = 78) 1200 dyn-s-cm^{-5}. Overall in-hospital mortality after PEA was 4%, with all deaths occurring in patients with a total pulmonary resistance of greater than 1200 dyn-s-cm^{-5} and decompensated right heart failure on presentation. Whether or not preoperative pulmonary hemodynamics affect the risk of developing other potential complications after PTE is the subject of ongoing investigation.

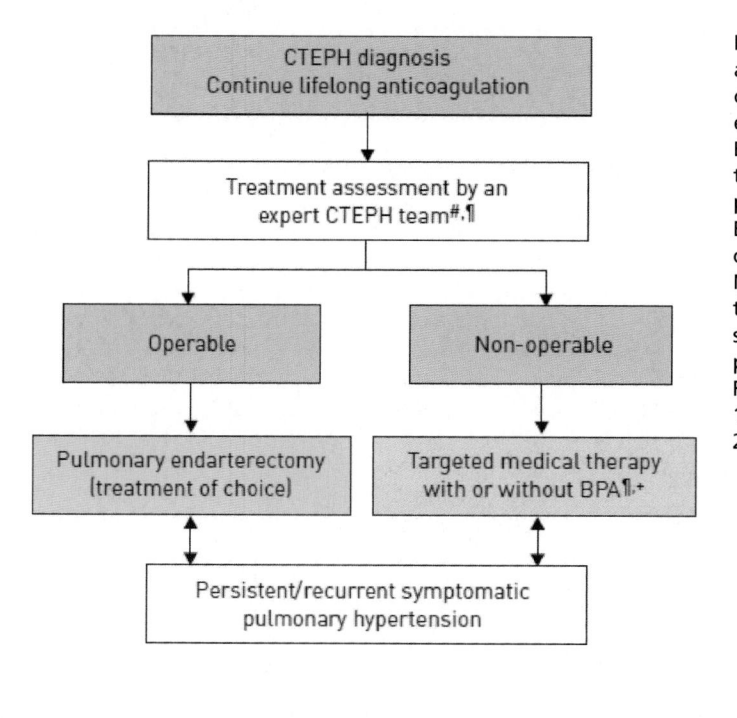

Fig. 1. Treatment algorithm for CTEPH adopted at the 6th World Symposium on PH. #, multidisciplinary: pulmonary endarterectomy surgeon, PH expert, BPA interventionalist and radiologist; ¶, treatment assessment may differ depending on the level of expertise; +, BPA without medical therapy can be considered in selected cases. (*From* Kim NH, Delcroix M, Jais X, et al. Chronic thromboembolic pulmonary hypertension. Eur Resp J 2019. Reproduced with permission of the © ERS 2020: European Respiratory Journal 53 (1) 1801915; DOI: 10.1183/13993003.01915-2018 Published 24 January 2019.)

There should also be the anticipation that a pulmonary thromboendarterectomy will have a meaningful outcome for the patient undergoing this complex and technically challenging procedure. Patients with significant comorbid conditions such as severe emphysema, or those with a life-limiting malignancy, are not only at considerable perioperative risk, but are unlikely to realize the functional status benefit that would be achieved with PTE surgery. And although surgery might be technically feasible, such an aggressive intervention might be considered ill advised. An additional consideration important to a positive surgical outcome is the determination that the thrombus burden observed on imaging correlates with degree of hemodynamic impairment observed during right heart catheterization. When the degree of PH seems to be out of proportion to the extent of accessible chronic thromboembolic disease apparent by angiography and surgical resection is not expected to result in a substantive improvement in pulmonary hemodynamics, avoidance of surgery is appropriate, and alternative approaches such as balloon angioplasty should be considered. Although this assessment is typically subjective, attempts at developing a more objective approach to assist in this decision making have been less than robust. Catheter techniques to distinguish upstream resistance owing to vessel obstruction on the basis of chronic thrombotic lesions from distal vascular resistance owing to concurrent small vessel vasculopathy known to contribute to the PH in patients with CTEPH have not been widely available and have proven difficult to reproduce.[19] It has also been hypothesized that fractional pulse pressure of the pulmonary artery, theoretically a reflection of small vessel arteriopathy, might be useful in predicting those patients with CTEPH with inoperable disease who might be at greater risk for a poor outcome after endarterectomy. Tanabe and colleagues[20] demonstrated that in a small number of patients undergoing endarterectomy, the fractional pulse pressure of the pulmonary artery was significantly higher in patients (n = 26) who survived the surgery than in those who did not survive (n = 6). Multivariate analysis, however, disclosed the fractional pulse pressure of the pulmonary artery to be a marginal predictor of mortality; a pulmonary vascular resistance of greater than 1100 dyn/s/cm^{-5} in this group proved to be a more significant predictor of a poor post-PTE hemodynamic outcome.

Difficulties with patient selection underscore the importance of collaborating with a center specializing in the evaluation and treatment of patients with chronic thromboembolic disease. As experience grows, the range of patients eligible to undergo PTE expands to the point that there are few absolute contraindications to surgery. Effective surgical intervention has been described in children,[21] in patients at the higher levels of body mass index,[22] patients with CTEPH with severe PH and right ventricular dysfunction,[18] and patients aged greater than 70 years,[23] as well as in those patients with various types of hemoglobinopathy.[24] In each of these patient subgroups, surgical strategies and unique risks may be involved, though manageable as experience grows at CTEPH centers of excellence.

PULMONARY THROMBOENDARTERECTOMY

The preferred treatment for patients with CTEPH, with the greatest chance for cure of their PH and right heart failure, is a PTE (also referred to as PEA). Pulmonary thromboendarterectomy is a unique surgical intervention to remove obstructive, adherent chronic thromboembolic lesions from within the pulmonary vascular bed. Details of the surgical procedure and intraoperative anesthesia care have been described and beyond the scope of this review.[25] However, the fundamental aspects of this unique surgical procedure have changed little over the past several decades. Performance of the surgery via a median sternotomy provides access to the central pulmonary vessels of both lungs, while avoiding disruption of what can be extensive systemic arterial collateral circulation and pleural adhesions that may develop following longstanding pulmonary arterial obstruction. Furthermore, if additional cardiac procedures are necessary, such as coronary artery bypass or valve surgery, this approach provides access to the heart.[26] The use of cardiopulmonary bypass with periods of hypothermic circulatory arrest is the unique feature of this cardiopulmonary surgical procedure. With endarterectomy of the adherent chronic thromboembolic material from the walls of the pulmonary vessel, establishment of an adequate dissection plane is critical to successful removal of clot. Intermittent circulatory arrest (absent cardiopulmonary bypass) periods avoid back-bleeding from a bronchial or systemic artery to pulmonary artery anastomoses and provides the necessary bloodless field to perform an optimal dissection, as well as providing the ideal environment to allow as complete an endarterectomy as possible. To safely extend circulatory arrest periods for up to 20 minutes, it is necessary to cool patients to 20°C (deep hypothermia) to provide for adequate tissue protection. The importance of this phase of the operation has grown as dissection from the segmental and subsegmental arteries has become technically feasible, making visualization of these more distal vessels possible.[27]

Published results have shown that the majority of patients undergoing PTE surgery experience both short- and long-term pulmonary hemodynamic improvement as a result of this operation. A decrease in the mean pulmonary artery pressure with augmentation in cardiac outcome is a consistent observation, although results vary between experienced centers.[17,28–32] In a report of the surgical outcomes in a series of 500 patients undergoing PTE between 2006 and 2010, Madani and colleagues[17] showed a reduction in pulmonary vascular resistance from a preoperative mean value of 719.0 ± 383.2 dyn/s/cm^{-5} to 253.4 ± 148.6 dyn/s/cm^{-5} postoperatively. The mean preoperative pulmonary artery pressure was 45.5 ± 11.6 mm Hg, decreasing to 26.0 ± 8.4 mm Hg after surgery, accompanied by an increase in cardiac output from 4.3 ± 1.4 L/min to 5.6 ± 1.4 L/min postoperatively.

Furthermore, mortality rates reported from centers performing PTE surgery have declined over the years, currently in the range of 2.2% to 11.4%[17,28–33]; the lower perioperative mortality figures are found at surgical centers with more extensive experience.[33] And as long-term data have become available, the hemodynamic and resultant functional status improvements are sustained in most patients, along with a favorable impact on long-term survivorship.[33–37]

Although endarterectomy surgery results in an entirely satisfactory outcome relating to pulmonary hemodynamics and functional status improvement, there are patients left with a degree of PH after surgery. Possible explanations for this postoperative outcome include residual chronic thromboembolic disease that could not be surgically resected, or a significant amount of coexisting distal vessel arteriopathy. The distinction between the 2 entities is important given the currently available targeted PH medical therapy as well as balloon pulmonary angioplasty. Difficulties reside in the varying definitions of residual PH between reporting centers and the paucity of long-term information available as to what level of residual PH negatively impacts functional status and survivorship. Over the past decades, estimates of postendarterectomy residual PH vary between 5% and 35% of operated patients, depending on the definition used, whether it is the standard PH definition of a mean pulmonary artery pressure of greater than 25 mm Hg, or an arbitrary pulmonary vascular resistance value.[34,36,38–40] A more comprehensive assessment of the prevalence and impact of residual

PH after surgery was reported by Cannon and colleagues[41] from the Papworth Group. In an analysis of 880 endarterectomy patients undergoing detailed hemodynamic assessment (right heart catheterization and noninvasive testing) at 3 to 6 months and annually after surgery as appropriate, this group found that only 28% of patients exhibited a mean pulmonary artery pressure of 20 mm Hg or less, whereas 51% had a mean pulmonary artery pressure of 25 mm Hg or greater measured by right heart catheterization at 3 to 6 months after PEA. One hundred eighty-seven patients were treated with PH targeted medical therapy during the period of follow-up (4.3 years); a mean pulmonary artery pressure of 30 mm Hg or greater correlated with initiation of pulmonary vasodilator therapy, whereas a mean pulmonary artery pressure of 38 mm Hg or greater and a pulmonary vascular resistance of 425 dyn/s/cm^{-5} or greater was associated with a survival disadvantage. Important to note that in this cohort there were only 2 cases of recurrent CTEPH.

One of the more significant advancements in the surgical approach to CTEPH over the past decade has been the achievement of successful endarterectomy of the distal pulmonary vascular bed to the level of the segmental and subsegmental vessels. Furthermore, the classification of surgical specimens has also been changed to more accurately reflect the vascular level at which an endarterectomy is initiated[2,27] (Fig. 2). In the initial report describing outcomes in this patient subgroup, D'Armini and colleagues[11] demonstrated a comparable decrease in pulmonary vascular resistance in the distal vessel endarterectomy group (n = 110) relative to the group undergoing more proximal endarterectomy (n = 221). The overall in-hospital mortality in this series was 6.9% (6.3% proximal, 8.1% distal), although 30% of the deaths were due to airway bleeding and 22% from persistent PH, without a reported difference in incidence between groups. The incidence of lung injury was not different between cohorts, and duration of mechanical ventilation and intensive care unit days was similar.

The early indications for PTE surgery focused on the treatment of patients with PH and right heart failure. As the experience in specialized CTEPH centers expands, the indications for surgical intervention has included those patients with symptomatic chronic thromboembolic disease without PH at rest. The proposed benefit of this intervention is to ameliorate dead space ventilation, retrieve pulmonary vascular reserve, and correct the pulmonary vascular response to exercise that is often demonstrated to be abnormal with carefully performed cardiopulmonary exercise

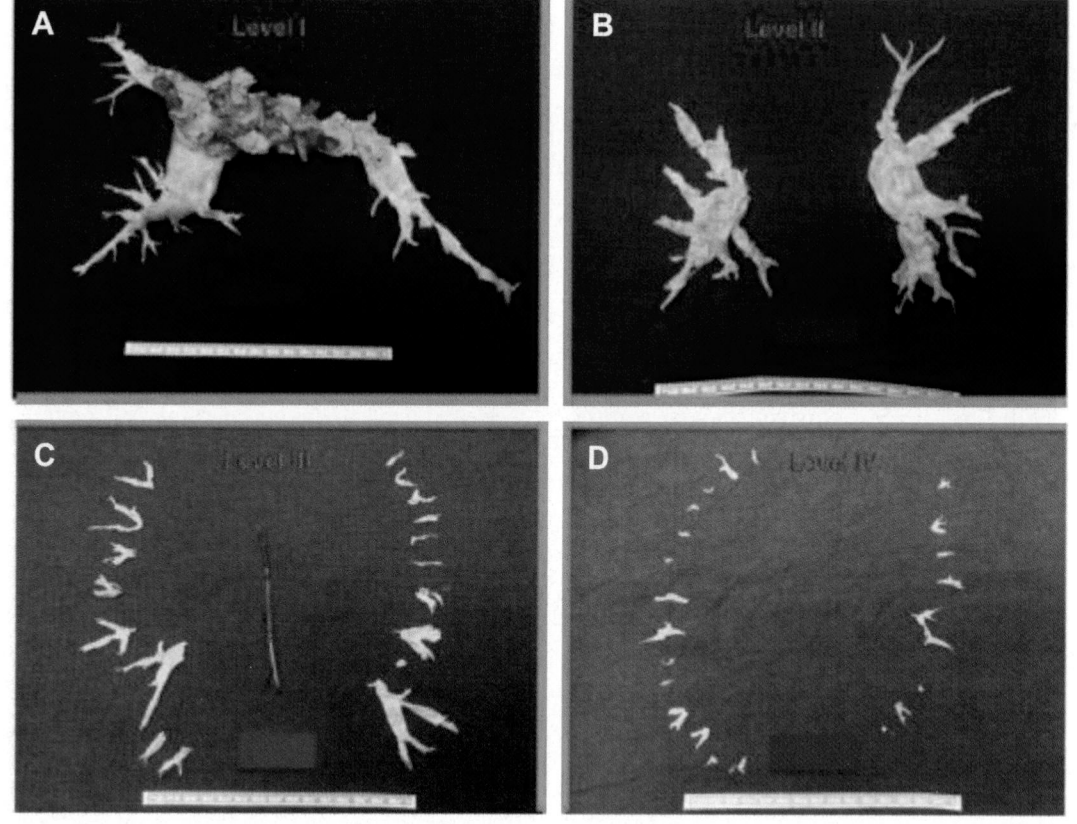

Fig. 2. University of California, San Diego, classification of PEA specimens. (*A*) Main pulmonary artery resection. (*B*) Lobar vessel resected material. (*C*) Segmental vessel resected material. (*D*) Subsegmental vessel resected material. (Reprinted with permission of the American Thoracic Society. Copyright © 2020 American Thoracic Society. Madani M, Mayer E, Fadel E, Jenkins DP. Jul 2016. Pulmonary Endarterectomy; Patient selection, Technical Challenges and Outcomes; Ann Am Thorac Soc Vol 13, Suppl 3; pp S240-S247. Annals of the American Thoracic Society is an official journal of the American Thoracic Society.)

studies.[42] Because the natural history of chronic thromboembolic disease is not fully understood, the prevention of CTEPH with early PEA surgery is only a theoretic consideration. A report from the Papworth Group of 42 patients with symptomatic chronic thromboembolic disease and a baseline mean pulmonary artery pressure of less than 25 mm Hg, PEA resulted in a significant improvement in functional status and quality of life. Although all survived to discharge, 17 patients (40%) experienced major complications from the endarterectomy consistent with the complex nature of this surgical intervention.[43]

Another group of patients with CTEPH that warrants discussion are those under consideration for a reoperative pulmonary thromboendarterectomy. Typically, these patients fall into 1 of 2 categories: either the first endarterectomy failed to remove what is demonstrably resectable chronic thromboembolic disease, or the patient has experienced recurrent CTEPH after a successful first PTE that

is again surgically amenable. Limited data as to patient selection and outcomes are available. A de novo evaluation as to intervention options is warranted to establish operability. If the basis for the patient's persistent symptoms and PH relates to inoperable chronic thromboembolic disease, PH-targeted medical therapy and/or balloon pulmonary angioplasty might be the best options. However, with recurrent operable CTEPH, 2 recent reports have shown that a second PTE can be efficacious,[44,45] although perhaps not to the same extent as that achieved with the initial endarterectomy.[45]

BALLOON PULMONARY ANGIOPLASTY

For a number of patients with CTEPH, endarterectomy surgery may not be feasible. Surgically inaccessible chronic thromboembolic disease, the presence of extensive comorbidities, or patient preference not to undergo PTE are among the primary reasons for not proceeding with PTE surgery. Over the past decade, balloon pulmonary angioplasty has evolved as a therapeutic option for the subgroup of patients with CTEPH. It is a percutaneous approach for the treatment of CTEPH relying on the use of telescoping catheters placed in a central vein, through which wires and balloons are guided to mechanically disrupt organized clot material and ameliorate the attendant pulmonary vascular obstruction (**Fig. 3**). The therapeutic intent is to decrease right ventricular afterload and thereby improve right ventricular function, to decrease pulmonary vascular resistance, and reperfuse lung parenchyma. Although this procedure was described as a potential treatment option for congenital pulmonary artery stenosis,[46] the first attempt in CTEPH, described in 1988, showed only marginal benefit.[47] A larger case series was reported in 2001 (18 patients with inoperable CTEPH), and although there were some favorable improvements in pulmonary hemodynamics, the rate and severity of complications, primarily reperfusion lung injury, slowed adoption of this intervention in this patient group.[48] However, beginning in 2012 as a result of a growing need for treatment options for patients with CTEPH, and with procedure refinements, several publications from medical centers in Japan and Norway demonstrated efficacy and a more favorable safety profile of balloon pulmonary angioplasty in those patients felt to have nonsurgical CTEPH.[49–53] With these early results, and with the potential to provide an effective treatment alternative or supplement to PH-targeted medical therapy, interest in and the

performance of balloon pulmonary angioplasty has rapidly expanded throughout the world, and has become a recognized treatment option for patients with surgically inoperable, distal vessel CTEPH (see **Fig. 1**).

Details of the procedure can be found in several of the Japanese publications and in recent reviews.[54–57] What is evident is that variation in the technical approach and patient selection is common among CTEPH centers performing balloon pulmonary angioplasty. Recent procedural descriptions and modifications of technique from that originally reported by several Japanese groups have been advocated to improve the safety profile of the procedure while at the same time maintaining efficacy. The observation has also been made by Brenot and colleagues[58] that, even within the same program, as experience expands, procedural safety and efficacy improves over time. Overall, there are some common guiding principles of the procedure. First, patient selection is critical to success. Not only is the determination that endarterectomy is not an option, but it is important to ensure that the type of chronic thrombotic lesions present is potentially amenable to angioplasty. Kawakami and colleagues[16] have characterized the vascular lesions that can be seen in distal vessel CTEPH (**Fig. 4**), and response to balloon pulmonary angioplasty varies among the lesions encountered. Ring-like stenoses and web lesions had the highest success rate with the lowest complication rates, whereas attempted angioplasty of total occlusion lesions was the least likely to be successful and the

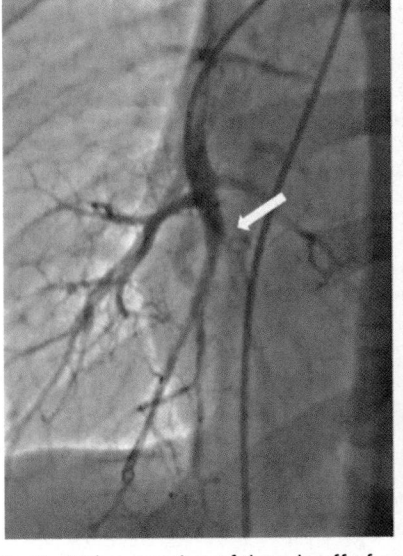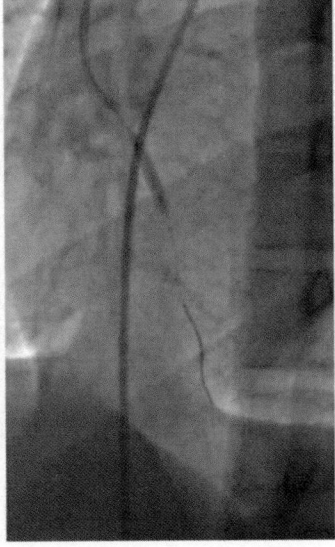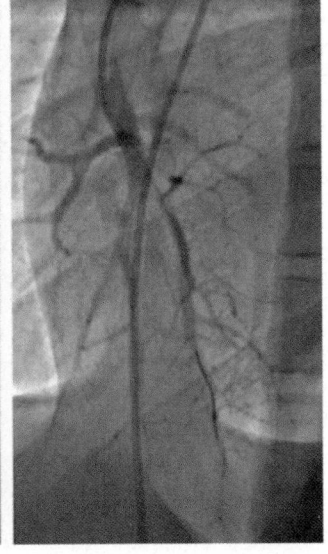

Fig. 3. Web narrowing of the takeoff of a segmental vessel leading to the right lower lobe from an organized clot (*arrow*). After balloon angioplasty, significant vessel opacification achieved with reperfusion of this lung segment.

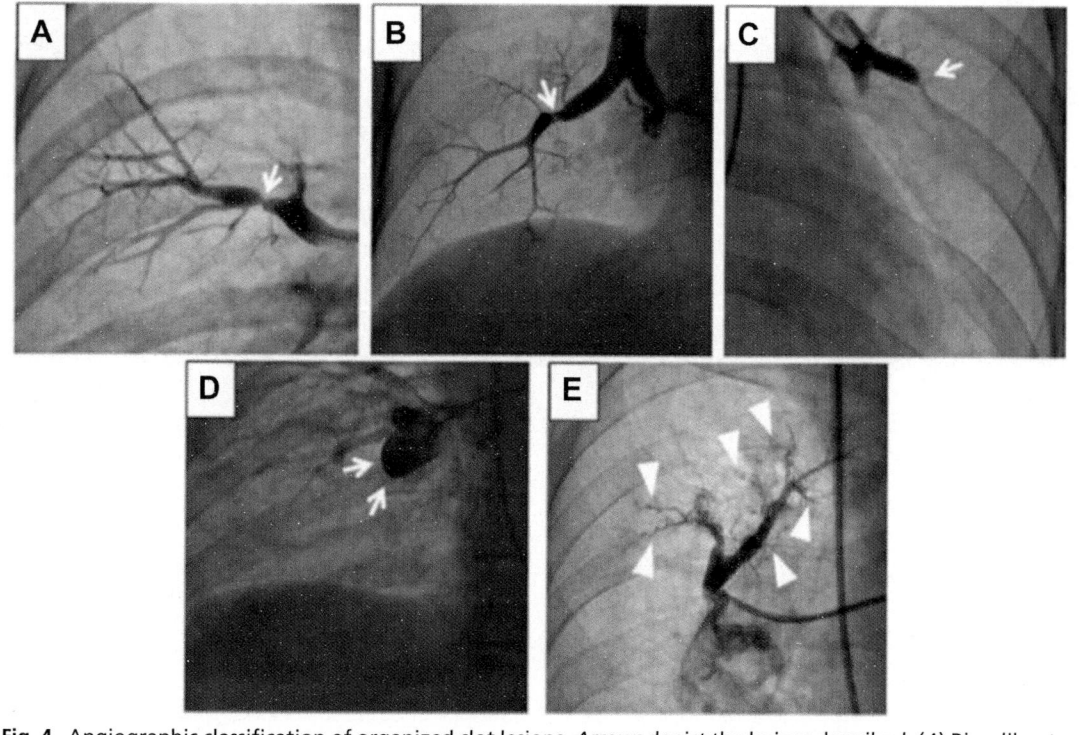

Fig. 4. Angiographic classification of organized clot lesions. *Arrows* depict the lesions described. (*A*) Ring-like stenosis lesion. (*B*) Web lesion. (*C*) Subtotal occlusion. (*D*) Total occlusion. (*E*) Tortuous lesion. Arrows point to the described lesions. (*From* Kawakami T, Ogawa A, Miyaji K, et al. Novel angiographic classification of each vascular lesion in chronic thromboembolic pulmonary hypertension based on selective angiogram and results of balloon pulmonary angioplasty. Cir Cardiovasc Interv 2016; with permission.)

manipulations of tortuous lesions was linked to a significant complication rate. Additionally, to achieve desired outcomes, balloon pulmonary angioplasty requires more than 1 interventional session. During each balloon pulmonary angioplasty session, attempts are made to maximize the number of segments treated while minimizing the risks of balloon pulmonary angioplasty-associated lung injury, noting that the improvement in the mean pulmonary artery pressure does not occur immediately after balloon pulmonary angioplasty.[50,59] Finally, patients with a higher mean pulmonary artery pressure (>35 mm Hg) before balloon pulmonary angioplasty and more severe PH may be at higher risk of balloon pulmonary angioplasty-associated lung injury.[50,53]

Following the encouraging reports from Japan, a number of CTEPH centers of excellence in Europe and North America have established balloon pulmonary angioplasty programs in response to the need to provide therapeutic options to patients with inoperable CTEPH. Despite differences in patient selection, differences in background use of PH-targeted therapies, and variations in the technical approach to balloon

pulmonary angioplasty, published series since 2012 have uniformly demonstrated substantial improvements in pulmonary hemodynamics, functional class, and markers of heart failure such as brain natriuretic peptide or *N*-terminal pro b-type natriuretic peptide. In a retrospective review of 308 patients (1408 sessions) enrolled in a multicenter Japanese registry (7 enrolling centers), Ogawa and colleagues[12] showed a decrease in the mean pulmonary artery pressure from 43.2 ± 11.0 to 24.3 ± 6.4 after final balloon pulmonary angioplasty, to 22.5 ± 5.4 at follow-up (n = 196). Accompanying this was a significant improvement in World Health Organization functional class, along with a decrease in PH-targeted medical therapy use (72.1% on at least 1 PH medication pre-balloon pulmonary angioplasty to 44.9% at follow-up) and supplemental oxygen (73.7% before balloon pulmonary angioplasty to 21.9% at follow-up). The overall survival was 96.8%, 96.8%, and 94.5% at 1, 2, and 3 years, respectively, after the initial balloon pulmonary angioplasty procedure for the 308 patients. Other high-volume balloon pulmonary angioplasty centers in Europe have recently reported similar

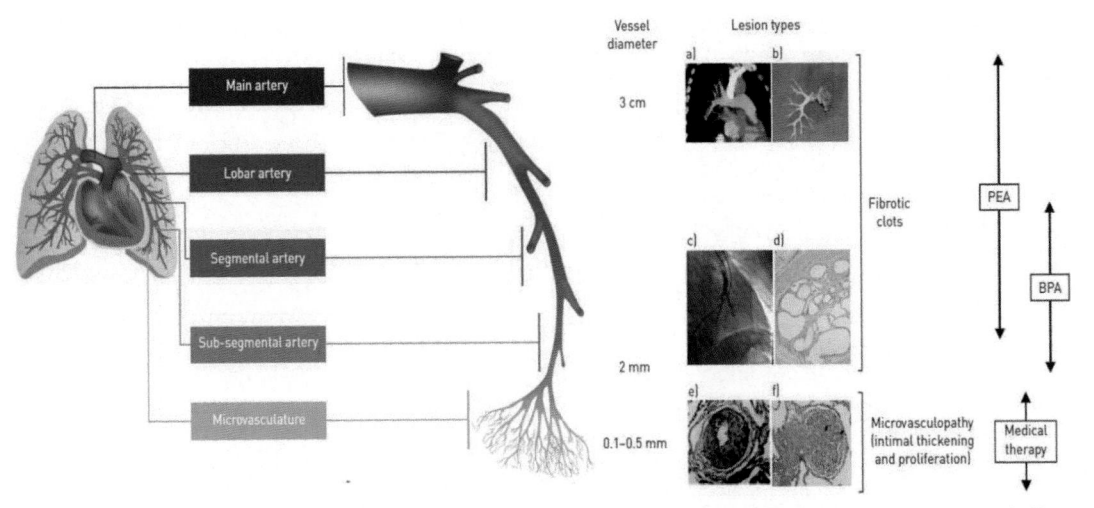

Fig. 5. Management options based on vascular level involved with chronic thromboembolic disease. BPA, balloon pulmonary angioplasty. (*From* Madani M, Ogo T, Simonneau G. The changing landscape of chronic thromboembolic pulmonary hypertension. Eur Respir Rev 2017. Reproduced with permission of the © ERS 2020: European Respiratory Review 26 (146) 170105; DOI: 10.1183/16000617.0105-2017 Published 20 December 2017.)

improvements in the short term, though not to the same extent hemodynamically as that seen above.[58,60]

Based on recent reports, the safety of balloon pulmonary angioplasty has improved from the first series reported in 2001. The rates of severe balloon pulmonary angioplasty-associated lung injury that required major interventions such as noninvasive ventilation and mechanical ventilation decreased from 16.7% in the initial series by Feinstein and colleagues[48] in 2001 to 6% in the large series by Mizoguchi and colleagues[49] in 2012. With technique changes and experience, much of the currently reported difficulties center on vascular injury and hemoptysis, with decreasing lung injury rates. In the Japanese Registry spanning the time period between 2004 and 2013, pulmonary injury was observed in 17.8% of patients, with pulmonary vascular injury in 3.4% and hemoptysis in 14.0%. Noted was the decrease in lung injury with experience and procedure modification.[12] Olsson and colleagues[60] in their series of 56 patients (266 balloon pulmonary angioplasty sessions) noted 25 procedure-related complications, mostly self-limited pulmonary vascular injury and hemoptysis, and only 1 fatal pulmonary hemorrhage. For the French group, procedure-related complications occurred in 113 of 1006 sessions, including lung injury (9.1% of all sessions), hemoptysis (7.1%), pulmonary artery perforation (2.8%), and pulmonary artery dissection (1.9%). Dividing their experience into initial and recent periods, Brenot and colleagues[58] were able to

demonstrate a decrease in severe lung injury rates from 10.4% to 1.8%.

The emergence of balloon pulmonary angioplasty has resulted in a new therapeutic option for patients with CTEPH. Ongoing challenges remain, however. Long-term efficacy is slowly being established[61] and, despite the advances in procedural techniques, there remains a standardized approach that is globally accepted and has been shown to minimize complications while optimizing results. Additionally, patient selection is not uniform and subjective, and patient phenotypes that will benefit the most from balloon pulmonary angioplasty have been difficult to define. Other issues such as the long-term consequences of radiation exposure and defining limits for the number of sessions that can safely be performed, the interplay between the use of PH-targeted medical therapy and balloon pulmonary angioplasty,[62] the role of combining PEA surgery and balloon pulmonary angioplasty for select patients with CTEPH and the sequencing of this approach,[63] and the proposed use of balloon pulmonary angioplasty in those patients with symptomatic chronic thromboembolic disease require careful scrutiny.[64]

SUMMARY

The treatment of CTEPH has expanded considerably over the past decade. The ability to endarterectomize chronic thromboembolic material from the distal pulmonary vascular bed, the availability of PH medical therapy to treat those patients with inoperable CTEPH and/or residual PH after PTE surgery, and the rebirth of pulmonary balloon angioplasty for nonsurgical patients with CTEPH have changed the management landscape for this unique patient population.[65] Although there are evident advantages to patient care with the increasing breadth of available therapies, the selection of patients who will optimally benefit from each of these interventions requires a multidisciplinary evaluation at a center experienced in CTEPH management. As shown in **Fig. 5**, the selection of surgical or catheter-based interventions to manage the pulmonary vascular obstructive component from chronic thromboembolic disease is not only a reflection of the experience of the cardiothoracic surgeons and interventional team at a specialized center, but also the capabilities of the diagnosticians to accurate assess the vascular level of disease. Simply stated, what is inoperable CTEPH to 1 group may be operable CTEPH to another. The ultimate challenge then becomes which intervention provides the optimal long-term outcome for any individual patient.

REFERENCES

1. Jenkins DP, Madani M, Mayer E, et al. Surgical treatment of chronic thromboembolic pulmonary hypertension. Eur Respir J 2013;41:735–42.
2. Kim NH, Delcroix M, Jais X, et al. Chronic thromboembolic pulmonary hypertension. Eur Respir J 2019; 53:1801915.
3. Fernandes TM, Auger WR, Fedullo PF. Epidemiology and risk factors for chronic thromboembolic pulmonary hypertension. Thromb Res 2018;164: 145–9.
4. Gall H, Hoeper MM, Richter MJ, et al. An epidemiological analysis of the burden of chronic thromboembolic pulmonary hypertension in the USA, Europe and Japan. Eur Respir Rev 2017;26:160121.
5. Klok FA, Dzikowska-Diduch O, Kostrubiec M, et al. Derivation of a clinical prediction score for chronic thromboembolic pulmonary hypertension after acute pulmonary embolism. J Thromb Haemost 2016; 14(1):121–8.
6. de Perrot M, Fadel E, McRae K, et al. Evaluation of persistent pulmonary hypertension after acute pulmonary embolism. Chest 2007;132(3):780–5.
7. Galiè N, Humbert M, Vachiery J-L, et al. 2015 ESC/ERS guidelines for the diagnosis and treatment of pulmonary hypertension. Eur Heart J 2016;37: 67–119.
8. Gopalan D, Delcroix M, Held M. Diagnosis of chronic thromboembolic pulmonary hypertension. Eur Respir Rev 2017;26:160108.
9. Auger WR, Fedullo PF, Moser KM, et al. Chronic major-vessel thromboembolic pulmonary artery

10. Rogberg AN, Gopalan D, Westerlund E, et al. Do radiologist detect chronic thromboembolic disease on computed tomography? Acta Radiol 2019; 60(11):1576–83.
11. D'Armini AM, Morsolini M, Mattiucci G, et al. Pulmonary endarterectomy for distal chronic thromboembolic pulmonary hypertension. J Thorac Cardiovasc Surg 2014;148:1005–12.
12. Ogawa A, Satoh T, Fukuda T, et al. Balloon pulmonary angioplasty for chronic thromboembolic pulmonary hypertension. Results of a multicenter registry. Circ Cardiovasc Qual Outcomes 2017;10: e004029.
13. Renapurkar RD, Bolen MA, Shrikanthan S, et al. Comparative assessment of qualitative and quantitative perfusion with dual-energy CT and planar and SPECT-CT V/Q scanning in patients with chronic thromboembolic pulmonary hypertension. Cardiovasc Diagn Ther 2018;8(4):414–22.
14. Dournes G, Verdier D, Montaudon M, et al. Dual-energy CT perfusion and angiography in chronic thromboembolic pulmonary hypertension: diagnostic accuracy and concordance with radionuclide scintigraphy. Eur Radiol 2014;24(1):42–51.
15. Sugimura K, Fukumoto Y, M13iura Y, et al. Three-dimensional-optical coherence tomography imaging of chronic thromboembolic pulmonary hypertension. Eur Heart J 2013;34(28):2121.
16. Kawakami T, Ogawa A, Miyaji K, et al. Novel angiographic classification of each vascular lesion in chronic thromboembolic pulmonary hypertension based on selective angiogram and results of balloon pulmonary angioplasty. Circ Cardiovasc Interv 2016; 9:e003318.
17. Madani MM, Auger WR, Pretorius V, et al. Pulmonary endarterectomy: recent changes in a single institution's experience of more than 2,700 patients. Ann Thorac Surg 2012;94:97–103.
18. De Perrot M, Thenganatt J, McRae K, et al. Pulmonary endarterectomy in severe chronic thromboembolic pulmonary hypertension. J Heart Lung Transplant 2015;34:369–75.
19. Toshner M, Suntharalingam J, Fesler P, et al. Occlusion pressure analysis role in partitioning of pulmonary vascular resistance in CTEPH. Eur Respir J 2012;40:612–7.
20. Tanabe N, Okada O, Abe Y, et al. The influence of fractional pulse pressure on the outcome of pulmonary thromboendarterectomy. Eur Respir J 2001;17:653–9.
21. Madani MM, Wittine LM, Auger WR, et al. Chronic thromboembolic pulmonary hypertension in pediatric patients. J Thorac Cardiovasc Surg 2011; 141(3):624–30.
22. Fernandes TM, Auger WR, Fedullo PF, et al. Baseline body mass index does not significantly affect

outcomes after pulmonary thromboendarterectomy. Ann Thorac Surg 2014;98:1776–81.

23. Berman M, Hardman G, Sharples L, et al. Pulmonary endarterectomy: outcomes in patients > 70. Eur J Cardiothorac Surg 2012;41:e154–60.

24. Balakrishman M, Besser M, Ravaglioli A, et al. Pulmonary endarterectomy is effective and safe in patients with haemoglobinopathies and abnormal red blood cells: the Papworth experience. Eur J Cardiothorac Surg 2016;50(3):537–41.

25. Ng O, Giménez-Milà M, Jenkins DP, et al. Perioperative management of pulmonary endarterectomy – perspective from the UK National Health Service. J Cardiothorac Vasc Anesth 2019;33:3101–9.

26. Thistlethwaite PA, Auger WR, Madani MM, et al. Pulmonary thromboendarterectomy combined with other cardiac operations: indications, surgical approach, and outcome. Ann Thorac Surg 2001; 72:13–9.

27. Madani M, Mayer E, Fadel E, et al. Pulmonary endarterectomy: patient selection, technical challenges, and outcomes. Ann Am Thorac Soc 2016;13(Suppl 3):S240–7.

28. Mayer E, Jenkins D, Lindner J, et al. Surgical management and outcome of patients with chronic thromboembolic pulmonary hypertension: results from an international prospective registry. J Thorac Cardiovasc Surg 2011;141:702–10.

29. Ogino H, Ando M, Matsuda H, et al. Japanese single-center experience of surgery for chronic thromboembolic pulmonary hypertension. Ann Thorac Surg 2006;82:630–6.

30. de Perrot M, McRae K, Shargall Y, et al. Pulmonary thromboendarterectomy for chronic thromboembolic pulmonary hypertension: the Toronto experience. Can J Cardiol 2011;27:692–7.

31. Maliyasena VA, Hopkins PMA, Thomson BM, et al. An Australian tertiary referral center experience of the management of chronic thromboembolic pulmonary hypertension. Pulm Circ 2012;2:359–64.

32. Raza F, Vaidya A, Lacharite-Roberge AS, et al. Initial clinical and hemodynamic results of a regional pulmonary thromboendarterectomy program. J Cardiovasc Surg (Torino) 2018;59(3):428–37.

33. Delcroix M, Lang I, Pepke-Zaba J, et al. Long-term outcome of patients with chronic thromboembolic pulmonary hypertension. Results from an International Prospective Registry. Circulation 2016;133: 859–71.

34. Condliffe R, Kiely DG, Gibbs JS, et al. Improved outcomes in medically and surgically treated chronic thromboembolic pulmonary hypertension. Am J Respir Crit Care Med 2008;177:1122–7.

35. Freed DH, Thomson BM, Tsui SSL, et al. Functional and haemodynamic outcome 1 year after pulmonary thromboendarterectomy. Eur J Cardiothorac Surg 2008;34:525–30.

36. Corsico AG, D'Armini AM, Cerveri I, et al. Long-term outcome after pulmonary thromboendarterectomy. Am J Respir Crit Care Med 2008;178:419–24.

37. Ishida K, Masuda M, Tanabe N, et al. Long-term outcome after pulmonary endarterectomy for chronic thromboembolic pulmonary hypertension. J Thorac Cardiovasc Surg 2012;144:321–6.

38. Bonderman D, Skoro-Sajer N, Jakowitsch J, et al. Predictors of outcome in chronic thromboembolic pulmonary hypertension. Circulation 2007;115: 2153–8.

39. Thistlethwaite PA, Kemp A, Du L, et al. Outcomes of pulmonary thromboendarterectomy for treatment of extreme thromboembolic pulmonary hypertension. J Thorac Cardiovasc Surg 2006;1 31:307–13.

40. Freed DH, Thomson BM, Berman M, et al. Survival after pulmonary thromboendarterectomy: effect of residual pulmonary hypertension. J Thorac Cardiovasc Surg 2011;141:383–7.

41. Cannon JE, Su L, Kiely DG, et al. Dynamic risk stratification of patient long-term outcome after pulmonary endarterectomy. Results from the United Kingdom National Cohort. Circulation 2016;133: 1761–71.

42. van Kan C, van der Plas MN, Reesink HJ, et al. Hemodynamic and ventilatory response during exercise in chronic thromboembolic disease. J Thorac Cardiovasc Surg 2016;152:763–71.

43. Taboada D, Pepke-Zaba J, Jenkins DP, et al. Outcome of pulmonary endarterectomy in symptomatic chronic thromboembolic disease. Eur Respir J 2014;44:1635–45.

44. Ali JM, Dunning J, Ng C, et al. The outcome of reoperative pulmonary endarterectomy surgery. Interact Cardiovasc Thorac Surg 2018;26:932–7.

45. Merli VN, Vistarini N, Grazioli V, et al. Pavia experience in reoperative pulmonary endarterectomy. Semin Thorac Cardiovasc Surg 2017;29:464–8.

46. Gentles TL, Lock JE, Perry SB. High pressure balloon angioplasty for branch pulmonary artery stenosis: early experience. J Am Coll Cardiol 1993; 22(3):867–72.

47. Voorburg JAI, Manger Cats V, Buis B, et al. Balloon angioplasty in the treatment of pulmonary hypertension caused by pulmonary embolism. Chest 1988; 94:1249–53.

48. Feinstein JA, Goldhaber SZ, Lock JE, et al. Balloon pulmonary angioplasty for treatment of chronic thromboembolic pulmonary hypertension. Circulation 2001;103:10–3.

49. Mizoguchi H, Ogawa A, Munemasa M, et al. Refined balloon pulmonary angioplasty for inoperable patients with chronic thromboembolic pulmonary hypertension. Circ Cardiovasc Interv 2012;5:748–55.

50. Katoaka M, Inami T, Hayashida K, et al. Percutaneous transluminal pulmonary angioplasty for the treatment of chronic thromboembolic pulmonary

hypertension. Circ Cardiovasc Interv 2012;5: 756–62.

51. Sugimura K, Fukumoto Y, Satoh K, et al. Percutaneous transluminal pulmonary angioplasty markedly improves pulmonary hemodynamics and long-term prognosis in patients with chronic thromboembolic pulmonary hypertension. Circ J 2012;76:485–8.

52. Andreassen AK, Ragnarsson A, Gude E, et al. Balloon pulmonary angioplasty in patients with inoperable chronic thromboembolic pulmonary hypertension. Heart 2013;99:1415–20.

53. Inami T, Kataoka M, Shimura N, et al. Pulmonary edema predictive scoring index (PEPSI), a new index to predict risk of reperfusion pulmonary edema and improvement of hemodynamics in percutaneous transluminal pulmonary angioplasty. JACC Cardiovasc Interv 2013;7:725–36.

54. Roik M, Wretowski D, Labyk A, et al. Refined balloon pulmonary angioplasty driven by combined assessment of intra-arterial anatomy and physiology-multimodal approach to treated lesions in patients with non-operable distal chronic thromboembolic pulmonary hypertension-technique, safety and efficacy of 50 consecutive angioplasties. Int J Cardiol 2016;203:228–35.

55. Rivers-Bowerman MD, Zener R, Jaberi A, et al. Balloon pulmonary angioplasty in chronic thromboembolic pulmonary hypertension: new horizons in the interventional management of pulmonary embolism. Tech Vasc Interv Radiol 2017;20:206–15.

56. Mahmud E, Behnamfar O, Ang L, et al. Balloon pulmonary angioplasty for chronic thromboembolic pulmonary hypertension. Interv Cardiol Clin 2018;7: 103–17.

57. Lang I, Meyer BC, Ogo T, et al. Balloon pulmonary angioplasty in chronic thromboembolic pulmonary hypertension. Eur Respir Rev 2017;26:160119.

58. Brenot P, Jais X, Taniguchi Y, et al. French experience of balloon pulmonary angioplasty for chronic thromboembolic pulmonary hypertension. Eur Respir J 2019;53:1802095.

59. Hosokawa K, Abe K, Oi K, et al. Negative acute hemodynamic response to balloon pulmonary angioplasty does not predicate the long-term outcome in patients with chronic thromboembolic pulmonary hypertension. Int J Cardiol 2015;188:81–3.

60. Olsson KM, Wiedenroth CB, Kamp J-C, et al. Balloon pulmonary angioplasty for inoperable patients with chronic thromboembolic pulmonary hypertension: the initial German experience. Eur Respir J 2017;49(6) [pii:1602409].

61. Aoki T, Sugimura K, Tatebe S, et al. Comprehensive evaluation of the effectiveness and safety of balloon pulmonary angioplasty for inoperable chronic thrombo-embolic pulmonary hypertension: long-term effects and procedure-related complications. Eur Heart J 2017;38:3152–9.

62. Wiedenroth CB, Ghofrani HA, Adameit MSD, et al. Sequential treatment with riociquat and balloon pulmonary angioplasty for patients with inoperable chronic thromboembolic pulmonary hypertension. Pulm Circ 2018;8(3):1–7.

63. Wiedenroth CB, Liebetrau C, Breithecker A, et al. Combined pulmonary endarterectomy and balloon pulmonary angioplasty in patients with chronic thromboembolic pulmonary hypertension. J Heart Lung Transplant 2016;35:591–6.

64. Wiedenroth CB, Olsson KM, Guth S, et al. Balloon pulmonary angioplasty for inoperable patients with chronic thromboembolic disease. Pulm Circ 2018; 8(1):1–6.

65. Madani M, Ogo T, Simonneau G. The changing landscape of chronic thromboembolic pulmonary hypertension. Eur Respir Rev 2017;26:170105.

Pulmonary Hypertension and Right Ventricular Failure
Lung Transplant Versus Heart-Lung Transplant

Jessica H. Huston, MD[a],*, Evan L. Brittain, MD, MSc[b], Ivan M. Robbins, MD[c]

KEYWORDS

- Lung transplant • Pulmonary arterial hypertension • Right ventricular failure • Heart-lung transplant

KEY POINTS

- Pulmonary arterial hypertension has limited therapeutic options that improve survival, transplantation is 1 option.
- Right ventricular failure improves after lung transplantation; however, postoperative management of fluid and hemodynamic shifts can be complex, especially with regard to left ventricular diastolic dysfunction.
- Heart-lung dual organ transplant should be reserved for patients with complex congenital heart disease or severe left ventricular systolic function.

Pulmonary hypertension can occur as a disorder primarily affecting the pulmonary arteries, or as a result of other disorders affecting the heart, postcapillary vasculature, or lung parenchyma. The most recent classification of pulmonary hypertension, from the 2018 World Health Symposium, defines 5 major groups, including pulmonary arterial hypertension (PAH), group 1 PH, defined as idiopathic or in association with other disorders, such as connective tissue disease or congenital heart disease (CHD), and pulmonary venous hypertension, group 2 PH, due to left ventricular (LV) systolic or diastolic dysfunction, left-sided valvular disease, or disorders affecting the pulmonary veins (**Box 1**).[1] PAH is a morbid disease with few, sustained effective therapeutic options and a high mortality even with advanced therapy.[2] Treatment includes oral, inhaled, continuous subcutaneous, and intravenous medications. Intravenous epoprostenol is the only medication that has been shown to improve mortality in group 1 PAH.[3] There are several diseases in which patients may develop associated precapillary pulmonary hypertension, such as sarcoidosis, idiopathic pulmonary fibrosis, and other parenchymal lung diseases; however, in this review we focus on patients with PAH, predominantly idiopathic or in association with CHD, and right ventricular (RV) failure, as these are the primary patients considered for lung or heart-lung transplant (HLT).

The decision to refer a patient with PAH for transplant evaluation is often made when, despite treatment with maximal medical therapies, the patient's functional status continues to decline as a result of progressive RV dysfunction. The

[a] Division of Cardiovascular Medicine, Department of Medicine, Vanderbilt University Medical Center, 1215 21st Avenue South, Suite 5037, Nashville, TN 37232, USA; [b] Division of Cardiovascular Medicine, Department of Medicine, Vanderbilt University Medical Center, 2525 West End Avenue, Suite 300A, Nashville, TN 37203, USA; [c] Division of Allergy, Pulmonary, and Critical Care Medicine, Vanderbilt University Medical Center, 1161 21st Avenue South, T1218 MCN, Nashville, TN, USA
* Corresponding author.
E-mail address: Jessica.h.huston@vumc.org

Cardiol Clin 38 (2020) 269–281
https://doi.org/10.1016/j.ccl.2020.01.002
0733-8651/20/© 2020 Elsevier Inc. All rights reserved.

1. PAH

    1.1 Idiopathic PAH

    1.2 Heritable PAH

    1.3 Drug-induced and toxin-induced PAH

    1.4 PAH associated with:

    1.4.1 Connective tissue disease

    1.4.2 HIV infection

    1.4.3 Portal hypertension

    1.4.4 Congenital heart disease

    1.4.5 Schistosomiasis

    1.5 PAH long-term responders to calcium channel blockers

    1.6 PAH with overt features of venous/capillaries (PVOD/PCH) involvement

    1.7 Persistent PH of the newborn syndrome

2. PH due to left heart disease

    2.1 PH due to heart failure with preserved LVEF

    2.2 PH due to heart failure with reduced LVEF

    2.3 Valvular heart disease

    2.4 Congenital/acquired cardiovascular conditions leading to postcapillary PH

3. PH due to lung disease and/or hypoxia

    3.1 Obstructive lung disease

    3.2 Restrictive lung disease

    3.3 Other lung disease with mixed restrictive/obstructive pattern

    3.4 Hypoxia without lung disease

    3.5 Developmental lung disorders

4. PH due to pulmonary artery obstructions

    4.1 Chronic thromboembolic PH

    4.2 Other pulmonary artery obstructions

5. PH with unclear and/or multifactorial mechanisms

    5.1 Hematological disorders

    5.2 Systemic and metabolic disorders

    5.3 Others

    5.4 Complex congenital heart disease

Abbreviations: LVEF, left ventricular ejection fraction; PAH, pulmonary arterial hypertension; PCH, pulmonary capillary hemangiomatosis; PH, pulmonary hypertension; PVOD, pulmonary veno-occlusive disease.
From Simonneau G, Montani D, Celermajer DS, et al. Haemodynamic definitions and updated clinical classification of pulmonary hypertension. Eur Respir J. 2019. Reproduced with permission of the © ERS 2020: European Respiratory Journal 53 (1) 1801913; DOI: 10.1183/13993003.01913-2018. Published 24 January 2019.

International Society for Heart and Lung Transplantation (ISHLT) guidelines for timing of referral advises that patients with New York Heart Association (NYHA) class III to IV symptoms and progressive disease despite optimal therapy should be considered for transplant.[4] The timing of transplantation should be based on clinical factors, including NYHA class while on maximal medical therapy, low or declining 6-minute walk distance, failure of parenteral therapy, cardiac index less than 2 L/min/m^2, and right atrial pressure greater than 15 mm Hg.[4] Here, we discuss key considerations in the evaluation of potential transplant candidates, including assessment of cardiac function, degree of RV and RV dysfunction, and differences between lung transplantation (LT) and HLT outcomes for this population.

RIGHT VENTRICULAR REMODELING AND FUNCTION

In contrast to the systemic vascular bed, the pulmonary vasculature is a low-resistance system with an RV that is more compliant than the left ventricle. Normally, mean pulmonary artery pressure (mPAP) is less than 20 mm Hg and pulmonary vascular resistance (PVR) is less than 3 Wood units.[1,5] In severe PAH, mPAP is frequently 60 mm Hg or greater and PVR is often greater than 10 Wood units. Early in the course of the disease, PAH is associated with RV pressure overload with volume overload developing as the resistance to pulmonary blood flow increases and RV function worsens. As a response, the RV remodels to compensate and accommodate the raised PVR (**Fig. 1**). Structural and functional changes in the RV due to adverse remodeling have therapeutic and prognostic importance in the PAH population. Both hemodynamic and echocardiographic RV dysfunction are associated with worse survival.[6,7] In patients with raised PVR the RV is the limiting component in functional capacity.[8] As the arterial resistance increases, the right ventricle is unable to proportionately increase contractility, leading to heart failure.[9,10] The initial response of the RV to increase in pulmonary pressures is predominantly hypertrophy, as an adaptive response to increased afterload and to maintain cardiac output without increasing wall stress.[11,12] RV hypertrophy and associated RV diastolic dysfunction also can cause subclinical RV dysfunction in this PAH population, although often not evaluated or discussed clinically.[13,14] Adaptive remodeling in the RV often manifests as concentric hypertrophy; however, with progression of RV-pulmonary arterial uncoupling maladaptive remodeling is seen when the RV is unable to adequately handle the afterload and

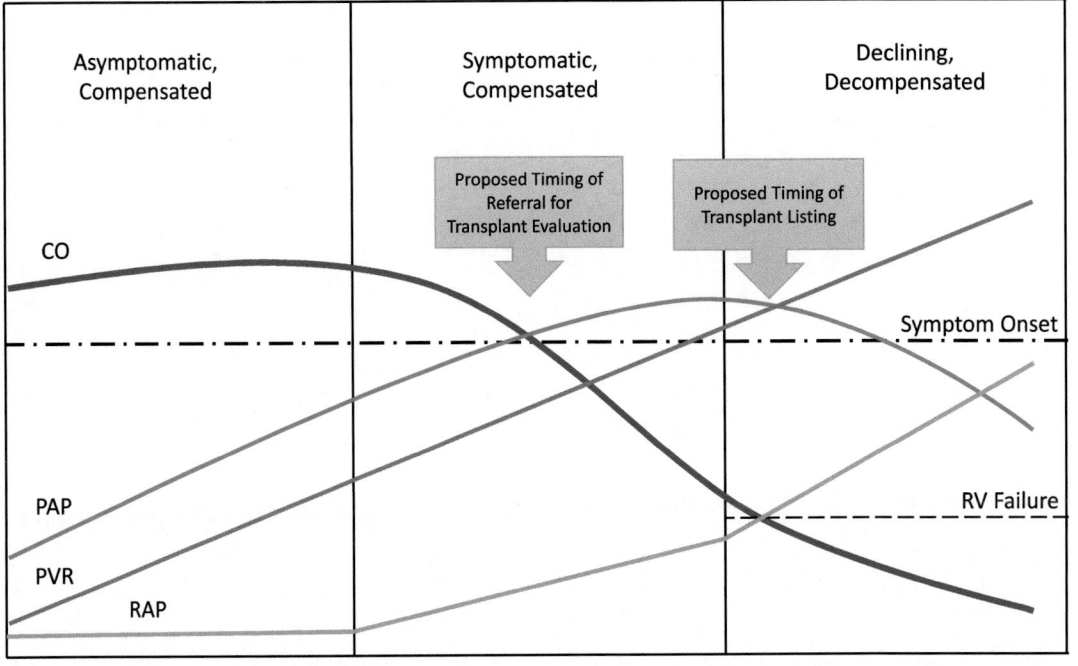

Fig. 1. The progression of pulmonary hypertension and right heart failure with proposed timing of transplant evaluation and listing. CO, cardiac output; PAP, pulmonary artery pressure; PVR, pulmonary vascular resistance; RAP, right atrial pressure; RV, right ventricle.

maintain cardiac output. Patients with PAH have higher RV mass, larger volume, and lower RV ejection fraction (EF) when compared with healthy controls.[15] In patients with PAH with a mismatch of mass to volume, RV mass/volume ratio $\leq$0.46, RV filling pressures were higher and cardiac index was reduced compared with healthy controls.[15] When myocardial wall stress in the RV, defined as (pressure × radius)/thickness, exceeds the adaptive remodeling ability, right heart failure and functional decline occur. Increased RV wall stress may drive myofibroblast proliferation and myocardial fibrosis, which is thought to have an adaptive role in reduction of RV dilatation and prevention of overstretching the myocytes. These structural alterations also lead to impairments in diastolic function and myocardial contraction.[16,17] Increased myocardial collagen deposition by myofibroblasts activates matrix metalloproteases and tissue inhibitors of metalloproteases, setting off a cascade of collagen turnover and extracellular membrane (ECM) remodeling leading to abnormal myocardial tissue structure.[18] Histologic assessments of the degree of RV fibrosis have been derived from RV biopsies in posttransplant or postmortem examinations; however, obtaining RV tissue in patients with PAH for clinical assessment of myocardial remodeling is rare and not part of routine clinical diagnostics. The challenge in differentiating adaptive versus maladaptive remodeling and fibrosis is that

it occurs on a continuum, without a clear threshold between the two. Despite hemodynamic and structural changes, the RV still has significant plasticity and the ability to recover from injury, although there currently are no accurate and reliable measures exist to determine RV reserve or capacity to recover.[19]

IMAGING MODALITIES

Assessment of both RV and LV function are essential to the pretransplant evaluation PAH. The primary noninvasive modalities used are echocardiography and MRI, both of which have benefits and limitations.

Echocardiography

In patients with PAH, multiple 2-dimensional measurements can be used to assess the RV (**Fig. 2**). Diastolic wall thickness greater than 5 mm and basal RV end diastolic diameter greater than 4.2 cm suggests pressure effects on the RV even without overt evidence of dysfunction.[20] The measurement of RV diameter can be significantly impacted by probe position and foreshortening, which often occurs due to the retrosternal location of the RV.[20,21] The RV is difficult to image in 2 dimensions due to the crescentic shape, bellows-like contraction, and dependence on the interventricular septum for

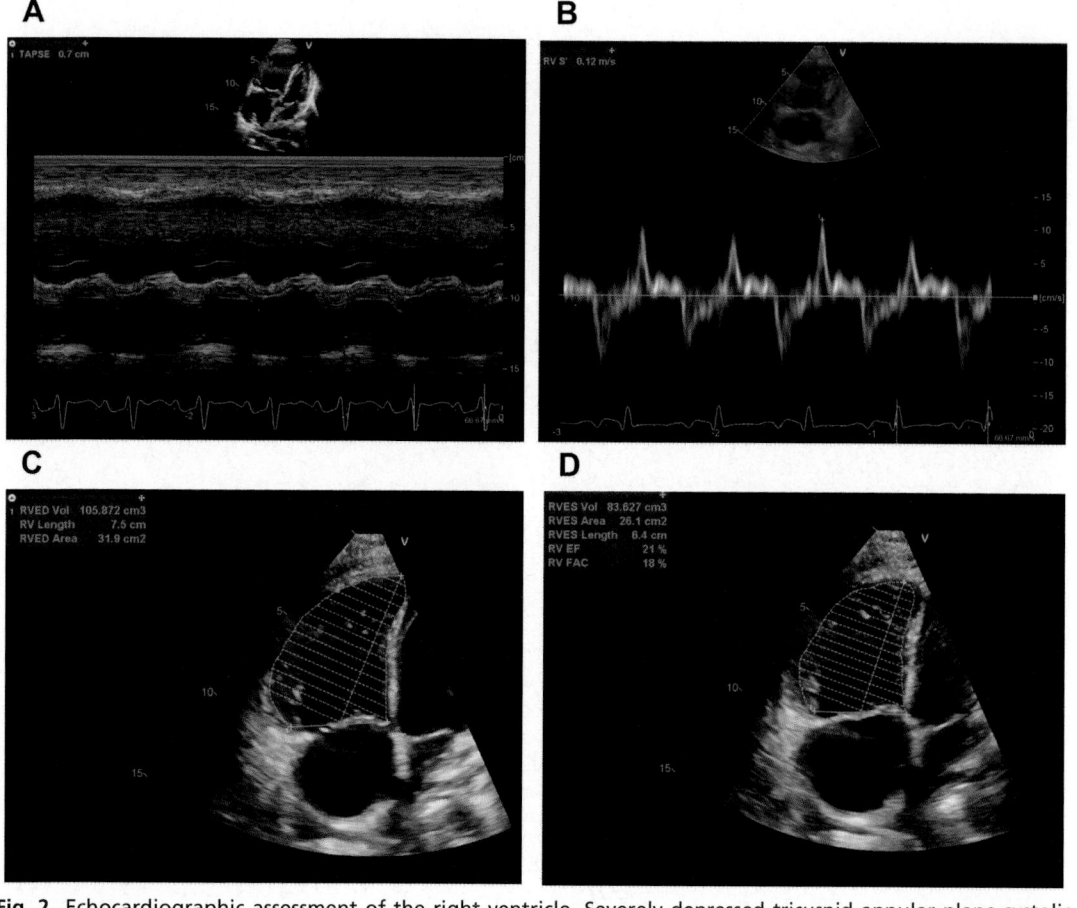

Fig. 2. Echocardiographic assessment of the right ventricle. Severely depressed tricuspid annular plane systolic excursion (*A*) (0.7 cm) in a patient with PAH. Tissue Doppler of the lateral tricuspid annulus showing a normal S′ value (*B*) (0.12 m/s). The RVFAC is calculated by the RV end diastolic area (*C*) minus the RV end systolic area (*D*), divided by the RV end diastolic area, multiplied by 100 (*D*) (RVFAC 18%). FAC, fractional area of change; PAH, pulmonary arterial hypertension; RV, right ventricular.

a large portion of systolic function.[22] Identifying the RV borders in a hypertrophied, dilated RV can also be difficult and make assessment of systolic function challenging.[23]

The initial imaging test for patients with suspected PAH is echocardiography to provide an estimation of RV systolic pressure (RVSP) using tricuspid regurgitant velocity.[20] In patients with known PAH, longitudinal imaging of the right ventricle is important in monitoring disease progression, where a reduction in echocardiographic estimated RVSP and worsening RV function should prompt concern for the inability of the RV to generate the previous degree of pressure and incipient RV failure. Conversely, reduction in estimated RVSP with preservation of RV function over time would suggest therapeutic response and improved prognosis.[24] Despite reliance on estimated RVSP, the measure is fraught with issues, such as the amplification of small degrees of error because

tricuspid regurgitant velocity is squared and multiplied by 4 then added to an estimated right atrial pressure to get the RVSP.[20] Echocardiographically measurable tricuspid regurgitant jets are absent in 47% of patients with pulmonary hypertension by right heart catheterizations and estimated right atrial pressure by echocardiography is known to be variable and unreliable.[25,26]

Most RV contractility and stroke volume is derived from longitudinal shortening as opposed to LV contractility, which arises predominantly from transverse shortening.[27] Improvement in RV contraction after initiation of PAH-specific therapy is seen primarily as improvement in longitudinal contraction, suggesting that this element is afterload responsive.[27] Longitudinal RV shortening is measured by tricuspid annular plane systolic excursion (TAPSE) with a TAPSE less than 1.6 cm considered abnormal, and less than 1.8 is a marker for poor prognosis in patients with

PAH.[20,28] Ventricular-arterial (VA) coupling is a measure of the RV contractile response to pulmonary arterial resistance, where uncoupling occurs when RV dilation progresses to preserve stroke volume at the expense of increased wall stress. This uncoupling leads to high metabolic demand and reduction in cardiac output.[29,30] Echocardiographic VA coupling, a surrogate of the invasively measured coupling, is represented by the ratio of TAPSE/RVSP.[31,32] Uncoupling occurs in end-stage disease and invasive measures of VA coupling have prognostic value, which has yet to be seen in noninvasive measures.[10,33] Systolic longitudinal RV contractility is represented by the peak systolic tricuspid lateral annular velocity (also called S′) by pulsed wave Doppler tissue imaging of the tricuspid annulus. A normal S′ peak velocity is $\geq$10 cm/s, in PAH an S′ peak velocity less than 9.7 cm/s portends poor prognosis.[20,34] RV-myocardial performance index (RV-MPI) incorporates both systolic and diastolic phases of the cardiac cycle by Doppler assessment of the lateral tricuspid annulus and is defined as the isovolumic time (isovolumic contraction time + isovolumic relaxation time) divided by ejection time. RV-MPI is used as an assessment of global RV function, where RV dysfunction is defined as greater than 0.4 by pulsed-wave Doppler or greater than 0.55 by tissue Doppler, both of which values are of prognostic value in PAH.[20,28,35] However, RV-MPI can be difficult to calculate due to image quality and short intervals, and can be falsely low when right atrial pressure is raised.[36] RV fractional area of change, a 2-dimensional iteration LVEF, less than 35% indicates RV systolic dysfunction.[20] This measure is different from TAPSE and S′ in that it incorporates the entire free wall into functional assessment, as opposed to just the basal RV or tricuspid annulus. The ability of the RV to adapt to increased workload and systemic oxygen demand can also be evaluated by dobutamine stress testing, this may expose RV reserve and exercise capacity in PAH.[37,38] Strain evaluation by speckle tracking echocardiography is another tool for evaluating RV systolic function.[39] Patients with PAH have significantly lower RV free wall and longitudinal strain than healthy controls.[40] Quantitative RV free wall systolic strain has prognostic importance across the spectrum of pulmonary hypertension syndromes, whereas longitudinal strain is predictive of development of right heart failure, clinical worsening, and mortality in PAH.[41,42] All of these measures rely on adequate imaging of the whole RV, specifically the free wall. The RV fractional area of change can be limited due to difficulties with endocardial definition; TAPSE and RV-MPI

can often be applied despite difficult acoustic windows.

The relationship between the RV and LV is important in the assessment of progression of disease and the understanding of hemodynamics in advanced PAH and RV failure. Diastolic septal shift, movement of the interventricular septum into the LV cavity, signals exceedingly high right heart pressures and impingement of the RV on LV filling. Ventricular interdependence is a byproduct of fixed intrapericardial volume in which RV pressure and volume overload leads to the interventricular septum bowing into the LV, disrupting LV geometry and early diastolic filling.[43] LV end systolic and diastolic eccentricity index is a measure of the effect of interventricular septal shift on LV function and has prognostic value in PAH.[35] The LV end systolic and diastolic eccentricity indices are the ratio of perpendicular transverse dimensions in the short axis of the heart where a normal eccentricity index approaches 1. In chronic PAH with RV volume and pressure overload the eccentricity ratio is greater than 1.[44,45] An LV eccentricity index $\geq$1.7 portends a poor prognosis for patients with PAH who also have RV dysfunction by TAPSE.[35] Pericardial effusion is another echo finding that suggests poor prognosis in patients with PAH, and likely reflects inhibition of lymphatic drainage but raised right-sided filling pressures.[44]

Assessment of LV function by echocardiography in PAH is important for decision making in the transplant evaluation process. It can be difficult to accurately assess the degree of LV dysfunction in the setting of interventricular septal flattening and leftward septal shift with chronic RV pressure and volume overload. Geometric changes in the RV-LV interaction can inhibit diastolic filling and systolic function due to septal dys-synchrony. There is echocardiographic evidence that both systolic and diastolic function of the LV decline in PAH.[46] Geometrically impaired left atrial and LV filling is exacerbated by decreased RV cardiac output and reduced stroke volume through the pulmonary vascular bed into the left atrium. These hemodynamic derangements can lead to LV myocardial dysfunction and atrophy.[47] Contractile dysfunction independent of hemodynamic distortions have also been found in the LV myocytes of patients with PAH contributing to diastolic dysfunction.[47,48] Echocardiographic evaluation of LV diastolic dysfunction is based on mitral annular velocity, left atrial size, tricuspid regurgitant velocity, and mitral inflow velocity.[49] These measures have been shown to be of modest correlation with direct hemodynamic measurements of diastolic dysfunction in patients with diastolic heart failure unrelated to pulmonary hypertension.[50] Septal mitral annular velocity is

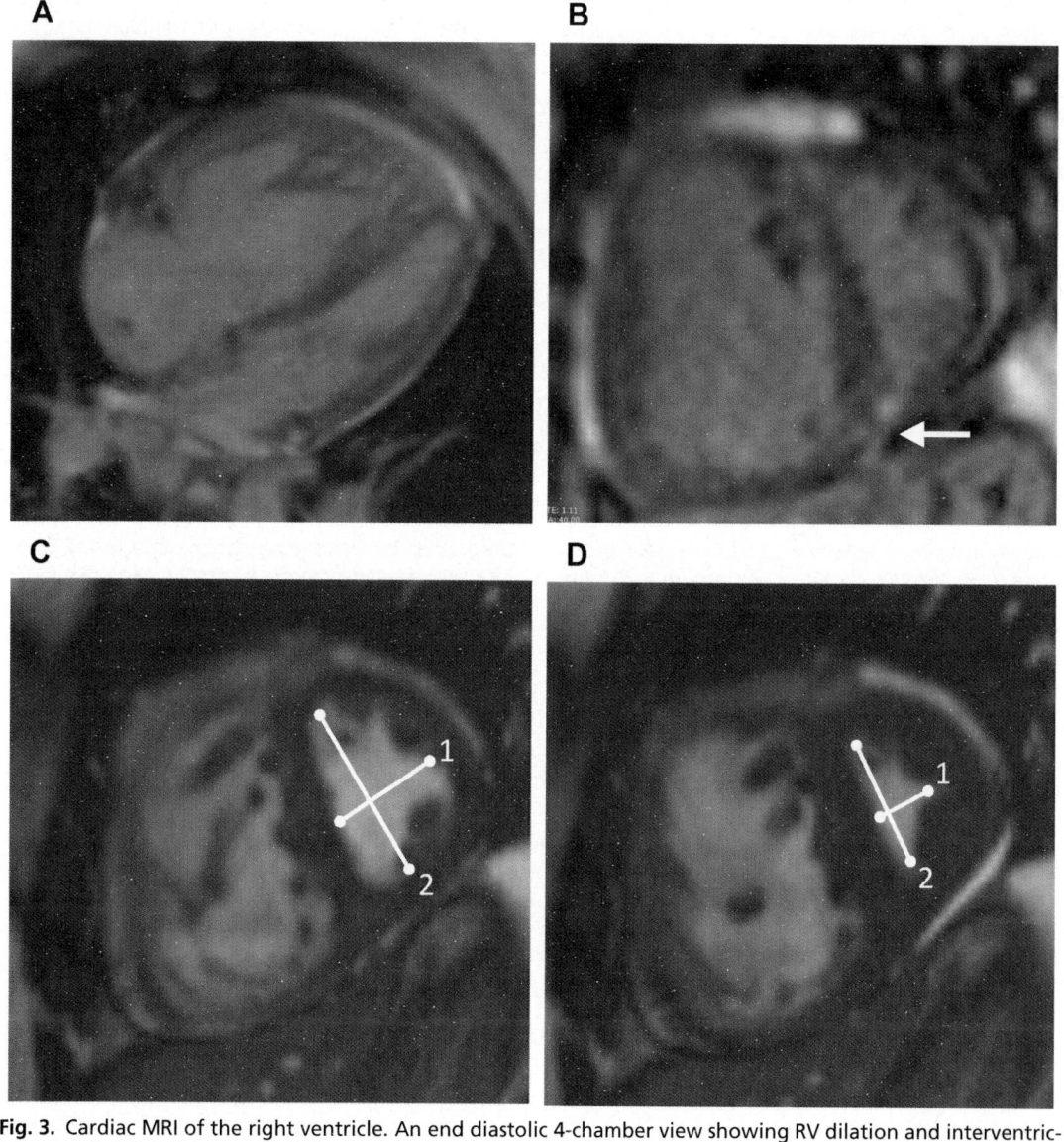

Fig. 3. Cardiac MRI of the right ventricle. An end diastolic 4-chamber view showing RV dilation and interventricular septal shift (*A*). Late gadolinium enhancement can be seen at RV insertion sites in PAH (*B, arrow*). Left ventricular eccentricity index can be calculated by the ratio of the transverse diameter (1) to the longitudinal (2) diameter of the LV during diastole (*C*) and systole (*D*). LV, left ventricle; PA, pulmonary artery; PAH, pulmonary arterial hypertension; RV, right ventricle.

universally reduced in patients with PAH, as a function of altered ventricular interdependence, and thus diastolic function in PAH may need to be evaluated by lateral mitral annular velocity alone.[49] There is uncertainty in the assessment of LV diastolic function in RV failure; specifically, what degree of diastolic dysfunction will exist if geometry is restored and RV pressure and volume overload is relieved is difficult to determine.

MRI

Cardiac MRI (cMRI) can provide important information on right and LV function in PAH different from that gleaned from echocardiography. cMRI is a 3-dimensional imaging modality specifically good at quantifying chamber volumes, providing a reliable EF, and quantifying stroke volume with a great degree of reproducibility (**Fig. 3**).[51,52] In a study of 64 patients with PAH who underwent cMRI, stroke volume index $\leq$25 mL/m^2, RV end diastolic volume index $\geq$84 mL/m^2, and LV end diastolic volume index $\leq$40 mL/m^2 were all predictors of increased mortality over a follow-up period of 32 months ($\pm$16 months).[53] Improvements in RV and LV end diastolic volumes as a response to treatment are predictors of better prognosis.[53,54]

Mauritz and colleagues[54] studied 42 treatment-naive patients with PAH who underwent cMRI at baseline and 1 year. Nonsurviving patients with PAH had lower baseline impaired longitudinal ($\leq 14 \pm 7$ mm) and transverse ($\leq 5.1 \pm 5.5$ mm) RV shortening, and worsening of transverse RV shortening with PAH-specific therapy was a negative prognostic sign. In another study of 110 patients with PAH, RVEF less than 35% by cMRI was associated with significantly worse prognosis than patients with PAH with normal RVEF.[24] Stroke volume has also emerged as a prognostic marker in PAH because maintenance of normal stroke volume indicates the ability of the RV to adapt to raised PVR and increased afterload.[55] cMRI is able to accurately measure chamber dimensions and volumes without the consideration of acoustic windows, which can be an issue in echocardiography with regard to defining RVEF more accurately. The ability to monitor mass, volume, dimensions, and function over time with this modality is highly reproducible.[56]

cMRI is an important tool in assessing LV function in patients with PAH. This modality can be used to evaluate mitral valve inflow and estimate LV diastolic dysfunction; however, this is not standard for clinical diastolic evaluation.[57] LV end diastolic volume on MRI also has prognostic value in PAH and changes in response to therapy.[58] LV systolic and diastolic eccentricity indices via MRI correlate with mPAP, and improvement of LV end diastolic volume index and LVEF with PAH-targeted therapy correlates with improved outcomes.[45,58] Specifically, the degree of improvement in LV end diastolic volume index correlates with improved functional capacity measured by 6-minute walk distance.[58] Despite the utility of cMRI in evaluating cardiac structure and function, this modality cannot reliably evaluate mPAP and does not offer an advantage over echocardiography in evaluation of LV diastolic function. However, cMRI after lung transplant has demonstrated normalization of both RV and LV function. Before and after lung transplant cMRI studies in a small cohort of 5 patients with PAH showed significant reverse RV remodeling, such that at 3 months after transplant RVEF improved to near normal and by 1 year both LV and RV mass were near normal.[59–61]

cMRI is often used to assess for scar and infiltrative disease in the case of left-sided heart failure. Current remodeling data suggest a significant component of fibrosis and structural changes of the ECM over time in PAH. In cMRI, injection of contrast can produce late gadolinium enhancement (LGE) of areas of myocardial scar or fibrosis. The presence of LGE at the RV insertion point on the interventricular septum in patients with PAH correlates with chronicity of disease, and extension of LGE into the interventricular septum has been seen in those with severe leftward septal shift.[62,63] A greater extent of LGE correlates with larger RV end diastolic volume index and lower RVEF.[63] The degree of LGE involvement of the RV insertion point and interventricular septum is a marker for advanced disease.[63,64] Overall, cMRI is an important imaging modality for assessing RV size and function; however, its use is limited by cost, availability, inadequate expertise, the inability to perform with cardiac implantable electronic devices, and requirement of a breath hold.[65]

INVASIVE HEMODYNAMICS

The diagnosis of PAH hinges on the demonstration of normal left-sided filling pressures, left ventricular end diastolic pressure or pulmonary artery wedge pressure (PWP) of less than 15 mm Hg, but the complexity of this assessment cannot be encompassed by one number. In the population with advanced PAH with RV failure there is septal shift into the LV. The resultant geometric changes in the LV can increase the PWP value, although rarely to a significant degree. Substantial increase of PWP should raise doubt about the diagnosis of PAH. In hemodynamic assessment of pulmonary hypertension, it is also important to use provocative maneuvers to uncover occult diastolic dysfunction, such as a 500-mL fluid challenge or the addition of exercise to right heart catheterization. The presence of raised PWP with these maneuvers indicates underlying LV diastolic dysfunction.[66] The difficulty lies in ascertaining to what degree the PWP increase can be attributed to the septal shift, especially given that these patients may have risk factors for LV systolic and diastolic dysfunction.

TRANSPLANT IN PULMONARY ARTERIAL HYPERTENSION

Transplantation for PAH was first undertaken as HLT, then evolved into the use of single LT (SLT), and subsequently double LT (DLT).[67] As expertise has advanced and our ability to manage postoperative hemodynamic complications has evolved, DLT has become the preferred procedure for patients with PAH given data that the RV recovers after relief of increased afterload.[68,69] Overall, the ISHLT registry reports improved median survival of DLT compared with SLT (7.4 versus 4.6 years), regardless of the underlying disease.[70] Raised PAP has consistently been shown to be associated with a higher incidence of primary graft dysfunction

(PGD) in LT, in patients with PAH, as well as in secondary pulmonary hypertension, regardless of procedure type.[71,72] Bando and colleagues[73] published their single-center transplant experience in PAH, consisting of patients with idiopathic PAH (IPAH) and those with Eisenmenger syndrome, in which the decision to perform LT or HLT depended on donor availability. Those undergoing DLT and HLT showed greater decrease in mPAP and increase in cardiac output early after transplant compared with SLT.[73] Graft-related mortality and NYHA functional status 1 year after transplant was also significantly worse with SLT compared with DLT or HLT.

A major factor in post-LT survival is the underlying cause for transplantation.[74,75] The legacy of lung transplant in IPAH has demonstrated one of the highest early mortality rates after transplant.[76] However, conditional 1-year survival is significantly better than in other disease cohorts.[76] This suggests that outcomes in this population depend on perioperative management of hemodynamic derangements and fluid shifts in the setting of pre-transplant RV dysfunction. Mechanical positive pressure ventilation poses a specifically high risk to this patient population who have poor RV function as well as more severe LV diastolic dysfunction than other disease cohorts undergoing LT.

Double-Lung Versus Heart-Lung

DLT is now favored as the procedure of choice for patients with PAH, particularly from the standpoint of organ availability and allocation equity. Therefore, HLT has generally been reserved for patients with evidence of left-sided cardiac dysfunction, although there is no consensus in the existing literature as to how to define this (**Table 1**). In a study by Bando and colleagues,[73] there was preference for HLT in patients with Eisenmenger syndrome with unrepairable cardiac defects, coronary artery disease, or an LVEF less than 35%. Simple cardiac lesions leading to Eisenmenger syndrome, such as an atrial or ventricular septal defect, have the potential for repair at the time of DLT, thus making the use of HLT less imperative. In patients with PAH, indications for HLT are less clear, especially when it comes to degree of RV failure, as there currently are no hemodynamic, echocardiographic, radiologic, or serologic predictors of irreversible RV failure. In a survey of 35 pulmonary hypertension and transplant centers, DLT was preferred by 83% of centers for patients with PAH, including patients with severe right heart failure and NYHA III or IV functional classes. Reported indications for HLT were severe LV failure (although LVEF for HLT patients ranged from 32% to 55%) in three-quarters of the respondents, severe RV failure criteria (RVEF of 10%–25%) in 45% of centers, and degree of tricuspid regurgitation in only 24% of centers.[77] Fadel and colleagues[78] stated preference for HLT over DLT in patients with severe RV dilation and dysfunction, low cardiac index (<2.2 L/min/m^2), inotrope-dependent RV failure, and renal failure, although it is clear that many patients with these hemodynamic derangements may do quite well with DLT.

Despite concerns about severe RV dysfunction and limitations of RV recovery, there are several small studies that have documented marked improvement of RV function after LT, even in patients with severe increases of PVR. As early as 1991, Pasque and colleagues[79] reported significant improvement in hemodynamics and RVEF by radionucleotide evaluation (22% $\pm$ 15% to 51% $\pm$ 11%, $P = .006$) in 7 patients with IPAH who underwent SLT. More recently, Gorter and colleagues[69] studied 10 patients with PAH before and after DLT with cMRI. After transplantation, significant improvement in RV function was seen: RVEF increased from 32% to 64% with a decrease in RV volume and mass each by over 50%. There

---

Table 1
Comparison of double-lung and heart-lung transplantation

	Double-Lung	Heart-Lung
Pros	• Better donor organ allocation equity • Less complex operative dissection	• Option for severe RV or LV dysfunction and complex congenital heart disease
Cons	• ↑Ischemic time • ↑Bypass time • Use of ECMO postoperatively • Longer mechanical ventilation	• ↑Wait list times • Scarce resource use Dual organ rejection surveillance
Median survival, y	7.1	6.5

Abbreviations: ECMO, extracorporeal membrane oxygenation; LV, left ventricular; RV, right ventricular.
  Data from Refs.[75,76,78,91,92]

was also significant improvement in LV eccentricity index (2.8–1.1, $P<.001$) and RV/LV volume ratio (2.3–0.8, $P<.001$). The bulk of the data suggest that, even in cases of severely impaired RV function as a result of pulmonary vascular disease, RV function improves substantially after lung transplant. By implication, then, HLT is not required for patients with PAH with RV dysfunction and no confounding factors, such as complex CHD or severe LV systolic function.[80,81]

Another, perhaps greater, concern in patients with PAH undergoing DLT is persistent, occult LV diastolic dysfunction, which can be unveiled by increased cardiac output to the left heart after LT. This can lead to pulmonary edema, prolonged mechanical ventilation, acute renal failure, and hypotension requiring use of vasopressors. This was first reported in 3 patients with PAH who developed LV dysfunction after SLT leading to respiratory insufficiency and hemodynamic decompensation.[82] More recently, Avriel and colleagues[83] studied LV diastolic dysfunction in 116 patients with PAH who underwent DLT. They defined LV diastolic dysfunction using echocardiographic measures of increased isovolumic relaxation time, reduced E:A ratio, and decreased mitral deceleration time. In this study, patients with PAH with grade 2 or greater LV diastolic dysfunction before transplant had significantly worse 1-year survival compared with those with normal LV diastolic function, and LV diastolic dysfunction was the only variable that correlated with overall survival (hazard ratio = 5.4; 95% CI, 1.3–22; $P = .02$).[83] Follow-up echocardiography at 1 month after transplant showed persistence of diastolic dysfunction in these patients.

The presence of LV dysfunction after LT has become more manageable in recent years as contemporary approaches to lung transplantation often incorporate preoperative, intraoperative, and posttransplant use of extracorporeal membrane oxygenation (ECMO).[84,85] The use of perioperative ECMO allows control of pulmonary perfusion, and RV and LV loading, and minimizes pulmonary edema and potential drivers of PGD, albeit at the expense of potential vascular, thrombotic, and bleeding complications.[86] The use of ECMO perioperatively seems to allow for incremental LV conditioning over time, shown by increased cardiac output, EF, and improved LV dimensions during the first postoperative week.[84] The configuration of the ECMO circuit (veno-arterial, veno-venous, PA to left atrium, or right atrium to left atrium) can alter hemodynamics favorably and aid in assessment of patient response to normalization of pulmonary pressures postoperatively.[85] This approach may facilitate the use of DLT and avoidance of HLT in patients with PAH

with severe RV failure, marginal LV systolic function, or significant LV diastolic dysfunction. No survival difference has been seen between DLT and HLT; however, significant differences in patient selection limit interpretation in this nonrandomized body of data.[67,87]

Practices and decisions about transplant procedure currently depend on local expertise and pathophysiologic understanding of disease. Synthesis of many factors is necessary to determine which patient may require HLT instead of DLT. Variability lies in individual transplant program thresholds of LV and RV dysfunction for DLT.[73,77] Part of this decision making is the consideration that wait times for HLT are longer than for DLT; in 1 study, HLT patients had more than double the waitlist time.[77,88] In addition many centers have younger age cutoffs for HLT as opposed to DLT.[77,88] With regard to outcome, in an older retrospective review of 219 patients with pulmonary hypertension (82% in RV failure, 57% with PAH) who underwent HLT or DLT, in-hospital mortality and long-term survival were not statistically different between the 2 groups. Rates of PGD and bronchial complications were higher in the DLT group and time on mechanical ventilation was significantly longer in the DLT patients.[78] Data from the ISHLT registry also show a similar outcome with HLT and LT, either SLT or DLT, for IPAH having similar 1 year (approximately 70%) and median survival of 9 years, contingent on surviving to 1 year.[89] Another consideration in comparing HLT versus DLT is that initial immunosuppression in patients receiving dual organ transplantation frequently includes more potent T cell suppression for induction therapy and higher levels of chronic immunosuppression.[75,89] In addition, the surveillance for rejection of dual- versus single-organ transplant requires HLT patients to have twice as many rejection surveillance procedures, including pulmonary function testing and echocardiograms, as well as serial lung and cardiac biopsies. Use of HLT has been declining in recent years and current practices indicate that, in PAH, HLT is reserved for patients with significant LV dysfunction or complex CHD.[80,90]

SUMMARY

Despite many available disease-specific therapies, the morbidity and mortality of PAH remains high. Therefore, transplantation is the only curative treatment of patients with severe pulmonary vascular disease. Clinical and imaging evidence of RV dysfunction should prompt escalation of therapy and potentially transplant evaluation referral. These patients frequently die of right heart failure even with medical treatment. Despite concerns over severe RV dysfunction in many patients with PAH, the current expert consensus is that the vast majority of transplant patients with PAH will have RV recovery with DLT. Complications related to posttransplant LV dysfunction is a potential issue in DLT of patients with PAH, but perioperative use of ECMO has mitigated this problem. In the absence of complex CHD or significant left-sided cardiac disease, DLT, in our opinion, is the method of choice for transplantation in PAH.

ACKNOWLEDGMENTS

The authors thank Matthew Bacchetta, MD, for his expertise and guidance with this review. Dr Brittain's research is supported by grants R01HL146588 from the National Institutes of Health, grants 13FTF16070002 and Gilead Scholars Program in Pulmonary Arterial Hypertension. Dr Robbins' research is supported by grants 1R01HL142720-01A1 and 5U01HL125212 from the National Institutes of Health.

DISCLOSURE

The authors have nothing to disclose.

REFERENCES

1. Simonneau G, Montani D, Celermajer DS, et al. Haemodynamic definitions and updated clinical classification of pulmonary hypertension. Eur Respir J 2019;53(1) [pii:1801913].
2. Hoeper MM, Kramer T, Pan Z, et al. Mortality in pulmonary arterial hypertension: prediction by the 2015 European pulmonary hypertension guidelines risk stratification model. Eur Respir J 2017;50(2) [pii: 1700740].
3. Barst RJ, Rubin LJ, Long WA, et al. A comparison of continuous intravenous epoprostenol (prostacyclin) with conventional therapy for primary pulmonary hypertension. N Engl J Med 1996;334(5):296–301.
4. Orens JB, Estenne M, Arcasoy S, et al. International guidelines for the selection of lung transplant candidates: 2006 update—a consensus report from the Pulmonary Scientific Council of the International Society for Heart and Lung Transplantation. J Heart Lung Transplant 2006;25(7):745–55.
5. Kovacs G, Berghold A, Scheidl S, et al. Pulmonary arterial pressure during rest and exercise in healthy subjects: a systematic review. Eur Respir J 2009; 34(4):888–94.
6. D'Alonzo GE, Barst RJ, Ayres SM, et al. Survival in patients with primary pulmonary hypertension. Results from a national prospective registry. Ann Intern Med 1991;115(5):343–9.
7. Le RJ, Fenstad ER, Maradit-Kremers H, et al. Syncope in adults with pulmonary arterial hypertension. J Am Coll Cardiol 2011;58(8):863–7.
8. Miyamoto S, Nagaya N, Satoh T, et al. Clinical correlates and prognostic significance of six-minute walk test in patients with primary pulmonary hypertension. Comparison with cardiopulmonary exercise testing. Am J Respir Crit Care Med 2000; 161(2 Pt 1):487–92.
9. Chantler PD, Lakatta EG, Najjar SS. Arterial-ventricular coupling: mechanistic insights into cardiovascular performance at rest and during exercise. J Appl Physiol (1985) 2008;105(4):1342–51.
10. Sanz J, Garcia-Alvarez A, Fernandez-Friera L, et al. Right ventriculo-arterial coupling in pulmonary hypertension: a magnetic resonance study. Heart 2012;98(3):238–43.
11. Vonk-Noordegraaf A, Haddad F, Chin KM, et al. Right heart adaptation to pulmonary arterial hypertension: physiology and pathobiology. J Am Coll Cardiol 2013;62(25 Suppl):D22–33.
12. Bogaard HJ, Abe K, Vonk Noordegraaf A, et al. The right ventricle under pressure: cellular and molecular mechanisms of right-heart failure in pulmonary hypertension. Chest 2009;135(3):794–804.
13. Rain S, Handoko ML, Trip P, et al. Right ventricular diastolic impairment in patients with pulmonary arterial hypertension. Circulation 2013;128(18):2016–25, 2011-2010.
14. Murch SD, La Gerche A, Roberts TJ, et al. Abnormal right ventricular relaxation in pulmonary hypertension. Pulm Circ 2015;5(2):370–5.
15. Badagliacca R, Poscia R, Pezzuto B, et al. Right ventricular remodeling in idiopathic pulmonary arterial hypertension: adaptive versus maladaptive morphology. J Heart Lung Transplant 2015;34(3):395–403.
16. Lopez B, Gonzalez A, Querejeta R, et al. Alterations in the pattern of collagen deposition may contribute to the deterioration of systolic function in hypertensive patients with heart failure. J Am Coll Cardiol 2006;48(1):89–96.
17. Stewart JA Jr, Massey EP, Fix C, et al. Temporal alterations in cardiac fibroblast function following induction of pressure overload. Cell Tissue Res 2010; 340(1):117–26.
18. Polyakova V, Hein S, Kostin S, et al. Matrix metalloproteinases and their tissue inhibitors in pressure-overloaded human myocardium during heart failure progression. J Am Coll Cardiol 2004;44(8):1609–18.
19. Brittain EL, Hemnes AR, Keebler M, et al. Right ventricular plasticity and functional imaging. Pulm Circ 2012;2(3):309–26.
20. Rudski LG, Lai WW, Afilalo J, et al. Guidelines for the echocardiographic assessment of the right heart in adults: a report from the American Society of Echocardiography endorsed by the European

Association of Echocardiography, a registered branch of the European Society of Cardiology, and the Canadian Society of Echocardiography. J Am Soc Echocardiogr 2010;23(7):685–713 [quiz: 786–8].

21. Mitchell C, Rahko PS, Blauwet LA, et al. Guidelines for performing a comprehensive transthoracic echocardiographic examination in adults: recommendations from the American Society of Echocardiography. J Am Soc Echocardiogr 2019;32(1):1–64.

22. Haddad F, Couture P, Tousignant C, et al. The right ventricle in cardiac surgery, a perioperative perspective: I. Anatomy, physiology, and assessment. Anesth Analg 2009;108(2):407–21.

23. Ho SY, Nihoyannopoulos P. Anatomy, echocardiography, and normal right ventricular dimensions. Heart 2006;92(Suppl 1):i2–13.

24. van de Veerdonk MC, Kind T, Marcus JT, et al. Progressive right ventricular dysfunction in patients with pulmonary arterial hypertension responding to therapy. J Am Coll Cardiol 2011; 58(24):2511–9.

25. O'Leary JM, Assad TR, Xu M, et al. Lack of a tricuspid regurgitation Doppler signal and pulmonary hypertension by invasive measurement. J Am Heart Assoc 2018;7(13) [pii:e009362].

26. Magnino C, Omede P, Avenatti E, et al. Inaccuracy of right atrial pressure estimates through inferior vena cava indices. Am J Cardiol 2017;120(9):1667–73.

27. Brown SB, Raina A, Katz D, et al. Longitudinal shortening accounts for the majority of right ventricular contraction and improves after pulmonary vasodilator therapy in normal subjects and patients with pulmonary arterial hypertension. Chest 2011; 140(1):27–33.

28. Forfia PR, Fisher MR, Mathai SC, et al. Tricuspid annular displacement predicts survival in pulmonary hypertension. Am J Respir Crit Care Med 2006; 174(9):1034–41.

29. Singh I, Rahaghi FN, Naeije R, et al. Dynamic right ventricular-pulmonary arterial uncoupling during maximum incremental exercise in exercise pulmonary hypertension and pulmonary arterial hypertension. Pulm Circ 2019;9(3). 2045894019862435.

30. Koop AC, Bossers GPL, Ploegstra MJ, et al. Metabolic remodeling in the pressure-loaded right ventricle: shifts in glucose and fatty acid metabolism-a systematic review and meta-analysis. J Am Heart Assoc 2019;8(21):e012086.

31. Guazzi M, Bandera F, Pelissero G, et al. Tricuspid annular plane systolic excursion and pulmonary arterial systolic pressure relationship in heart failure: an index of right ventricular contractile function and prognosis. Am J Physiol Heart Circ Physiol 2013; 305(9):H1373–81.

32. French S, Amsallem M, Ouazani N, et al. Non-invasive right ventricular load adaptability indices in patients with scleroderma-associated pulmonary arterial hypertension. Pulm Circ 2018;8(3). 2045894018788268.

33. Vanderpool RR, Pinsky MR, Naeije R, et al. RV-pulmonary arterial coupling predicts outcome in patients referred for pulmonary hypertension. Heart 2015;101(1):37–43.

34. Ernande L, Cottin V, Leroux PY, et al. Right isovolumic contraction velocity predicts survival in pulmonary hypertension. J Am Soc Echocardiogr 2013; 26(3):297–306.

35. Ghio S, Klersy C, Magrini G, et al. Prognostic relevance of the echocardiographic assessment of right ventricular function in patients with idiopathic pulmonary arterial hypertension. Int J Cardiol 2010;140(3):272–8.

36. Tei C, Dujardin KS, Hodge DO, et al. Doppler echocardiographic index for assessment of global right ventricular function. J Am Soc Echocardiogr 1996; 9(6):838–47.

37. Ghio S, Fortuni F, Greco A, et al. Dobutamine stress echocardiography in pulmonary arterial hypertension. Int J Cardiol 2018;270:331–5.

38. Sharma T, Lau EM, Choudhary P, et al. Dobutamine stress for evaluation of right ventricular reserve in pulmonary arterial hypertension. Eur Respir J 2015;45(3):700–8.

39. Shukla M, Park JH, Thomas JD, et al. Prognostic value of right ventricular strain using speckle-tracking echocardiography in pulmonary hypertension: a systematic review and meta-analysis. Can J Cardiol 2018;34(8):1069–78.

40. Fukuda Y, Tanaka H, Sugiyama D, et al. Utility of right ventricular free wall speckle-tracking strain for evaluation of right ventricular performance in patients with pulmonary hypertension. J Am Soc Echocardiogr 2011;24(10):1101–8.

41. Fine NM, Chen L, Bastiansen PM, et al. Outcome prediction by quantitative right ventricular function assessment in 575 subjects evaluated for pulmonary hypertension. Circ Cardiovasc Imaging 2013;6(5): 711–21.

42. Sachdev A, Villarraga HR, Frantz RP, et al. Right ventricular strain for prediction of survival in patients with pulmonary arterial hypertension. Chest 2011; 139(6):1299–309.

43. Gan C, Lankhaar JW, Marcus JT, et al. Impaired left ventricular filling due to right-to-left ventricular interaction in patients with pulmonary arterial hypertension. Am J Physiol Heart Circ Physiol 2006;290(4): H1528–33.

44. Raymond RJ, Hinderliter AL, Willis PW, et al. Echocardiographic predictors of adverse outcomes in primary pulmonary hypertension. J Am Coll Cardiol 2002;39(7):1214–9.

45. Ryan T, Petrovic O, Dillon JC, et al. An echocardiographic index for separation of right ventricular volume and pressure overload. J Am Coll Cardiol 1985;5(4):918–27.

46. Chang SM, Lin CC, Hsiao SH, et al. Pulmonary hypertension and left heart function: insights from tissue Doppler imaging and myocardial performance index. Echocardiography 2007;24(4):366–73.

47. Manders E, Bogaard HJ, Handoko ML, et al. Contractile dysfunction of left ventricular cardiomyocytes in patients with pulmonary arterial hypertension. J Am Coll Cardiol 2014;64(1):28–37.

48. Hsu S, Kokkonen-Simon KM, Kirk JA, et al. Right ventricular myofilament functional differences in humans with systemic sclerosis-associated versus idiopathic pulmonary arterial hypertension. Circulation 2018;137(22):2360–70.

49. Nagueh SF, Smiseth OA, Appleton CP, et al. Recommendations for the evaluation of left ventricular diastolic function by echocardiography: an update from the American Society of Echocardiography and the European Association of Cardiovascular Imaging. Eur Heart J Cardiovasc Imaging 2016;17(12):1321–60.

50. Nauta JF, Hummel YM, van der Meer P, et al. Correlation with invasive left ventricular filling pressures and prognostic relevance of the echocardiographic diastolic parameters used in the 2016 ESC heart failure guidelines and in the 2016 ASE/EACVI recommendations: a systematic review in patients with heart failure with preserved ejection fraction. Eur J Heart Fail 2018;20(9):1303–11.

51. Swift AJ, Rajaram S, Campbell MJ, et al. Prognostic value of cardiovascular magnetic resonance imaging measurements corrected for age and sex in idiopathic pulmonary arterial hypertension. Circ Cardiovasc Imaging 2014;7(1):100–6.

52. Swift AJ, Rajaram S, Condliffe R, et al. Diagnostic accuracy of cardiovascular magnetic resonance imaging of right ventricular morphology and function in the assessment of suspected pulmonary hypertension results from the ASPIRE registry. J Cardiovasc Magn Reson 2012;14:40.

53. van Wolferen SA, Marcus JT, Boonstra A, et al. Prognostic value of right ventricular mass, volume, and function in idiopathic pulmonary arterial hypertension. Eur Heart J 2007;28(10):1250–7.

54. Mauritz GJ, Kind T, Marcus JT, et al. Progressive changes in right ventricular geometric shortening and long-term survival in pulmonary arterial hypertension. Chest 2012;141(4):935–43.

55. van Wolferen SA, van de Veerdonk MC, Mauritz GJ, et al. Clinically significant change in stroke volume in pulmonary hypertension. Chest 2011;139(5):1003–9.

56. Grothues F, Smith GC, Moon JC, et al. Comparison of interstudy reproducibility of cardiovascular magnetic resonance with two-dimensional echocardiography in normal subjects and in patients with heart failure or left ventricular hypertrophy. Am J Cardiol 2002;90(1):29–34.

57. Rathi VK, Doyle M, Yamrozik J, et al. Routine evaluation of left ventricular diastolic function by cardiovascular magnetic resonance: a practical approach. J Cardiovasc Magn Reson 2008;10:36.

58. Peacock AJ, Crawley S, McLure L, et al. Changes in right ventricular function measured by cardiac magnetic resonance imaging in patients receiving pulmonary arterial hypertension-targeted therapy: the EURO-MR study. Circ Cardiovasc Imaging 2014;7(1):107–14.

59. Frist WH, Lorenz CH, Walker ES, et al. MRI complements standard assessment of right ventricular function after lung transplantation. Ann Thorac Surg 1995;60(2):268–71.

60. Globits S, Burghuber OC, Koller J, et al. Effect of lung transplantation on right and left ventricular volumes and function measured by magnetic resonance imaging. Am J Respir Crit Care Med 1994;149(4 Pt 1):1000–4.

61. Moulton MJ, Creswell LL, Ungacta FF, et al. Magnetic resonance imaging provides evidence for remodeling of the right ventricle after single-lung transplantation for pulmonary hypertension. Circulation 1996;94(9 Suppl):II312–9.

62. Junqueira FP, Macedo R, Coutinho AC, et al. Myocardial delayed enhancement in patients with pulmonary hypertension and right ventricular failure: evaluation by cardiac MRI. Br J Radiol 2009;82(982):821–6.

63. Blyth KG, Groenning BA, Martin TN, et al. Contrast enhanced-cardiovascular magnetic resonance imaging in patients with pulmonary hypertension. Eur Heart J 2005;26(19):1993–9.

64. Freed BH, Gomberg-Maitland M, Chandra S, et al. Late gadolinium enhancement cardiovascular magnetic resonance predicts clinical worsening in patients with pulmonary hypertension. J Cardiovasc Magn Reson 2012;14:11.

65. Benza R, Biederman R, Murali S, et al. Role of cardiac magnetic resonance imaging in the management of patients with pulmonary arterial hypertension. J Am Coll Cardiol 2008;52(21):1683–92.

66. Vachiery JL, Adir Y, Barbera JA, et al. Pulmonary hypertension due to left heart diseases. J Am Coll Cardiol 2013;62(25 Suppl):D100–8.

67. Christie JD, Edwards LB, Kucheryavaya AY, et al. The Registry of the International Society for Heart and Lung Transplantation: twenty-seventh official adult lung and heart-lung transplant report–2010. J Heart Lung Transplant 2010;29(10):1104–18.

68. Long J, Russo MJ, Muller C, et al. Surgical treatment of pulmonary hypertension: lung transplantation. Pulm Circ 2011;1(3):327–33.

69. Gorter TM, Verschuuren EAM, van Veldhuisen DJ, et al. Right ventricular recovery after bilateral lung transplantation for pulmonary arterial

hypertensiondagger. Interact Cardiovasc Thorac Surg 2017;24(6):890–7.

70. Chambers DC, Yusen RD, Cherikh WS, et al. The registry of the International Society for Heart and Lung Transplantation: thirty-fourth adult lung and heart-lung transplantation report—2017; focus theme: allograft ischemic time. J Heart Lung Transplant 2017;36(10):1047–59.

71. Christie JD, Carby M, Bag R, et al. Report of the ISHLT working group on primary lung graft dysfunction part II: definition. A consensus statement of the International Society for Heart and Lung Transplantation. J Heart Lung Transplant 2005;24(10):1454–9.

72. Diamond JM, Lee JC, Kawut SM, et al. Clinical risk factors for primary graft dysfunction after lung transplantation. Am J Respir Crit Care Med 2013;187(5):527–34.

73. Bando K, Armitage JM, Paradis IL, et al. Indications for and results of single, bilateral, and heart-lung transplantation for pulmonary hypertension. J Thorac Cardiovasc Surg 1994;108(6):1056–65.

74. Studer SM, Levy RD, McNeil K, et al. Lung transplant outcomes: a review of survival, graft function, physiology, health-related quality of life and cost-effectiveness. Eur Respir J 2004;24(4):674–85.

75. Chambers DC, Cherikh WS, Harhay MO, et al. The International Thoracic Organ Transplant Registry of the International Society for Heart and Lung Transplantation: thirty-sixth adult lung and heart-lung transplantation report—2019; focus theme: donor and recipient size match. J Heart Lung Transplant 2019;38(10):1042–55.

76. Yusen RD, Edwards LB, Kucheryavaya AY, et al. The Registry of the International Society for Heart and Lung Transplantation: thirty-second official adult lung and heart-lung transplantation report—2015; focus theme: early graft failure. J Heart Lung Transplant 2015;34(10):1264–77.

77. Pielsticker EJ, Martinez FJ, Rubenfire M. Lung and heart-lung transplant practice patterns in pulmonary hypertension centers. J Heart Lung Transplant 2001;20(12):1297–304.

78. Fadel E, Mercier O, Mussot S, et al. Long-term outcome of double-lung and heart-lung transplantation for pulmonary hypertension: a comparative retrospective study of 219 patients. Eur J Cardiothorac Surg 2010;38(3):277–84.

79. Pasque MK, Trulock EP, Kaiser LR, et al. Single-lung transplantation for pulmonary hypertension. Three-month hemodynamic follow-up. Circulation 1991;84(6):2275–9.

80. Toyoda Y, Toyoda Y. Heart-lung transplantation: adult indications and outcomes. J Thorac Dis 2014;6(8):1138–42.

81. Weill D, Benden C, Corris PA, et al. A consensus document for the selection of lung transplant candidates: 2014—an update from the Pulmonary Transplantation Council of the International Society for Heart and Lung Transplantation. J Heart Lung Transplant 2015;34(1):1–15.

82. Birsan T, Kranz A, Mares P, et al. Transient left ventricular failure following bilateral lung transplantation for pulmonary hypertension. J Heart Lung Transplant 1999;18(4):304–9.

83. Avriel A, Klement AH, Johnson SR, et al. Impact of left ventricular diastolic dysfunction on lung transplantation outcome in patients with pulmonary arterial hypertension. Am J Transplant 2017;17(10):2705–11.

84. Tudorache I, Sommer W, Kuhn C, et al. Lung transplantation for severe pulmonary hypertension—awake extracorporeal membrane oxygenation for postoperative left ventricular remodelling. Transplantation 2015;99(2):451–8.

85. Tipograf Y, Salna M, Minko E, et al. Outcomes of extracorporeal membrane oxygenation as a bridge to lung transplantation. Ann Thorac Surg 2019;107(5):1456–63.

86. Van Raemdonck D, Hartwig MG, Hertz MI, et al. Report of the ISHLT working group on primary lung graft dysfunction Part IV: prevention and treatment: a 2016 consensus group statement of the International Society for Heart and Lung Transplantation. J Heart Lung Transplant 2017;36(10):1121–36.

87. Olland A, Falcoz PE, Canuet M, et al. Should we perform bilateral-lung or heart-lung transplantation for patients with pulmonary hypertension? Interact Cardiovasc Thorac Surg 2013;17(1):166–70.

88. Brouckaert J, Verleden SE, Verbelen T, et al. Double-lung versus heart-lung transplantation for precapillary pulmonary arterial hypertension: a 24-year single-center retrospective study. Transpl Int 2019;32(7):717–29.

89. Christie JD, Edwards LB, Aurora P, et al. The registry of the International Society for Heart and Lung Transplantation: twenty-sixth official adult lung and heart-lung transplantation report—2009. J Heart Lung Transplant 2009;28(10):1031–49.

90. Chambers DC, Cherikh WS, Goldfarb SB, et al. The International Thoracic Organ Transplant Registry of the International Society for Heart and Lung Transplantation: thirty-fifth adult lung and heart-lung transplant report—2018; focus theme: multiorgan transplantation. J Heart Lung Transplant 2018;37(10):1169–83.

91. Sultan S, Tseng S, Stanziola AA, et al. Pulmonary hypertension: the role of lung transplantation. Heart Fail Clin 2018;14(3):327–31.

92. George MP, Champion HC, Pilewski JM. Lung transplantation for pulmonary hypertension. Pulm Circ 2011;1(2):182–91.